The Anaesthesia Science Viva Book
Second Edition

The Anaesthesia Science Viva Book

SECOND EDITION

Clinical science as applied to anaesthesia,
intensive therapy and chronic pain
A guide to the oral questions

SIMON BRICKER MA, MB ChB, FRCA

Examiner in the Final FRCA
Consultant Anaesthetist
The Countess of Chester Hospital
Chester, UK

Medical illustrations by
CELYN BRICKER

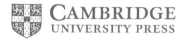

CAMBRIDGE
UNIVERSITY PRESS

CAMBRIDGE
UNIVERSITY PRESS

University Printing House, Cambridge CB2 8BS, United Kingdom

Published in the United States of America by Cambridge University Press, New York

Cambridge University Press is part of the University of Cambridge.

It furthers the University's mission by disseminating knowledge in the pursuit of education, learning and research at the highest international levels of excellence.

www.cambridge.org
Information on this title: www.cambridge.org/9780521726443

First edition © Greenwich Medical Media 2004
Second edition © S. Bricker 2009

First published 2004
Second edition 2009
7th printing 2016

Printed in the United Kingdom by Bell and Bain Ltd

A catalogue record for this publication is available from the British Library

Library of Congress Cataloguing in Publication data
Bricker, Simon.
  The anaesthesia science viva book : clinical science as applied to anaesthesia,
  intensive therapy, and chronic pain : a guide to the oral questions / Simon Bricker ;
  medical illustrations by Celyn Bricker. – 2nd ed.
    p. ; cm.
  Includes index.
  ISBN 978-0-521-72644-3 (pbk.)
  1. Anesthesia–Examinations–Study guides.   I. Title.
  [DNLM: 1. Anesthesia.   2. Clinical Medicine.   WO 200 B849a 2009]
  RD82.3.B75 2009
  617.9′6076–dc22   2008028638

ISBN 978-0-521-72644-3 Paperback

Contents

Contents

Contents

Preface to the Second Edition

The emphasis, if not the content, of the Final FRCA science viva is changing. In response to muted criticism that an otherwise good exam has been diminished by a basic science viva that at times seemed to be little more than 'Primary Lite', the College has introduced greater clinical focus. This has meant that many of the answers that appeared in the first edition needed some reorientation. Yet, as before, this book's prime purpose remains to give you a wide range of potential questions presented in a way that is relevant to the exam that you are facing, and organized so that the information is manageable. As before, the introduction still aims to give you some insight into how the clinical science viva works, together with some revised general guidance as to how to improve your chances of success.

The examination questions continue to be divided broadly into the four subject areas of anatomy, physiology, pharmacology and physics, although the increased clinical emphasis can mean that the distinction between the subject areas can be somewhat blurred. The anatomy question on the internal jugular vein, for example, may well include some discussion of the physiology of central venous pressure. Equally, some questions on pharmacology may encompass aspects of physiology with which there is obvious potential for overlap. This means that you may not always find all the necessary information within one single answer, but should find most of it covered in other sections. The basic format of the book remains unchanged, although the content has been updated where appropriate. A new feature of this edition is the inclusion of some illustrations and diagrams which should make the material more accessible.

My family, as always, offered no objection to the project; and, as always, my thanks and love to them for their support. The anatomical drawings were produced by a student who is studying Fine Art at Edinburgh University and who happens to be my eldest son Celyn. To him are due especial thanks.

Simon Bricker
2008

Preface to the First Edition

The Final FRCA examination has a daunting syllabus which is tested by a multiple choice paper, by written short answer questions, by one oral examination in clinical anaesthesia, and finally by another in applied basic clinical science. This book is intended to give you some insight into how the clinical science viva works, along with some general guidance as to how to improve your chances of passing. More importantly it aims to provide you with a wide range of potential questions that contain, nonetheless, a manageable amount of information.

The introduction explains the format of the viva, outlines how the questions are constructed, conducted and marked, and offers some advice about technique. The questions then follow, which are typical of those which have appeared, are divided broadly into the four areas which the exam is designed to cover, namely applied anatomy, physiology, pharmacology and clinical measurement. One section, entitled 'Miscellaneous Science and Medicine' includes a number of subjects which do not fall readily into any of the other categories.

You may notice that there is some overlap in content with the companion volume, 'Short Answer Questions in Anaesthesia'. Where this has happened I have reworked the answers both to give more detail and to focus the topic more specifically towards the oral part of the exam, but a degree of duplication in one or two of the questions is inevitable.

The answers have been constructed to provide you with enough information to pass the viva, but as I have had to be selective in the detail that has been included they do not claim to be complete accounts of the subjects. This means that in some areas you may notice various omissions, but none I hope so egregious that your chances of success will be ruined. Each of the questions is prefaced by a short commentary on the relevance (or otherwise) of the subject that is being asked. There follows the body of the answer to the likely areas of questioning. This is presented mainly in the form of bulleted, but detailed points, which include supporting explanation. These are written in text rather than as lists, because I felt that this format would make the book easier to read. If some of the questions seem long, then it is either because the background information is complex, or because they contain enough material for more than one viva topic.

Even in a structured examination a viva may take an unforeseen course, and so the answers also include some possible directions which the questioning might follow. Although each one is intended to provide background details more than sufficient to allow you to pass, in many cases they are simplified, and it is always possible that some examiners may ask at least part of the question in more depth than can be covered in a book of this size. There are 150 specimen questions in this book, and on the day of the exam you will be asked only four. Odds of about 40 to 1 or less do not provide a huge incentive for study, but I should hope that at least some of the material would be relevant to your anaesthetic practice. The material that is irrelevant, and there is certainly some, may at least prove of some future use as in due course you guide less experienced colleagues through the FRCA.

I promised my family that I would never again succumb to the temptation of writing a book. I lied. To my wife and three boys, therefore, my love and thanks for their unfailing patience and support.

Simon Bricker
2004

Advice on answering clinical science viva questions

The clinical science viva

The format of the Final FRCA examination has remained materially unchanged since its inception in 1996, and the clinical science viva continues to test 'the understanding of basic science to the practice of anaesthesia, intensive therapy and pain management'. The College has always included the proviso that 'it is accepted that candidates will not have acquired a detailed knowledge of every topic during the period of recognised training', but this has on occasion contrasted uneasily with the bitter perception of at least some candidates that they had been examined almost to destruction on scientific minutiae. This perception, against a background of muted unease about this section of the exam, has been acknowledged by the College, which has decided therefore to introduce greater clinical emphasis into the science oral. The change of emphasis is relatively subtle, because both the College and its examiners remain reluctant to dilute the rigour of what for most candidates will be the last examination in anaesthesia that they are likely to take. Nevertheless, the tenor of many of the questions has now altered so that the clinical applications of the underlying science have more prominence than hitherto. The questions continue to have two parts: the basic scientific principles and their clinical application, but many of the topics will now be introduced via a clinically orientated question that is intended to reassure you that the subject does have anaesthetic relevance. The viva, or 'structured oral examination', as the College prefers to call it, lasts 30 minutes, during which time you will be asked questions on four different and unrelated subjects. The time spent on each should be around 7–8 minutes.

The marking system

The marking system continues to evolve. In the past, a 'close marking' system has been used, which meant that instead of being given a numerical mark a candidate was awarded one of four grades, which ranged from '1' to '2+'. A '1' represented a poor fail and '1+' a fail; a '2' was a pass and a '2+' was an outstanding pass. One of the justifications for the close marking system was that it did force examiners to make a definite choice between a pass and a fail, which a numerical marking system might otherwise allow them to avoid. A '1' mark in any part of the exam meant that the candidate was judged either to be potentially dangerous or to be too ignorant of the fundamentals of anaesthetic practice to pass, even should their other marks include three '2+'s. A '2+' represented an outstanding pass, indicative of a potential prize-winner. (The award of a prize may be considered if a candidate achieves a '2+' in each of the four parts of the exam at their first attempt.) For most candidates, therefore, the '1' and the '2+' marks were largely theoretical: what was much more important for them was the distinction between a '1+' and a '2'. What is now proposed is a system in which each of the four questions in the science oral will be marked independently by each examiner. Instead of receiving a single close mark, agreed by the two examiners after conferring, you will receive eight separate marks. Examiners have a choice of '0' (poor fail), '1' (fail) and '2' (pass). This is intended to reduce bias and variability further. At the time of writing it is not exactly clear how these marks will be translated into a final grade; nor how this system will be adjusted to allow feedback to unsuccessful candidates; nor how it will identify the exceptional candidate.

You will be aware that the FRCA is a structured examination. The material on which candidates are to be tested is made available to the examiners only on each morning of the exam. The questions are changed after each session to avoid any possibility of later candidates obtaining unfair advantage. Each pair of examiners will decide between themselves which two of the four questions they are going to ask. This is broadly the extent of the choice that they are able to make because the scope of each question is limited both by the guidance answer and by the relatively short time available for each topic. The first examiner will spend 7 or 8 minutes on the first subject before changing to the second. At the first bell (after 15 minutes), the other examiner will repeat the process. The examiner who is not asking questions will usually be making detailed notes which inform the marking process. Previously, at the end of the viva, each examiner used to record an independent mark before conferring and agreeing a final mark. The system that is currently envisaged is one in which the examiners will independently assess performance in each one of the four questions. The two will no longer confer; with this practice will disappear any accusation that one examiner may exert undue pressure on the other during the marking process. Importantly, this system also means that you must not allow yourself to become demoralized should a question go particularly badly. You must leave it behind you, conscious that the four questions are unrelated and that your other answers may well redeem it. In that respect it is not unlike the short answer question paper, in which a good answer can outweigh a poor one.

Appearance and affect

You cannot fail the Final FRCA because of your appearance or because of poor taste in clothes, and most examiners will be able to recollect candidates whose personal presentation could at best be described as unconventional. It rarely matters. At worst, however, an unkempt or casual appearance may convey the subliminal impression that you are unprofessional, and at the least it is likely to be a distraction. You should therefore wear something neutral and reasonably smart, which is comfortable and which you have worn before. The examination areas can be hot and there is no need to increase your stress levels further by forcing yourself into a three-piece suit or other outfit that sees the light of day only rarely.

Nor can you fail the FRCA because of inappropriate behaviour alone. Examiners are well aware of the stress that candidates are enduring, and most will make every attempt to put you at your ease. They are also likely to assume that aggressive or facile responses are a manifestation of stress and will make allowances accordingly. I have been answered with hostility: 'For God's sake don't ask me that – I've never even thought about it', and with fatuity: 'I'll probably know the answer when you tell me it.' I have also been subject to what might be described as the Bertie Wooster approach: the candidate didn't quite call me Jeeves but did say that 'it blocks the 1,2 hydroxy-whatsit, oh I don't know, you give the stuff and the atom bings off.' I have been patronized: 'Forgive me, but what I think that you are trying to ask is', and have even had to resist the obvious retort to the candidate who asked: 'Can I interest you in the concept of context-sensitive half-time?' None of it much matters. Yet examiners can be indulgent only up to a point, and the overall impression that you are creating will not be reassuring. If an inappropriate manner is also accompanied by a weak performance then you will stand little chance of being given the benefit of the doubt. Take issue with examiners, by all means: it is stimulating for both sides to develop a considered discussion of a topic, but avoid getting into an argument because the rules of this particular enterprise are not written in your favour.

Oral questions

On average you will have about 7 minutes on the topic. Should a question have somewhat limited scope, or if your knowledge is thin, you may spend a bit less time on it, but consistency demands that the examiners divide the time more or less equally. As explained above, these vivas are structured and the examiners have no choice of question. Although it would be logical, given the avowed purpose of the clinical science oral, to subdivide the questions into anaesthesia, intensive therapy and pain management, in practice they do not fit readily into these categories. In the past, the four questions could be somewhat random: it is now usual to have one question which relates to applied anatomy, one to physiology, one to pharmacology and one to physics, clinical measurement, equipment and statistics. This classification is not absolute (topics such as jaundice or latex allergy do not fit strictly into any one of these groups), but it does indicate the broad division of the available questions. The structured nature of the exam minimizes the likelihood of an examiner being able to question you in excessive depth on a subject which happens to be an area of special interest or expertise. It also increases the likelihood of an examiner having to ask questions about a subject in which they do not even have a current generalist interest. The sub-specialty interests of examiners change as retiring examiners are replaced but, at any one time, only about 15–20% will have an interest in intensive care medicine, in paediatric anaesthesia or in neuroanaesthesia, while a much smaller number will work in chronic pain management. Thus a paediatric cardiac anaesthetist may have to ask about adult ophthalmic applied anatomy, a neuroanaesthetist about neonatal fluid requirements, or an obstetric anaesthetist about intensive therapy ventilatory strategies. These examiners will not necessarily be ignorant on these topics, but it is certainly possible that your own clinical experience will be more recent and well informed than theirs. This should give you confidence, and you should not let the stress of the exam situation override it. Many candidates, for example, will have performed percutaneous tracheostomies in intensive care. However, unless your examiner is an intensivist, it is possible (if not probable) that he or she has performed not even one, and so your own clinical experience in this area is already much wider than his or hers. Draw confidence from this, and do not be intimidated. The examiner guidance may even be dated and say, for instance, that the approach should be through the first and second tracheal rings, whereas your own experience may reflect the increasing tendency to site the tracheostomy lower, between the second and third. So, if you do get the sense that the examiner is unhappy with your answer mainly because it does not accord with what is written on the sheet, then have the confidence to explain the current thinking. Do not be argumentative, but simply offer your considered reasoning of the issue. This is likely to increase your own credibility while perhaps denting that of the examiner. So, if you have recently seen an innovative technique used in the operating theatre, in the chronic pain clinic or in intensive care, do not be hesitant about citing it during the discussion.

The other consequence of the format of the structured oral is that it may lack fluency. It is partly a reflection of examining technique. Some examiners simply introduce the question before initiating a discussion, with only occasional reference to their paperwork. This is usually because they are familiar with the material and can allow the viva to run a more spontaneous course because they have confidence enough in their own ability to assess the answers. An examiner who is less comfortable with the topic and who is less certain of the criteria against which the answers are to be judged is likely to spend much more time referring to the answer sheet. Alternatively, of course, they might just be particularly pedantic in their interpretation of how a structured viva should be conducted. You may get a clue as to which of these you are facing by the way that they introduce the topic. The one type of examiner will try to put you more at ease by phrasing the question in a way which emphasizes the clinical context. Other examiners may simply look down at the sheet and intone 'What is an inotrope?' This second examiner is likely to want facts, and ideally the facts that are listed on the answer paper. He or she clearly has not realized that you are not telepathic. If, however, you have some confidence both in your knowledge and in your clinical experience, you may be able to get him or her on the defensive. Remember that such an examiner may never have initiated the use of dopexamine or enoximone, and if you sense a slight uncertainty which confirms that suspicion, then expound as freely as they will let you. Remember also that this may be the limit of the manipulation that you are able to employ, unless you can muster the bravado of the candidate who, when his examiner tried to interrupt his fluent and detailed answer, paused briefly to announce 'No, thank you, but I wish to finish.' The examiner, by his own confession somewhat intimidated by the intellectual onslaught, allowed the candidate to continue to the bell. That candidate passed; however, this is not a strategy for the faint-hearted.

What you may be able to do, however, is to refine your viva technique to improve the overall impression that you create. Take, for example, two imaginary candidates who have been asked about the Poiseuille–Hagen equation. The examiner initiates the questioning: 'Does this have any clinical relevance?' Candidate: 'Yes'. Examiner: 'Can you give me some examples?' Candidate: 'It affects fluid flow through tubes.' Examiner: 'In what way?' Candidate: 'If you increase the driving pressure, then you increase the flow' . . . and so it goes on, with more abbreviated answers prompted by the examiner from a candidate who gives no real sense of mastery of the subject. Could it be done better? The examiner asks the same question: 'Does this have any clinical relevance?' Candidate: 'The equation strictly applies only to Newtonian or ideal fluids, but in practice it still has cardiorespiratory implications. The relationship means that gas or liquid flow though a tube is inversely proportional to the length and viscosity of the fluid, and is directly proportional to the pressure gradient down the tube and, crucially, to the fourth power of its diameter.' This candidate, in contrast, requires no prompting, but demonstrates instead an orderly and logical approach that conveys the impression of obvious understanding of the topic.

Only the occasional candidate achieves the fluency of the second example, whereas rather more candidates behave like the first and require a little help. Yet if you do have some knowledge of the subject asked, you can train yourself, with practice, to deliver the information both with more facility and more enthusiasm. This applies particularly to the clinical areas of the viva in which you can make your experience count.

You do not need to worry about trying to pace the viva. It is the responsibility of the examiners to ensure that the requisite points are covered, and the guided answer sheets from which they are working contain more information than all but the most exceptional candidate will cover in the time. The clinical science questions continue broadly to have two parts, the basic science and its clinical application. However, this is still none the less a science oral and, despite the aspiration to increase the clinical relevance, the reality remains that in many of the questions it is the basic science that will be seen as the more important. Take for example the humidification of inspired gases. The clinical benefits of humidification are obvious: inhaled dry gases inspissate secretions, affect ciliary function and may cause impaired gas exchange due to atelectasis. However, these benefits can be summarized in a sentence; a sentence moreover that does not contain concepts that are especially complex. In contrast, the physical principles of latent heat of vaporization and saturated vapour pressure (which may be introduced by the subject of humidification) are topics which may warrant more detailed discussion. Equally, the anatomy of the nerves supplying the lower abdominal wall will take much longer to discuss than the description of a field block.

The viva on each subject lasts less than 8 minutes. The examiner will take up at least 20% of this time in framing the questions. That leaves you, therefore, with only about 5 or 6 minutes during which you have to talk. Were you to read out steadily, fluently and without hesitation one of the average length answers in this book, it would probably take you twice that long. There are few candidates, moreover, who can answer viva questions as rapidly as they can read. You should find this reassuring, because it means that you cannot be expected to convey more than a proportion of the information that appears in each of the specimen questions.

Why do they have to ask these kinds of question?

When your examiner looks up with an air of benign amusement from the question paper and invites you to discuss 'cytochrome P450' or 'chirality', your initial instinct may be to leap across the table to transfix them with your free Royal College examinations pencil. Some examiners, at least, will ask these questions with at least a hint of apology, which may raise your spirits marginally as you sense that these individuals might be on your side. Other examiners alas will be completely bereft of irony.

The difference between them should be obvious, but it might be of interest, if little consolation, were you to be aware of some of the reasons why such questions can arise.

A brief history of anaesthesia's inferiority complex

Anaesthesia had its humble origins in mid nineteenth century dentistry, and although hospital-based anaesthesia did become more sophisticated, in the early twentieth century simple general anaesthesia in the UK was still being delivered by individuals who were not only without medical qualifications but in many instances were without even a rudimentary education. In contrast, however, physicians and surgeons of that era had high social and intellectual standing that had been established for centuries. As the specialty evolved over succeeding decades it continued to enjoy only very modest status. There were, however, some politically astute individuals who recognized the potential perils of anaesthetic humility and who thought it unwise to succumb to anaesthesia's inferiority complex. In particular they recognized the truth that anaesthetists could achieve equality of status with surgeons only if they had a qualification that was equivalent to the Fellowship of the Royal College of Surgeons, the FRCS. It was this realization which explained the early two-part exams, first the Diploma of Anaesthesia, and then the FFARCS which was the immediate forerunner of the FRCA. These examinations were modelled on the FRCS, had a low pass mark in the region of 25–30% and, by including in the syllabus detailed anatomy and pathology, established the precedent for rigour in the basic sciences.

The establishment of a difficult anaesthetic exam with a low pass rate actually played a crucial role in the development of the specialty. When you are tempted, therefore, to curse the College for erecting the hurdles of the Primary and Final FRCA, you could at least reflect that the difficulty of these examinations may in some oblique way ensure that you get paid the same as your colleagues in surgery and medicine. Anaesthesia has a reputation for having amongst the most difficult postgraduate exams and, superficial though this may sound, it does remain one of the ways in which the specialty safeguards its standing.

Did this attempt to mirror the FRCS take the process too far? At times it can certainly seem so, and you may have to console yourself with the familiar, yet no less true, observation that 'Examinations are formidable even to the best prepared ... for the greatest fool may ask more than the wisest man can answer.' (Rev. Charles Colton 1780–1832). A more recent perspective was provided by a distinguished professor of medicine and scientist from Oxford. During his valedictory speech to the faculty of medicine he commented that in 30 years of clinical medicine his intimate knowledge of the Krebs cycle had influenced his management 'of not one single patient'. Medicine is as often pragmatic and empirical as it is intellectual. Some, but not all, examiners agree with that view, and do not accept that a detailed knowledge of scientific minutiae is necessary for the safe and effective practice of clinical anaesthesia. It may be obvious at your viva into which category the examiner falls.

Strategies for answering clinical science questions

Anatomy

Some candidates demonstrate a very detailed knowledge of areas of human anatomy, which allows them to embark on a thorough description of all the relevant structures and their immediate relations. Others have a more modest working knowledge and there is a final group which includes candidates who are able to demonstrate that they have only a very vague idea of where these structures lie. You will know as soon as the question is asked of you which of these types you most closely match. One obvious strategy for passing questions on applied anatomy is just to learn it, or at least develop enough confidence to be able to launch into a rapid account of the area in question. The speed of delivery is of some importance. Not every examiner will be able to recall the precise anatomical details that are found in the questions in this book. This means that they will probably have to make repeated reference to their answer sheet to check that what you are saying is true. Yet if they were to ask you to clarify more than one or two of your descriptions then too much of the time in the viva would be lost. There is a tendency, therefore, for the examiner to listen to what you are saying, rather than making frequent interruptions. At the end of your account he or she may simply judge their overall impression of its accuracy. Confident presentation may, in this instance, allow you to mask some gaps in your knowledge.

What if you are the candidate whose recollection of an area is vague? Your chances of success in the question will depend on whether it is what could be termed 'theoretical anatomy' or 'practical anatomy'. The coronary arterial and venous circulation is an example of theoretical anatomy. Certainly it is important, and of course it is true that anaesthesia may influence it, but it remains a visual construct which is neither seen nor felt. One tactic, which may salvage something from this part of the viva, is to move swiftly to the functional anatomy of the circulation. 'The main importance for anaesthetists of the right and left coronary circulations', you could state airily, 'lies in the way that we can influence oxygen supply and demand.' The examiner will take you back to check that you are indeed ignorant of the anatomy, but you will at least have initiated the physiological discussion which is the clinical part of the question and which, in any case, is generally of greater interest to both candidates and examiners alike. Other examples of theoretical anatomy are the cerebral circulation and the blood supply to the spinal cord.

Questions on 'practical anatomy' should be rather easier to handle because they relate to areas such as the internal jugular vein and the brachial plexus, detailed knowledge of which is of direct and self-evident importance. You can also reinforce this knowledge by disciplining yourself to visualize the relevant structures each time that you perform or observe a procedure relating to such an area. If you rehearse in your mind the nerves that are being blocked for an awake carotid endarterectomy as you see it being done, or describe the anatomy of the sacrum to a less experienced colleague to whom you are teaching a caudal block, it will not be long before the details are secure in your mind without recourse to yet more evening study. In other words, you can revise for the Final FRCA during the course of your daily work. This does not of course apply only to anatomy, but is true of other areas of the examination as well.

The examiner may ask you if you have performed a particular procedure, or may even give you a question that allows you to discuss, for example, an upper or lower limb block of your choosing. In respect of practical procedures that you claim to have undertaken, you should be aware that the threshold for a pass shifts sharply upwards. If you say that you regularly perform caudal blocks in children or interscalene blocks in adults, but then go on to reveal that your knowledge either of the anatomy or of the appropriate drug doses is at best hazy, then you will fail the viva badly. In examination anaesthesia, as in real life anaesthesia, whenever you are in any doubt you should choose the safest option. Better in both situations to admit that you have done very few caudal or interscalene blocks and that you would seek experienced help.

Finally, anatomy questions do lend themselves readily to diagrammatic answers. Many candidates seem to benefit from being allowed to describe the anatomy while they draw; producing the diagram acts as a stimulus to recollection. It is worth practising this technique because the number of anatomy topics is relatively small and it is almost certain that one of them will appear as a question.

Physiology

Anatomy, pharmacology and physics are all large scientific disciplines, yet in the context of the Final FRCA their scope is restricted, and the areas of specific relevance to anaesthetic practice are finite. Physiology, in contrast, is very wide-ranging, and questions appear which are related to all the systems, including renal, gastrointestinal and endocrine.

When the oral was marked as a whole entity it was almost inevitable that examiners would give more weight to core topics related to respiratory and cardiac physiology. The change in the marking system is probably intended to mean that this is no longer the case, with topics such as 'plasma proteins' and 'thyroid hormones' ranked equally with 'oxygen delivery' and 'pulmonary oedema'. However, it is likely that examiners will mark less stringently those subjects which they do not regard as central. You may need to do less, in other words, to pass a question on gut hormones than on assessment of cardiac function. So, as before, what this means in practice is that your grasp of core areas needs to be more secure than your knowledge of more peripheral aspects of physiology. It is not that you will not get asked a question on the latter, but that you will disadvantage yourself much more by ignorance of the former.

Pharmacology

The number of core anaesthetic drugs is limited. The sum of the regularly used induction agents, neuromuscular blockers, volatiles, analgesic drugs and local anaesthetics exceeds barely 20. The pharmacology of these substances is almost by definition applied science, and so you will find examiners much less forgiving of deficiencies in anaesthetic pharmacological knowledge than they would be of ignorance of lasers or medical statistics. You may feel somewhat aggrieved if the viva concentrates on GABA and NMDA receptor theory, but you should recognize that there is only so far that such a topic can be pursued, and you should be able to acknowledge finally that questioning about the scientific foundation of your everyday anaesthetic practice is a legitimate area of enquiry. Given the restricted numbers of drugs, however, it should not be an insuperable task to acquire the necessary amount of information. Some of the questions can be straightforward and lend themselves readily to a structured answer that you can adapt across the range of anaesthetic drugs. One such question, for instance, may ask you to enumerate the properties of an ideal volatile agent, and to compare desflurane and sevoflurane against that ideal. You will see that this same question could be asked of local anaesthetics, neuromuscular blockers, inotropes, anti-emetics and any number of classes of agents. You will also need to have some understanding of subjects such as pharmacokinetics and receptor theory. Other areas of relevance to anaesthetists are the non-anaesthetic drugs that patients may commonly take. The potential list is quite long and includes anti-hypertensive agents, drugs to treat asthma, drugs to treat diabetes and drugs which affect mood. Much of the knowledge that you may have acquired in working for the Primary FRCA will stand you in good stead for the Final. One final piece of advice: if you are asked the dose of a drug and you are unsure, then do not guess. Both in anaesthetic exams and in anaesthetic practice it is safer by far to admit that you would look it up.

Clinical measurement and equipment

You might have hoped to have left much of the physics and clinical measurement behind, but as also applies to pharmacology questions, much of the knowledge that you may have acquired in working for the Primary FRCA will be helpful for the Final. Some Final examiners are mesmerized by the physics involved in some of the questions that appear: others are less beguiled. If you are examined by one of the former group then expect to be asked to define, for example, the SI units that are appropriate to the particular question, and try not to worry if you get so immersed in the science that you only touch briefly on its clinical application. This is less likely than once it was now that there is an explicit emphasis on the clinical applications. At the other extreme lies the examiner who takes the view that complex anaesthetic devices are essentially black boxes whose inner workings can safely be left a mystery. In this case the viva will follow a rather different course, and it is probable that the emphasis will be more on clinical uses and on sources of error in interpretation of the information that is delivered. You will still need, therefore, to be prepared for both. Yet even those examiners who have considerable enthusiasm for this subject will recognize that there is a limit to how far it can reasonably be taken. The detailed physics underlying magnetic resonance imaging, for example, is too formidable to be covered in an oral such as this. If you can articulate the basic principles of the topic, whether it be magnetic resonance scanning or lasers, and if you can demonstrate that you are aware of its clinical and safety implications, then in most cases that should be enough to ensure you a pass.

Statistics

There are doctors who have an intuitive gift for statistics, which is a subject that they find very straightforward. Included amongst such doctors are some examiners and some candidates, and they do not therefore understand the collective groan that goes up when the prospect emerges either of having to ask or to answer a question on medical statistics. The fact remains, however, that the topic is unpopular with the majority of anaesthetists. Yet paradoxically this may be of some benefit to those who are uncomfortable with the concepts. Most examiners are conditioned by their own experience of asking about statistics to expect less than brilliant answers. What this means in practice is twofold. First, that the questions are not especially demanding and, second, that as long as you are able to enunciate some basic principles and definitions then you are more likely to get a bare pass than you would were you to offer the same level of information about, say, the anatomy of the epidural space. So as a minimum make sure, for example, that you know the difference between parametric and non-parametric data and tests, between paired and unpaired *t*-tests, about degrees of freedom and about the null hypothesis. Be prepared to discuss briefly the principles which underlie meta-analysis and be familiar with the results of at least one meta-analysis which is of clinical importance. Questions on statistics are unlikely now to stand alone but may be linked to subjects such as the design of clinical trials.

And finally: information, understanding and 'buzz words'

It is only a few years since one particularly ferocious examiner, having encountered some hapless candidate or other, argued that no one should be allowed to pass the FRCA if they did not know the structure of ether. Although she said 'structure' it is likely that she really meant 'formula' (which as it happens is $CH_3—CH_2-O-CH_2-CH_3$). Either way the proposition is absurd. Yet it does raise interesting issues in relation to postgraduate examinations. What is their primary purpose? What are they actually for?

Some have argued that, in addition to providing a test of knowledge and a core syllabus, examinations also act as an incentive to learn, and perhaps less urgently, as an incentive to teach. They are used as a hurdle to promotion, and success indicates to colleagues that a standard of training has been achieved. This may also offer a measure of reassurance to an increasingly suspicious public, particularly if the examination is perceived as conferring a title of distinction.

Only two of these functions are of immediate relevance to you. The first is the suggestion that the possession of the diploma of FRCA is a title of distinction. That may sound somewhat grandiose, but in fact it is in everyone's interest that it should be such. The diploma should not be easily won: it should feel like an exam that is difficult to pass yet one that is worth passing. Were it not so, then examiners and candidates alike would rapidly become demotivated and the standing of the specialty would slide. This thought may offer some solace as you lose many months of your life to the book work that is necessary. The second relevant factor is the exam's function as a test of knowledge. It is relatively simple to test for information, harder to assess understanding, and more difficult still to provide an objective test of judgement. So as a particular exam evolves, its structure and content elide to create what in effect becomes an examination game. Yet it is a game whose rules curiously do seem to become clear both to candidates and to examiners as independently they develop a broad appreciation of the level of knowledge that the exam expects.

This is partly because with many topics which appear as examination questions there is what could be described as a hierarchy of information. Take, for instance, 5-hydroxytryptamine (5-HT). At one end of its continuum of knowledge is the straightforward fact that it is an aminergic neurotransmitter. At the more difficult end are details such as the significance of the inositol triphosphate pathway for 5-HT_2 receptor function. In between these two extremes is the information about drugs which act at 5-HT receptors, the classes of 5-HT receptors, the subsets of those receptors and the physiological functions that they mediate. Somewhere along that scale is the boundary between a pass and a fail. So how much do you have to know about 5-HT to pass the question? Ask yourself. Should you know that ondansetron is a 5-HT_3 antagonist? Probably. Should you know the exact details of the fourteen 5-HT receptors that have been identified? Probably not, particularly as their functions have not been fully elaborated. Should you know that all bar 5-HT_3 receptors are coupled to G proteins? Possibly. Should you know that cerebrospinal fluid production is mediated via 5-HT_{2C} receptors? Not unless you are heading for the prize. Strange to say most examiners would probably give much the same replies. Both parties seem to understand the rules which dictate that the viva will start at the simpler end of the spectrum and move towards that fail/pass boundary. It is inevitable that it will take some time to cover the basic information, so how do you then convince the examiners that you deserve to pass? Facile though it may seem, some of the time you do it by producing the appropriate buzz words. They can be described as buzz words because, unless you are a potential prizewinner who has swept the core knowledge aside, there is unlikely to be much time to discuss the more complex information in any detail. By producing the key words and phrases you will, however, have given the examiner at least the subliminal impression that you know more about the subject than just basic information. So what are the buzz words in the example above? One of them would be G protein-coupling. This has a nice echo of Primary FRCA basic science about it and its mention alone may well satisfy the examiner who is unlikely then to explore your knowledge of ligand-gated ion channels. Similarly, it might help were you to mention that there were seven main 5-HT receptor types. What about a question, say, on atracurium or sevoflurane: how much should you know? Clearly you will have to display sufficient knowledge to show that your use of these agents is safe and effective. But beyond that it will help if you happen to refer to atracurium as a 'benzylisoquinolinium' and sevoflurane as a 'halogenated ether'. The examiners are not going to start asking about benzylisoquinolinium chemistry, although they might perhaps want to know what you mean by a 'halogenated ether'. Were you to reply that it is a hexafluorinated methyl isopropyl ether then that line of questioning would end. That is because it is actually a complete dead end down which, were you to have the knowledge, you could continue with the information that sevoflurane is fluoromethyl 1,1,1,3,3,3–hexafluoroisopropyl ether and that it can be synthesized by a reaction that involves formaldehyde and hydrogen fluoride. By this point even the most astringent examiner would recognize that you had both left anaesthesia far behind in the hot pursuit of irrelevant facts.

So, as you revise topics it is worth bearing this advice in mind because it should not be too difficult to identify those small additional pieces of information that may add further credibility to your answers. Another supplementary tactic that may stall a particular line of questioning is to throw in some entertaining piece of information about which the examiner is almost certainly ignorant. The MAC_{50} of sevoflurane, for example, is 3.3 in the sheep but only 2.3 in the horse; the oxygen concentration of the air expired by the sperm whale is 1.5% . . . This may seem dispiritingly reductive yet it does reflect the reality of a standardized exam in which basic knowledge has to be explored in a relatively rigid way. However, if your grasp of that basic knowledge is sound then you deserve to pass, and it would be unfortunate to fail the examination for want of a few of these simple strategies.

Good luck

Anatomy and its applications

The cerebral circulation

Commentary

This is a standard question but one which contains a lot of anatomical detail. It may be helpful to practise drawing a simple explanatory diagram. The viva may be linked to intracranial aneurysms and their management, and it may also touch on physiological aspects of cerebral perfusion, on the problem of cerebral vasospasm or briefly on the subject of intracranial pressure.

The viva

You will be asked about the arterial supply to the brain. The venous drainage is included below but is less likely to feature prominently in the oral.

Arterial supply (Figure 2.1)

- The brain is supplied by four major vessels: two internal carotid arteries which provide two-thirds of the arterial supply, and the two vertebral arteries which deliver the remaining third. (Some texts quote an 80:20 distribution.)
- The vertebral arteries give off the posterior inferior cerebellar arteries, before joining to form the basilar artery. This also provides the anterior inferior cerebellar and the superior cerebellar arteries.
- The basilar artery then gives off the two posterior cerebral arteries, which supply the medial side of the temporal lobe and the occipital lobe.
- The artery then anastomoses with the carotid arteries via two posterior communicating arteries.
- The internal carotid arteries meanwhile give rise to the middle cerebral arteries which supply the lateral parts of the cerebral hemispheres. They also provide much of the supply to the internal capsule, through which pass a large number of cortical afferent and efferent fibres.

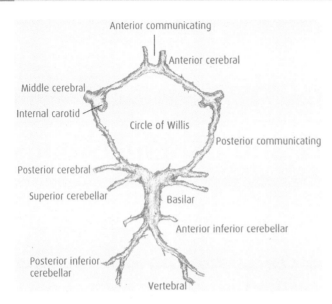

Fig. 2.1 Arterial supply of the brain.

- The carotids also give rise to the anterior cerebral arteries, which are connected by the anterior communicating artery and which supply the medial and superior aspects of the hemispheres.
- The three arterial stems (basilar and carotid arteries), linked by the anterior and posterior communicating arteries, comprise the arterial circle of Willis. This is said to be incomplete in up to 15% of normal asymptomatic subjects.

Venous system

- The cerebral and cerebellar cortices, which are relatively superficial structures, drain into the dural sinuses. These venous sinuses lie between the two layers of the cranial dura mater. The superior sagittal sinus lies along the attached edge of the falx cerebri, dividing the hemispheres, and usually drains into the right transverse sinus. The inferior sagittal sinus lies along the free edge of the falx and drains via the straight sinus into the left transverse sinus. (The straight sinus lies in the tentorium cerebelli.) The transverse sinuses merge into the sigmoid sinuses before emerging from the cranium as the internal jugular veins.
- Deeper cranial structures drain via the two internal cerebral veins, which join to form the great cerebral vein (of Galen). This also drains into the inferior sagittal sinus.
- The cavernous sinuses lie on either side of the pituitary fossa and drain eventually into the transverse sinuses.

Direction the viva may take

You may be asked about aneurysmal subarachnoid haemorrhage (SAH).

- Intracranial aneurysms account for about 75% of cases of spontaneous SAH; the incidence is 1 in 10–12 000 persons per year. The overall mortality rate approaches 50%.
- Aneurysms are associated with a weakening of the tunica media of the arterial wall and develop most commonly at vascular bifurcations. Only 10–20% of aneurysms

form in the posterior vertebrobasilar circulation. Most are found in the anterior carotid circulation, in the middle cerebral artery and in the anterior and posterior communicating arteries.

- **Cerebral vasospasm:** this is the major cause of morbidity and mortality following SAH. Its onset may be delayed for some days after the acute event and it may persist for 2 weeks. There are various theories for its aetiology which the viva will be most unlikely to explore, but it is worth noting that a large volume of subarachnoid blood (as seen on CT) is a consistent predictor of its development.
- **Prevention and management:** there will not be time to cover this in any detail, so an understanding of the broad principles will suffice. The calcium channel blocker nimodipine is given routinely for prophylaxis and improves outcome. Established or incipient cerebral vasospasm is managed with so-called 'Triple-H' therapy, **H**ypertension, **H**ypervolaemia and **H**aemodilution, the combination of which aims to increase perfusion pressure, decrease blood viscosity and maximize cerebral blood flow.

Further direction the viva may take

The direct anaesthetic implications of the anatomy described above are modest. You may be asked briefly about cerebral perfusion (page 147) or intracranial pressure (page 143). Below are some miscellaneous facts which may prove useful during the discussion.

- The circle of Willis provides effective collateral blood supply in the presence of arterial occlusion. Three out of four of the main arteries can be occluded as long as the process is gradual, without producing cerebral ischaemia. The normal intracranial blood volume is around 150 ml.
- The middle cerebral artery has been described as 'the artery of cerebral haemorrhage'. This is mainly because it supplies the internal capsule, where a large number of important cortical afferent and efferent fibres congregate.
- The superficial areas of the cerebral (and cerebellar) cortex drain to the venous sinuses via thin-walled veins. These are vulnerable to rupture, with the formation of subdural haematomas, particularly in the elderly in whom there is a loss of brain mass.
- Other potential intracranial catastrophes include cavernous sinus thrombosis, sagittal sinus thrombosis and cortical vein thrombosis (CVT). CVT is associated with pregnancy, and is reported as occurring in between 1 in 3000 and 1 in 6000 deliveries. If this figure is accurate, then CVT is being under-diagnosed, because very few obstetric anaesthetists encounter the one or two cases a year that this incidence would suggest.

The internal jugular vein

Commentary

The right internal jugular vein is probably the first site of choice for central venous cannulation, although in many intensive care units the subclavian route remains popular. The vein is readily accessible and the technique has a relatively low complication rate.

The ability to cannulate the vessel is a core skill. Questions on its anatomy may be preceded by a more general discussion about central venous pressure monitoring.

The viva

You may be asked about the principles of, and indications for, central venous cannulation.

- **Principle:** the central venous pressure (CVP) gives information both about a patient's volaemic status and about the function of the right ventricle.
- **Intravascular volume:** the CVP is the hydrostatic pressure generated by the blood within the right atrium (RA) or the great veins of the thorax. It provides an indication of volaemic status because the capacitance system, which includes all the large veins of the thorax, abdomen and proximal extremities, forms a large compliant reservoir for two-thirds of the total blood volume.
- **Right ventricular function:** CVP measurements also provide an indication of right ventricular (RV) function. Any impairment of RV function will be reflected by the higher filling pressures that are needed to maintain the same stroke volume (SV).
- **Normal values:** the normal range is 0–8 mmHg, measured at the level of the tricuspid valve. The tip of the catheter should lie just above the right atrium in the superior vena cava. CVP measurements are sometimes recorded as negative values. Sustained mean negative values can occur only if the transducer has been placed above the level of the right atrium. Transient negative values may be recorded in conditions such as severe acute asthma in which partial respiratory obstruction generates high negative intrathoracic pressures which are transmitted to the central veins.
- **Indications:** CVP catheters are used for the monitoring of CVP, for the insertion of pulmonary artery catheters (much less commonly in current practice), and to provide access for haemofiltration and transvenous cardiac pacing. They also allow the administration of drugs that cannot be given peripherally, such as inotropes and cytotoxic agents, and the infusion of total parenteral nutrition. In massive air embolism they can be used to aspirate air from the right side of the heart, although few anaesthetists have ever used them for this purpose.

Direction the viva will take

You may then be asked to describe the anatomy of the **internal jugular vein** (Figure 2.2)

- The internal jugular vein originates at the jugular foramen in the skull (the foramen drains the sigmoid sinus) and is a continuation of the jugular bulb.
- It follows a relatively straight course in the neck to terminate behind the sterno-clavicular joint where it joins the subclavian vein.
- Throughout its course it lies with the carotid artery and the vagus nerve within the carotid sheath, but it changes position in relation to the artery, lying first posteriorly before moving laterally and then anterolaterally.
- The vein is superficial in the upper part of the neck and then descends deep to the sternocleidomastoid muscle. The structures through which a cannulating needle passes are skin and subcutaneous tissue, the platysma muscle, sternocleidomastoid (in the lower neck) and the loose fascia of the carotid sheath.

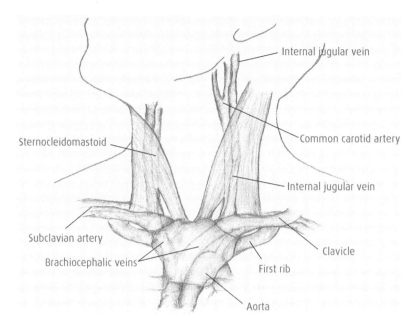

Fig. 2.2 The great veins of the neck.

- Anterior to the vein at the top of its course lie the internal carotid artery and the vagus nerve.
- Posterior to the vein (from above downwards) are the lateral part of C_1, the prevertebral fascia and vertebral muscles, the cervical transverse processes, the sympathetic chain and, at the root of the neck, the dome of the pleura. On the left side the jugular vein lies anterior to the thoracic duct.
- Medial to the vein are the carotid arteries (internal and common) and four cranial nerves: the ninth (glossopharyngeal, IX), the tenth (vagus, X), the eleventh (accessory, XI) and the twelfth (hypoglossal, XII).

Further direction the viva may take

You may be asked briefly to describe a technique for venous cannulation.

You will have had experience of this technique. Describe the one with which you are most familiar. The use of ultrasound-guided cannulation is now widespread but does not absolve you of the need to know the basic anatomy (for the 'landmark' approach).

- As an example: the high approach. A fine 'seeking' needle (25G or similar) is inserted at the level of the superior border of the thyroid cartilage (at about C_4) and on the medial border of sternocleidomastoid.
- The needle is directed caudally at an angle of 30° in the direction of the ipsilateral nipple. The vein is usually quite superficial, although this will depend on the body habitus of the patient.
- Once the vein is located, the Seldinger technique (catheter over guidewire) can be used to establish definitive central access.

You might also be asked what other site you would choose were internal jugular cannulation to be impossible (for example, in major head and neck surgery or in a patient with neck and facial burns).

- The alternatives are the **subclavian**, **femoral** and the **median cubital** and **basilic** veins of the antecubital fossa. A peripheral long line can be inserted via the latter (page 76). This technique has few complications but the catheter tip may fail to pass beyond the acute curve at the clavipectoral fascia and the catheter length means that fluid cannot be infused rapidly. The femoral vein is commonly overlaid by the superficial femoral artery and the variable anatomy means that femoral access can sometimes be difficult. The route is used commonly in children but is more of a last resort in adults, in whom the subclavian veins are usually a better alternative.
- **Anatomy of the subclavian veins:** the right and left subclavian veins are relatively short, extending from the outer border of the first rib to the medial border of the scalenus anterior muscle. Here they unite with the internal jugular veins to form the brachiocephalic veins. The important relations are anteriorly the clavicle, posteriorly the subclavian artery and inferiorly the dome of the pleura. The insertion point of the cannula is usually 1 cm below the clavicle at its midpoint, directed towards the suprasternal notch.

Further direction the viva could take

You may be asked about complications associated with the technique and how these may be avoided. The following is a compilation of the most common; the literature is full of others which range from spinal accessory nerve injury to cardiac tamponade. Cite one or two of these by all means, but you will be unlikely to have the opportunity to discuss them in any detail.

- **Complications:** some of these can be minimized by the use of an ultrasound-guided needle. The National Institute of Clinical Excellence (NICE) report of September 2002 recommended the routine use of ultrasound for locating the internal jugular vein. Evidence to support its use for other sites is not yet robust but experience is widening to the point at which ultrasound-guided cannulation will be routine.
- **Carotid artery puncture or cannulation:** the risk is reduced if the artery is palpated continuously throughout cannulation, and it is minimized by the use of an ultrasound-guided needle.
- **Pneumothorax (and haemothorax):** this is less likely if a high approach is used, which avoids the dome of the pleura.
- **Thoracic duct injury (chylothorax):** the thoracic duct cannot be damaged if the left side is not used. Otherwise the risk is minimized by using a high approach.
- **Intrapleural placement:** here too the risk is minimized by using a high approach which avoids the pleura. A check X-ray will prevent inadvertent intrapleural infusion.
- **Air embolism:** positioning the patient head down during insertion (and removal) decreases the risk.
- **Cardiac arrhythmias:** these may occur should the guidewire or catheter reach the heart.

- **Infection:** central line infection can be disastrous. Significant infection is said occur in around 12% of insertions, although the rate of bacterial colonization is likely to be higher. The risks are reduced by scrupulous aseptic technique as well as meticulous aftercare (page 106).

Ocular anatomy

Commentary

Questions on the eye seem to be over-represented in the Final FRCA. It may be owing to the fact that considerable anatomical detail is concentrated in a small well-circumscribed area, and that the oral can go in a number of directions, including pupillary and eye signs and intraocular pressure. You will not be expected to cover the entire anatomy of the eye, but the account which follows should prepare you for most eventualities.

The viva

You may be asked about methods of anaesthetizing the eye for intraocular surgery. Although retrobulbar and peribulbar blocks are being supplanted by sub-Tenon's block and by topical local anaesthesia, they allow some discussion of the anatomy. You will only have to discuss one or two of these methods, usually the one(s) with which you are familiar, and so there is more detail below than you will need.

- **Topical:** the anterior structures can be anaesthetized using topical amethocaine 0.5% or 1.0%, oxybuprocaine 0.4% and proxymetacaine 0.5%. Topical anaesthesia is simple and (mostly) safe and effective, although the lack of akinesia of the eye and eyelids means that the surgeon has to control eye movement via the intraocular instruments. Anaesthesia can be supplemented by the addition of lignocaine to the irrigation fluid, or by further instillation of drops. These can cause oedema of the cornea and excessive doses may exacerbate the problem.
- **Retrobulbar block:** this is performed by a single injection that is made either percutaneously or transconjunctivally. The axial length of the eye gives a guide to needle depth and, if the percutaneous approach is used, a 25-mm needle is long enough to reach the retrobulbar muscular cone. The injection (3–4 ml) is made at the junction of the lateral and middle thirds of the orbital margin in the inferotemporal quadrant. Complications include retrobulbar haemorrhage, penetration of the globe, damage to the optic nerve or ophthalmic vessels, and central spread of local anaesthetic (1 in 500). Retrobulbar block is very effective, but potential complications have led many to abandon it in favour of other techniques.
- **Peribulbar block:** this has been cited as a safe and effective alternative to retrobulbar block, but it too is not without its problems. Larger volumes of local anaesthetic are required (8–10 ml), which increases the intraorbital pressure and causes periorbital chemosis. The onset of block is also considerably slower and the failure rate higher. The risk of scleral perforation is not removed because the technique requires one inferotemporal and one superonasal injection, both of which are directed beyond the

equator of the globe. (Some include a third injection, made at the extreme medial side of the palpebral fissure).

- **Sub-Tenon's block:** the popularity of this technique has increased because it is viewed as safer than the sharp needle approaches. It is, however, more invasive, in that a modest amount of surgical dissection is necessary. After topical anaesthesia to the conjunctiva the patient is asked to look upwards and outwards (in the direction of the operator). This improves access to the inferonasal quadrant where the injection is made, as posteriorly as possible. A fold of conjunctiva is drawn upwards with forceps. A small nick at the base of this fold with surgical scissors opens the sub-Tenon's fascia. A blunt cannula is then inserted gently into this space and guided backwards following the contour of the globe. Injection of 4–5 ml of local anaesthetic solution will provide analgesia and adequate akinesia. The globe can in theory be perforated, and central spread of local anaesthetic has been described, but these complications are sufficiently rare for sub-Tenon's block to be considered suitable for administration by trained, but non-medical, practitioners.

Direction the viva may take

You may be asked to describe the anatomy of the orbit or you may be invited to concentrate on one aspect, such as the extraocular muscles or the structures passing through the main orbital fissures.

- The bony orbit has been described variously as a pyramid whose apex is directed inwards and upwards; as a cone; and as a pear whose stem points towards the optic canal. Its roof consists of the orbital plate of the frontal bone, with the anterior cranial fossa above, while its floor is formed by the zygoma and the maxilla, with the maxillary sinus beneath. Its medial wall is formed by parts of the maxilla, lacrimal bone, ethmoid and sphenoid, and beyond it lie the ethmoid air cells and the nasal cavity. The zygoma and the greater wing of the sphenoid make up its lateral wall.
- The bony orbit contains the globe, together with the muscles, nerves and blood vessels that subserve the normal functions of the eye.
- The normal globe has an axial length of around 24 mm (as measured in the anteroposterior diameter). An eye longer than 26 mm is usually myopic. Its outer layer comprises sclera and cornea, the middle vascular layer contains the choroid, the ciliary body and the iris, and the innermost layer comprises neural tissue in the form of the retina.
- The movements of the globe are controlled by the six extraocular striated muscles. The four recti (lateral, medial, superior and inferior) originate from the annulus of Zinn, the tendinous ring which encircles the optic foramen, and insert beyond the equator of the globe. The lateral and medial recti have two heads. The superior oblique muscle originates above and medial to the annulus, curves round the trochlea (which acts like a pulley) before inserting behind the equator and beneath the superior rectus. The inferior oblique originates from the lacrimal bone and inserts posterolaterally on the globe, having passed beneath the inferior rectus muscle.
- **Motor innervation:** the lateral rectus is supplied by the sixth cranial nerve, the abducens (VI), and the superior oblique is supplied by the fourth, the trochlear (IV).

The remaining muscles are supplied by the third cranial nerve, the oculomotor (III). (This also supplies levator palpebrae superioris, which elevates the eyelid).

- **Autonomic innervation:** sympathetic innervation is by the long and short ciliary nerves via the superior cervical ganglion. Nerve impulses dilate the pupil via the dilators of the iris. Parasympathetic innervation is by the short postganglionic ciliary nerves via the ciliary ganglion. The pre-ganglionic supply comes from the oculomotor nerve, and its impulses constrict the pupil.
- **Sensory supply:** this is derived mainly from the ophthalmic branch of the fifth cranial nerve, the trigeminal (V), although branches of the maxillary division make some contribution to lateral structures and to the nasolacrimal apparatus. There are a large number of sensory nerves for such an anatomically confined area. The examiner is unlikely to dwell on these in any detail but, in summary, the innervation that may have relevance for ocular surgery can be outlined as follows. The ophthalmic division V^1 branches into the frontal nerve, which then subdivides into the supratrochlear nerves (medial upper conjunctiva), the supraorbital nerve (upper conjunctiva) and the long ciliary nerve (cornea, iris and ciliary muscle). V^1 also forms the nasociliary nerve, which in turn branches into the infratrochlear nerve (inner canthus and lacrimal sac), and the long sensory root to the ciliary ganglion (thence to the cornea and iris). The lacrimal branch of V^1 supplies the rest of the conjunctiva.
- **Foramina:** the orbit contains nine fissures and foramina, of which three are particularly important: the optic foramen (canal), and the superior and inferior orbital fissures.
- **Optic canal.** The optic nerve and ophthalmic artery traverse the optic foramen.
- **Superior orbital fissure:** through this fissure run the oculomotor, trochlear and abducens nerves to the extraocular muscles, together with the frontal, nasociliary and lacrimal nerves, and the superior and inferior ophthalmic veins. The oculomotor, abducens and nasociliary nerves traverse the lower part of the fissure and enter the muscular cone between the two heads of the lateral rectus. The trochlear, frontal and lacrimal nerves remain outside the cone.
- **Inferior orbital fissure:** through the inferior fissure run the zygomatic and infraorbital nerves (branches of V^2), the infraorbital artery and the inferior ophthalmic vein.

Further direction the viva may take
You could be asked about intraocular pressure (page 150).

The autonomic nervous system

Commentary
This potentially is a large question which, were you to address it in even moderate detail, would exceed the time available. The account below is simplified, but it should

prove adequate. Discussion of the core anatomy may be preceded by a more clinically orientated question on, for example, autonomic neuropathy. Other topics may include sympathetic blocks, vagal reflexes or sympathetically maintained pain. There is unlikely to be time to explore these topics in any depth, and you will probably have to convey only the headline details.

The viva

There are a number of routes into this anatomical question.

You may be asked about autonomic neuropathy.

- **Autonomic neuropathy:** this may be associated with conditions such as diabetes, chronic alcoholism, nutritional deficiency, Guillain–Barré syndrome, Parkinson's disease and AIDS. Rarely, it is seen as a primary condition in the Shy–Drager syndrome or familial dysautonomia. Its clinical features include disordered cardiovascular responses and orthostatic hypotension, the absence of sinus arrhythmia and inability to compensate during the Valsalva manoeuvre. Patients may complain of flushing, erratic temperature control with night sweats, episodic diarrhoea and nocturnal diuresis. The normal response to hypoglycaemia is lost, as are normal diurnal rhythms.

Alternatively, you may be asked about sympathetic blocks.

- **Sympathetic blocks:** examples include lumbar sympathectomy (page 63), stellate ganglion block (page 46) and coeliac plexus block (page 59). Chemical or surgical sympathectomy has been used to improve the blood supply in vasospastic or atherosclerotic disorders of the peripheral circulation, to control hyperhydrosis, and to treat pain associated with myocardial ischaemia. Sympathetic blocks also have a place in the management of sympathetically maintained pain (pages 24, 386).

You may be asked to describe the anatomy of the autonomic nervous system.

Sympathetic division

- Pre-ganglionic myelinated efferents from the hypothalamus, medulla oblongata and spinal cord leave the cord with the ventral nerve roots of the first thoracic nerve down to the second, third and, in some subjects, the fourth lumbar spinal nerves (T_1–L_{2-4}).
- These efferents pass via the white rami communicantes to synapse in the sympathetic ganglia lying in the paravertebral sympathetic trunk, which is closely related throughout its length to the spinal column.
- They synapse with post-ganglionic neurons, usually non-myelinated, some of which pass directly to viscera. Others pass back via the grey rami communicantes to rejoin the spinal nerves with which they travel to their effector sites. A number of pre-ganglionic fibres (from T_5 and below) synapse in collateral ganglia which are close to the viscera that they innervate. These collateral ganglia include the coeliac ganglion (receiving fibres from the greater and lesser splanchnic nerves) and the superior and inferior mesenteric ganglia. The adrenal medulla is innervated directly by pre-ganglionic fibres via the splanchnic nerves, which pass without relay through the coeliac ganglion.

- The sympathetic supply to the head originates from three structures: the superior cervical ganglion, the middle cervical ganglion and the stellate ganglion.
- Distribution of the sympathetic supply to the viscera occurs via a series of sympathetic plexuses. The main three are the cardiac, the coeliac and the hypogastric plexuses.
- The segmental sympathetic supply to the head and neck is from T_1 to T_5; to the upper limb from T_2 to T_5; to the lower limb from T_{10} to L_2; and to the heart from T_1 to T_5.
- The anatomy of the sympathetic division is such that it can function better as a mass unit. The parasympathetic division, in contrast, comprises relatively independent components.

Parasympathetic division

- The parasympathetic nervous system has a cranial and a sacral outflow. The cranial efferents originate in the brain stem and travel with the third (oculomotor), seventh (facial), and ninth (glossopharyngeal) cranial nerves. These pass via the ciliary, sphenopalatine, submaxillary and otic ganglia to subserve parasympathetic function in the head. The most important cranial efferent is the tenth (vagus) cranial nerve, which supplies the thoracic and abdominal viscera. Its fibres synapse with short post-ganglionic neurons that are on or near the effector organs.
- The sacral outflow originates from the second, third and fourth sacral spinal nerves to supply the pelvic viscera. As with the vagus nerve, the fibres synapse with short post-ganglionic neurons that are close to the effector organs.

Autonomic afferents

- These mediate the afferent arc of autonomic reflexes and conduct visceral pain stimuli. The vagus has a substantial visceral afferent component, the importance of which is well recognized by anaesthetists who commonly have to deal with vagally mediated bradycardia or laryngeal spasm. Sympathetic afferent fibres are also involved in the transmission of visceral pain impulses, including those originating from the myocardium. This is the rationale for using stellate ganglion block to treat refractory angina pectoris. Sympathetic afferents are also involved in sympathetically maintained pain states such as the complex regional pain syndrome. There is usually no direct communication between afferent neurons and sympathetic post-ganglionic fibres, but following injury there is some form of sympathetic–afferent coupling.

Neurotransmitters

- **Sympathetic:** acetylcholine is the neurotransmitter at sympathetic pre-ganglionic fibres (at nicotinic receptors). Noradrenaline is the neurotransmitter at most post-ganglionic fibres, apart from those to sweat glands and to some vasodilator fibres in skeletal muscle.
- **Parasympathetic:** acetylcholine is the neurotransmitter throughout the parasympathetic division, acting at nicotinic receptors in autonomic ganglia, and at muscarinic post-ganglionic receptors thereafter.

Direction the viva may take

Diverse supplementary topics could include vagal reflexes or sympathetically maintained pain.

- **Vagal reflexes:** the word 'vagus' comes from the Latin, meaning 'wandering'. (Had it been derived instead from Greek, then the nerve – improbably – would have been called the 'plankton'). It distributes widely, and sources of stimulation that can lead to bradycardia and sometimes to asystolic cardiac arrest include the dura, the zygoma, the extraocular muscles, particularly the medial rectus, the carotid sinus, the pharynx, the glottis, the bronchial tree, the heart, the mesentery and peritoneum, the bladder and urethra, the testis and the rectum and anus. The Brewer–Luckhardt reflex describes laryngospasm that is provoked by a distant stimulus. Vagal reflexes can be attenuated by the use of an anticholinergic such as atropine, but in low doses this can stimulate the vagus before it blocks it (the Bezold–Jarisch reflex).
- **Sympathetically maintained pain:** in some pain syndromes it appears that efferent noradrenergic sympathetic activity and circulating catecholamines have a role in maintaining chronic pain. There is usually no communication between sympathetic efferent and afferent fibres, but following nerve injury it is apparent that modulation of nociceptive impulses can occur not only at the site of injury, but also in distal undamaged fibres and the dorsal root ganglion itself (page 386).

The trigeminal nerve

Commentary

The applied anatomy of the trigeminal nerve is relevant mainly for those working in the management of chronic pain. Trigeminal neuralgia is described classically as one of the most extreme pains in human experience, one which is reported to have driven some patients even to suicide. It is a dramatic condition, and one that is amenable to a range of treatments. You should have some familiarity with it.

The viva

You may be asked about trigeminal neuralgia: its definition, its clinical features and its management. It is during the discussion of non-pharmacological management that you will be asked to describe its anatomy.

- **Definition:** trigeminal neuralgia is a severe neuropathic pain with a reputation as one of the worst pains in human experience.
- **Clinical features:** the peak onset of the condition is in middle age. The pain typically is intermittent, lancinating, and extremely severe. Attacks are spasmodic, lasting only seconds. Patients are pain-free in the interim, but episodes may be very frequent. Pain is limited usually to one (occasionally two) of the branches of the trigeminal nerve, which supplies sensation to the face. It occurs least commonly in the ophthalmic

division, which accounts for only around 5% of cases, and more frequently in the maxillary or mandibular divisions. The distribution is always unilateral. Paroxysmal pain can be precipitated by trigger points around the face which react to the lightest of stimuli, such as a light breeze or touch, and by actions such as chewing or shaving.

- **Pathogenesis:** this remains speculative. It may be caused centrally, with abnormal neurons in the pons exhibiting spontaneous and uncontrolled discharge in the nerve. It may also be caused by peripheral factors: due either to demyelination (in younger patients trigeminal neuralgia may be a first symptom of multiple sclerosis) or to compression by abnormal blood vessels in the posterior fossa.
- **Pharmacological treatment:** (in an anatomy viva you will not be asked about this in any detail; it is included below for completeness.)
  — *Carbamazepine* is effective in more than 90% of cases of true trigeminal neuralgia (100 mg b.d. up to maintenance of 600–1200 mg day^{-1}). The full blood count must be monitored because the drug can cause bone marrow suppression.
  — *Phenytoin* is effective in a smaller proportion (around 60%) and can be given intravenously for acute intractable pain (the starting dose is 300–500 mg day^{-1}).
  — *Baclofen* is an antispasmodic γ-amino butyric acid (GABA) analogue, which binds to GABA$_B$ receptors (the dose is up to 80 mg day^{-1}).
  — *Gabapentin* is a GABA analogue, which does not, however, act on GABA receptors. Its mechanism of action is unclear. It is an anticonvulsant which clinicians increasingly are using to treat neuropathic pain. The dose is titrated against response to a maximum of 1800 mg daily.

Direction the viva will take

You will be asked to describe the anatomy of the trigeminal nerve.

- The trigeminal (fifth cranial nerve, V) is the largest of the 12, and provides the sensory supply to the face, nose and mouth as well as much of the scalp. Its motor branches include the supply to the muscles of mastication.
- It has a single motor nucleus and three sensory nuclei in the brain. The motor nucleus is in the upper pons, and lying lateral to it is the principal sensory nucleus, which subserves touch sensation. The mesencephalic nucleus is sited in the midbrain and subserves proprioception. Pain and temperature sensation are subserved by the nucleus of the spinal tract of the trigeminal nerve. This lies deep to a tract of descending fibres which run from the pons to the substantia gelatinosa of the spinal cord.
- Sensory fibres pass through the trigeminal (Gasserian) ganglion. It is crescent-shaped (hence its alternative description as the semilunar ganglion), and lies within an invagination of dura mater near the apex of the petrous temporal bone, and at the posterior extremity of the zygomatic arch. The motor fibres of the trigeminal nerve pass below the ganglion.
- From this ganglion pass the three divisions of the nerve: the ophthalmic (V^1), which is the smallest of the three, the maxillary (V^2) and the mandibular (V^3).
- **Ophthalmic division:** this passes along the lateral wall of the cavernous sinus before dividing just before the superior orbital fissure into the lacrimal, nasociliary and

frontal branches. The frontal branch divides further into the supraorbital and supratrochlear nerves.

- **Maxillary division:** This runs below the ophthalmic division before leaving the base of the skull via the foramen rotundum. It crosses the pterygopalatine fossa, giving off superior alveolar dental nerves, zygomatic nerves and sphenopalatine nerves before entering the infraorbital canal and emerging through the infraorbital foramen as the infraorbital nerve.
- **Mandibular division:** this is the largest of the three branches and is the only one to have both motor and sensory components. Its large sensory root passes through the foramen ovale to join with the smaller motor root, which runs beneath the ganglion. Its branches include the sensory lingual, auriculotemporal and buccal nerves; the inferior dental nerve, which is mixed motor and sensory; and motor nerves to the muscles of mastication, the masseteric and lateral pterygoid nerves.

Further direction the viva may take

You may be asked about non-pharmacological methods of management of trigeminal neuralgia.

Destructive

- **Radiofrequency ablation:** a needle is passed percutaneously and under X-ray control through the foramen ovale to the trigeminal ganglion. The entry point of the needle is below the posterior third of the zygoma. Chemical ablation may also be used. This technique can be complicated by anaesthesia dolorosa, in which the patient loses not only the pain, but also most of the sensation to that side of the face, which feels dead and 'woody'. The patient needs to be awake and cooperative during part of the procedure but needs to be 'deeply sedated' – transiently – for the ablation itself. This can be challenging.

Surgical

- **Surgical decompression:** this is the most invasive therapeutic technique because it requires formal neurosurgical exploration of the posterior fossa to identify the aberrant vessel(s) which are compressing the nerve near its emergence from the pons.

The nose

Commentary

The nose has never featured highly in the anatomical canon of most anaesthetists. Perhaps it deserves greater prominence, acting as it does as a conduit for devices such as nasopharyngeal airways, nasotracheal tubes, nasogastric tubes and fibreoptic bronchoscopes. Be that as it may, the anatomy of the nose is part of the syllabus and so you will need to have a passing acquaintance with its main features. Potentially this subject could incorporate a considerable amount of information which would take too long to convey and so the examiner is unlikely to expect fine detail. The account below is simplified but should be sufficient for your purpose.

The viva

By way of introduction you may be asked about the important functions of the nose.

- **Functions:** it is the organ of olfaction; as part of the respiratory apparatus it warms and humidifies inspired gases; it has a secondary function as a resonator in speech and it filters inspired pathogens and irritants. In infants and small children the small degree of expiratory resistance which it provides combines with partial adduction of the vocal cords during expiration to produce the continuous positive airways pressure (CPAP) which opposes premature airway closure.

You will then be asked about the anatomy.

- **Framework of the nose:** the anatomy is not limited to the external nose but also includes the extensive nasal cavity which is composed of several bones of the skull. Each side of the nose comprises, in summary, the roof, medial and lateral walls, and floor.
  — *Roof:* this is formed from the nasal and frontal bones which make up the bridge of the nose: the cribriform plate of the ethmoid which forms the middle flat section; and the body of the sphenoid which slopes backwards and downwards to complete the posterior part of the cavity.
  — *Medial wall:* medially is the nasal septum – the lower part is cartilaginous; the upper is formed from the perpendicular plate of the ethmoid and from the vomer.
  — *Lateral wall:* this comprises the ethmoid above, the nasal maxilla below and in front, and the perpendicular plate of the palatine bone behind. This lateral wall contains the three turbinate bones, also known as the conchae (pronounced 'con-kee'). ('Turbinate' comes from the Latin word for 'spinning top', while 'concha' derives from the Latin word for 'mussel shell', reflecting the scrolled shape of the bones.) Each of the upper, middle and inferior conchae curves over a meatus. The shape of the conchae increases the flow of inspired air over as large a surface area as possible, thereby maximizing the humidifying, warming and filtering functions of the nose.
  — *Floor:* this surface is slightly curved and is formed from part of the maxilla and the palatine bone. Anteriorly is the nasal vestibule.
- **Blood supply:** the upper part of the nose is supplied by branches of the ophthalmic artery (anterior and posterior ethmoidal), while the lower is supplied by branches of the maxillary artery (sphenopalatine) and the facial artery (superior labial). Venous drainage is via the facial and ophthalmic veins, some tributaries of which drain into the cavernous sinus.
- **Olfaction:** olfactory receptors are found in a small area of the upper part of the nasal septum and the lateral walls. The fibres of the olfactory (first cranial) nerve pass through the cribriform plate of the ethmoid bone to synapse directly with cells in the olfactory bulb. Unlike other visceral afferents, these fibres do not synapse in

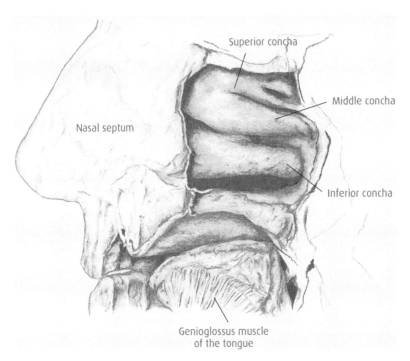

Fig. 2.3 The nose.

ganglia. As they pass through the cribriform plate, the nerve bundles become invested in a sleeve of dura, thereby providing a route of infection from the nasal cavity to the central nervous system.

- **Sensation:** branches of the trigeminal (V) nerve supply the nose. The septum is innervated mainly by the long sphenopalatine nerve (a branch of the maxillary division, V^2), with a contribution from the anterior ethmoidal nerve (a branch of the nasociliary nerve from V^1). The upper lateral wall is innervated by the short sphenopalatine nerve (also from V^2). The inferior part is innervated by the superior dental nerve and the greater palatine nerve (which are also branches of V^2).

Direction the viva may take
The nose is a conduit for various devices but you are likely to be asked about aspects which are relevant to airway management.

- **Instrumentation:** the nose is a passage for nasotracheal tubes, nasopharyngeal airways, nasogastric tubes, fibreoptic bronchoscopes, temperature probes and oesophageal Doppler monitoring probes. The technique for their insertion does not differ: each device should be directed straight backwards along the floor of the nose and beneath the inferior concha (Figure 2.3). It is not necessary to use any force: firm pressure is the most that is needed for an appropriate sized tube. The rich blood supply to the turbinates is under reflex control and the vessels engorge and empty in response to factors such as airflow pressure and temperature. Sustained but gentle pressure may be enough to allow vascular engorgement to subside and prevent the copious bleeding that can follow nasal instrumentation.

- **Indications for nasotracheal intubation:** nasal intubation allows surgeons optimal access to the oral cavity. Awake fibreoptic nasal intubation may be indicated in patients whose mouth opening is limited, but is also the route preferred by most anaesthetists for cases of predicted difficult intubation. Fibreoptic intubation has superseded blind nasal intubation, which is a technique that is no longer routinely taught. Nasal tubes are used in patients who require prolonged intubation. This applies more to children than to adults in whom tracheostomy is a more common option.

- **Contraindications for nasotracheal intubation:** midface deformity, congenital or acquired, may make nasal intubation impossible. Coagulopathy may be accompanied by significant nasal haemorrhage and traditional teaching always held, for example, that nasal intubation should be avoided in patients with haemophilia. One of the primary contraindications is basal skull fracture the clinical features of which can include cerebrospinal fluid (CSF) rhinorrhoea, so-called 'raccoon' eyes, and mastoid bruising (Battle's sign).

- **Complications:** brisk bleeding can occur following trauma to the rich blood supply. The nasopharyngeal mucosa is not robust and a nasal or nasogastric tube can breach the mucosa of the posterior pharyngeal wall. Nasal instrumentation is associated with bacteraemia, and some anaesthetists even give prophylactic antibiotics when using a nasotracheal tube. Intracranial placement has been described following procedures such as trans-sphenoidal neurosurgery, which leaves a small bony defect that can be penetrated inadvertently.

- **Which nostril should you use?** Most anaesthetists favour the right side, which is appropriate if the nares are symmetrical but more problematic if they are not. Asymmetrical nostrils indicate that the nasal septum is probably deviated. The naris that is narrower anteriorly is actually wider posteriorly and so, paradoxically, it is the narrower nostril that should be chosen.

- **Local anaesthesia:** the nasal mucosa is most effectively and easily blocked by topical solutions of local anaesthetic. Common options are cocaine 10% and lignocaine 5%/phenylephrine 0.5% mixtures. Xylometazoline (Otrivine) is a nasal decongestant which causes vasoconstriction of mucosal blood vessels. Its effect is short-lived and it usually causes rebound hyperaemia.

Sensory nerve supply to the face

Commentary

The major sensory supply to the face is easy to describe: it is the numerous terminal branches that may give you more difficulty. Equally, the examiner may not immediately be intimate with the 25 or more named nerves which originate from the trigeminal nerve, and so your detailed knowledge need extend only to those branches which can be blocked with local anaesthetic to allow minor surgery on the face or to provide postoperative analgesia.

The viva

This topic is basically applied anatomy. It may be introduced by means of a brief discussion about nerves which are at risk from pressure (such as the supraorbital nerves) or which may be affected by disease processes (such as herpes zoster affecting branches of the trigeminal nerve; or trigeminal neuralgia.) This will move quickly on to description of the anatomy.

- **Sensory supply:** the sensory supply to the face is provided mainly by the three divisions of the fifth cranial nerve, the trigeminal. (As the largest cranial nerve it also supplies much of the scalp, the mouth, teeth and the nasal cavity.) The skin over the parotid gland and the angle of the mandible is, however, supplied by the greater auricular nerve, which arises from the ventral rami of the second and third cervical nerves.
- **Trigeminal nerve divisions:** at the trigeminal (Gasserian) ganglion the nerve separates into the ophthalmic (V^1), the maxillary (V^2) and the mandibular (V^3) divisions.
  — *Ophthalmic (V^1):* the ophthalmic nerve supplies the skin of the nose, the forehead, eyelids and the scalp. (It also supplies the globe, the lacrimal apparatus and the conjunctiva). The nerve divides just before the superior orbital fissure into the lacrimal, nasociliary and frontal branches. The large frontal branch divides further into the supraorbital and supratrochlear nerves. The supraorbital nerve supplies the skin of the forehead and scalp sometimes as far back as the lambdoid suture. The supratrochlear nerve supplies part of the upper eyelid and the skin of the lower part of the forehead near the midline. The lacrimal nerve supplies the skin adjacent to the medial canthus of the eye, while the nasociliary nerve and its branches supply the skin of the nose down as far as the alae nasae.
  — *Maxillary (V^2):* this runs below the ophthalmic branch before leaving the base of the skull via the foramen rotundum to divide into its various branches. The zygomatic nerve divides further on the lateral wall of the orbit into a zygomaticotemporal branch which supplies the skin of the temple, and a zygomaticofacial branch which supplies the skin over the cheek bones. The maxillary nerve proper crosses the pterygopalatine fossa to enter the infraorbital canal from which it emerges through the infraorbital foramen as the infraorbital nerve. This supplies the skin of the lower eyelid, of the cheek and upper lip.
  — *Mandibular (V^3):* its large sensory root passes through the foramen ovale with branches that include the auriculotemporal, lingual and buccal nerves. The auriculotemporal nerve emerges from behind the temporomandibular joint to supply the skin over the tragus and meatus of the ear as well as the skin over the temporal region. The mandibular division also provides the inferior dental nerve, and one of its terminal branches, the mental nerve, emerges through the mental foramen in the mandible to supply the skin of the chin and lower lip.

Direction the viva may take

You will be asked how you could provide local anaesthesia for superficial surgery on the face. In practice it is easier by far to use local infiltration, but for the purposes of the question you will need to offer a more formal approach.

- The *supraorbital* and *supratrochlear* nerves can be blocked a few millimetres above the supraorbital ridge. If the injection is made too close to the eyebrow it increases the risk of periorbital haematoma. Alternatively, a single insertion point can be used in the midbrow region to allow bilateral blocks.

- The *infratrochlear* nerve can be blocked by a needle directed along the medial wall of the orbit via an insertion site about 1 cm above the inner canthus.
- The *infraorbital* nerve can be blocked as it exits the infraorbital foramen, which lies about 1.5 cm (a finger's breadth) below the inferior orbital margin in line with the pupil. The nerve can also be blocked by an intra-oral approach, injecting above the canine (3rd) tooth.
- The mental foramen, conveniently, is also in line with the pupil and the *mental* nerve can be blocked in the midpoint of the mandible (although the height of the foramen varies with age, being nearer the alveolar margin in the elderly).
- The superficial branches of the *zygomatic* nerve can be blocked by subcutaneous infiltration or by injection at their sites of emergence from the zygoma.
- The *auriculotemporal* nerve is blocked over the posterior aspect of the zygoma, and the *greater auricular* nerve by infiltration over the mastoid process behind the ear.
- Relatively small volumes of 3–5 ml of local anaesthetic will usually be sufficient to block all these nerves described.

Further direction the viva could take
The viva could continue with the subject of the trigeminal nerve and trigeminal neuralgia (pages 24–26).

Cervical plexus

Commentary
The clinical choice to offer a patient general or local anaesthesia for carotid endarter-ectomy (CEA) will in due course be informed by the GALA study. At the time of writing, this multicentre trial of general vs. local anaesthesia has recruited 3000 patients out of the planned sample size of 5000 and so it may be some years before the final results are published. Meanwhile, this remains a topical and practical question. Carotid surgery in patients who are awake is both interesting and challenging, and you will find it much easier to give a credible account if you have been able to see, and better still perform, some of the blocks that are required.

The viva
You may be asked to comment on the relative merits of general and local anaesthesia for CEA. It is inevitable that the answers may be somewhat reciprocal, in that the advantages of one mean that you avoid the disadvantages of the other.

- **Advantages of CEA under local anaesthesia:** normal cerebration depends upon adequate cerebral perfusion, and in the awake patient it is usually obvious whether or not this is being preserved. In effect the patient acts as their own cerebral function monitor, and signs of cerebral ischaemia are an indication for surgical shunt insertion. Local anaesthesia does not interfere with cerebral autoregulation, and the requirement for vasoactive drugs is less. Proponents of the technique claim lower morbidity and mortality rates, but robust outcome data await the results of the trial.

- **Disadvantages of CEA under local anaesthesia:** cerebral oxygen consumption does not fall (the cerebral metabolic rate for oxygen, $CMRO_2$, decreases under general anaesthesia) and a higher pulse and blood pressure during surgery results in higher myocardial oxygen demand than would otherwise be the case. It does also mean, however, that cerebral perfusion pressure is higher. Cooperation can on occasion be a problem; immobility during extended surgery may be very uncomfortable for the patient and, should their cerebration be obtunded by ischaemia, they may become restless and agitated. The nerve blocks may sometimes prove inadequate as surgery proceeds, but local supplementation by the surgeon can circumvent this problem.
- **Advantages of CEA under general anaesthesia:** general anaesthesia allows more control, can be extended indefinitely if necessary and during long procedures is more comfortable for the patient. At concentrations up to 1.0 MAC, sevoflurane decreases cerebral blood flow and $CMRO_2$. Experimental evidence suggests that general anaesthetic agents may confer a degree of neuroprotection, but the data are not robust enough to mandate their use.
- **Disadvantages of CEA under general anaesthesia:** it is clearly more difficult to assess cerebral oxygenation and, although low concentrations of volatile agents do reduce $CMRO_2$, they may still impair dynamic cerebral autoregulation at MAC levels below 1.0. In addition, there are the generic complications of general anaesthesia (in which your examiner will have little interest) and those of anaesthesia for head and neck surgery, such as restricted access to the airway.

Direction the viva will take

You will be asked to describe the anatomy relevant to the superficial and deep cervical plexus blocks that are performed for this procedure.

- The nerves which supply the lateral aspect of the neck all derive from the ventral rami of the second, third and fourth cervical spinal nerves ($C_{2,3,4}$). The first cervical nerve has no sensory distribution to skin.
- **Superficial cervical plexus anatomy:** the cutaneous supply to the anterolateral aspect of the neck is via the anterior primary rami of C_2, C_3 and C_4. These nerves emerge from the posterior border of the sternocleidomastoid muscle midway between the mastoid and the sternum. The accessory nerve is immediately superior at this point. The lesser occipital nerve (the first branch) supplies the skin of the upper and posterior ear; the greater auricular nerve (the second branch) supplies the lower third of the ear and the skin over the angle of the mandible; the anterior cutaneous nerve (the third branch) supplies the skin from the chin down to the suprasternal notch; and the supraclavicular nerves (the fourth branch) supply the skin over the lower neck, clavicle and upper chest.

- **Superficial cervical plexus block:** all these nerves can be blocked at the midpoint of the sternocleidomastoid by infiltrating up to 20 ml of local anaesthetic solution between the skin and the muscle. The external jugular vein crosses the muscle at this point and can be a useful landmark.
- **Deep cervical plexus anatomy:** the ventral ramus of the second nerve emerges from between the vertebral arches of the atlas and axis and runs forward between their transverse processes to exit between longus capitis and levator scapulae. The ventral ramus of the third nerve exits the intervertebral foramen lying in a sulcus in the transverse process, and emerges between the longus capitis and scalenus medius muscles. The ventral rami of the fourth and remaining cervical nerves appear between the scalenus anterior and the scalenus medius.
- **Deep cervical plexus block:** deep cervical plexus block in effect is a paravertebral block of C_2, C_3 and C_4. Needles are inserted at each of the three levels, using as landmarks a line between the mastoid process and the prominent tubercle of the sixth cervical vertebra (which is palpable as Chassaignac's tubercle at the level of the cricoid cartilage). The C_2 transverse process is approximately one finger's breadth below the mastoid process along this line with C_3 and C_4 following at similar intervals caudad. After encountering the transverse process, 5–8 ml of local anaesthetic can be injected with due precautions. Because there is little resistance to the spread of solutions through the paravertebral space in the cervical region, adequate anaesthesia can also be obtained using a single needle technique and a larger volume (15–20 ml) at a single level, usually C_3.

Further direction the viva could take

You may be asked about the complications of the blocks.

- **Complications:** superficial cervical plexus block risks mainly what can be described as generic complications of local anaesthesia, namely intravascular injection and systemic toxicity. The complications of deep cervical block are much the same as those associated with interscalene block, which is not surprising given the anatomical similarities, and include injection into the vertebral artery, extension of the block either extradurally or intrathecally, phrenic nerve block and cervical sympathetic block, which will manifest as Horner's syndrome (miosis, ptosis, anhidrosis and enophthalmos). The recurrent laryngeal nerve may also be affected with resultant hoarseness.

The larynx

Commentary

You will read in some textbooks that the competent anaesthetist should know as much about the anatomy of the larynx as an ENT surgeon. Examiners do not necessarily make the same assumption because in reality the clinical applications of such detailed knowledge are quite limited. You will, however, be expected to give a reasonably assured account of the main anatomical features. The account below should provide you with more than enough information, although it is simplified.

The viva

You may be asked about the factors which may influence your view at laryngoscopy. This does not mean that this is a question about difficult intubation, but it will provide a clinical introduction to the anatomical question.

Factors affecting the ease of laryngoscopy

- You will be aware that anaesthetists have long sought a test or a combination of tests that have a high sensitivity and specificity for predicting difficult intubation. None has yet been found. The simplest means of classifying the degree of difficulty is by using the Cormack and Lehane classification. (This describes the best view that is obtained at laryngoscopy: grade I, full view; grade II, posterior part of the glottis only; grade III, epiglottis only; grade IV, soft palate only).
- The larynx can be seen directly only if there is a single plane of view. This means that the three axes of the oral cavity, the pharynx and the larynx must be brought into alignment. In practice this is done by opening the mouth wide, flexing the neck, extending the head at the atlanto-occipital joint and lifting the base of the tongue and epiglottis upwards and forwards.
- Any factor which impedes this alignment will make direct laryngoscopy and intubation more difficult. Such factors include limited (<4 cm) mouth opening, prominent upper incisors, maxillary prognathism and the inability to protrude the lower incisors in front of the upper, limited neck mobility with restricted extension (thyromental distance of <6.5 cm), a high anterior larynx and obesity (weight >110 kg). Many other predictors of difficulty have been described, such as the radiological assessment of the atlanto-occipital gap, the C_1–C_2 gap and the AP depth of the mandible. However, a logical approach as outlined above will be more than enough to satisfy the examiner.

Direction the viva will take

You will be asked to describe the function and anatomy of the larynx.

- The larynx has a crucial role in protecting the airway from contamination. It does this by invoking what is one of the most powerful physiological reflexes, and one to which every anaesthetist who has managed intractable laryngospasm will attest. The larynx has also evolved into an organ of phonation.
- The larynx extends from the base of the tongue above, to the trachea below, and in the adult male it lies opposite the third to sixth cervical vertebrae. In the adult female and in children it lies higher.
- The larynx comprises a number of articulating cartilages which are joined by ligaments and which are subject to the action of various muscles which move these cartilages in relation to each other.

Cartilaginous framework

- The cartilaginous framework comprises the thyroid, cricoid and arytenoid cartilages. (The smaller corniculate and cuneiform cartilages contribute little to this structure.)
- The thyroid cartilage comprises two quadrilateral laminae which are fused anteriorly to form the laryngeal prominence. It articulates inferiorly with the cricoid. The thyroid notch lies at the level of C_4.
- The cricoid cartilage is a continuous ring with a narrow anterior arch and a deeper posterior lamina. It articulates on each side with the inferior cornu of the thyroid cartilage and with the base of the arytenoid cartilage.
- Each of the paired arytenoid cartilages is pyramidal in shape. The smooth concave base articulates with the cricoid cartilage. The lateral angle, or muscular process, projects backwards, while the anterior angle, or vocal process, projects forwards. The apex articulates with the corniculate cartilage.
- The two corniculate cartilages are small nodules which are sometimes fused with the arytenoids and which lie in the posterior aryepiglottic folds of mucous membrane. The two cuneiform cartilages lie anterior to the corniculate cartilages, also within the aryepiglottic fold.
- There are a number of intrinsic and extrinsic ligaments. Those of anaesthetic interest include the thyrohyoid membrane, which joins the upper border of the thyroid cartilage to the hyoid bone, and the cricothyroid ligament between the cricoid and thyroid cartilages.
- The vocal cords (also known as the vocal folds) are opalescent folds of mucous membrane which extend from the anterior vocal processes of the arytenoid cartilages as far as the middle of the angle of the thyroid cartilage. The vestibular folds, or false cords, lie lateral to the cords and comprise thicker folds of mucous membrane which also extend from the thyroid cartilage to the arytenoids.

Laryngeal muscles

- There are a number of extrinsic and intrinsic muscles of the larynx. The extrinsic muscles (the sternothyroid, the thyrohyoid and the inferior constrictor of the pharynx) attach the larynx to adjacent structures. The intrinsic muscles are of more immediate interest to the anaesthetist because they control the opening of the cords during inspiration, the closure of the cords and laryngeal inlet during swallowing, and the tension of the cords during speech.
- **Abduction:** Abduction of the cords is performed by the posterior cricoarytenoid muscles.
- **Adduction:** Adduction of the cords is performed by the lateral cricoarytenoids and the unpaired interarytenoid muscle.
- **Tensors:** the main tensors of the vocal cords are the cricothyroid muscles.
- **Relaxors:** the main relaxors of the vocal cords are the thyroarytenoid muscles.
- **Innervation:** All the muscles of the larynx, with one exception, are innervated by the recurrent laryngeal nerve. The exception is the cricothyroid muscle, which is supplied by the external branch of the superior laryngeal nerve.

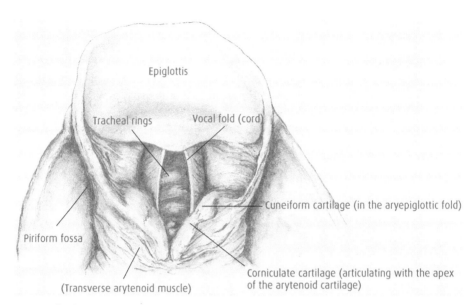

Fig. 2.4 The larynx.

Further direction the viva may take

You may be asked about the clinical relevance of this information.

- It is important to be able to recognize structures that are seen at laryngoscopy. Beyond the elevated epiglottis are the false and the true vocal cords. Posteriorly are the arytenoid cartilages (together with the bulges of the corniculate and cuneiform cartilages). Between the cords is the laryngeal inlet, or rima glottidis, beyond which may be visible the upper rings of the trachea (Figure 2.4).
- The arytenoids can be dislocated or subluxed during tracheal intubation or laryngeal mask insertion. This will interfere with the function of some of the intrinsic muscles and may compromise the airway. The cricoarytenoid joint may also be affected by systemic inflammatory arthropathies, particularly rheumatoid arthritis, and by the tissue changes associated with acromegaly.
- The anatomy of the cricoid cartilage is relevant both for rapid sequence induction of anaesthesia, and also for emergency access to the airway (page 44).
- It is also important to be able to recognize the airway signs of injury to the recurrent laryngeal nerve (page 38).

Innervation of the larynx

Commentary

The innervation of the larynx is another area that is regarded as core anatomy, and it does have immediate relevance for awake fibreoptic intubation. The other traditional question about the laryngeal nerves relates to the consequences of injury and, although anaesthetists see this very rarely, you may find yourself being questioned as though it were an everyday occurrence.

The viva
As a means of introducing the subject you may be asked how you would provide anaesthesia for awake fibreoptic intubation.

Nebulized lignocaine
- Nebulized local anaesthetic (such as lignocaine 4%) will provide adequate surface anaesthesia of the airway, although the procedure takes some time and patients may find it claustrophobic and uncomfortable. It may not anaesthetize the nasal mucosa adequately.

Topical anaesthetic
- The nasal mucosa can be anaesthetized with local anaesthetic plus vasoconstrictor to minimize risk of bleeding. Topical cocaine can be used to a maximum dose of 1.5 mg kg^{-1}. If oral intubation is planned, the tongue and posterior pharynx can be anaesthetized using lignocaine 4% or a lignocaine 10% metered pump which delivers 10 mg with each spray.

'Spray as you go' technique
- This is another simple method of anaesthetizing the airway, in which local anaesthetic (usually lignocaine 4%) is introduced under direct vision via the injector channel in the fibreoptic endoscope.

As none of the above techniques requires much anatomical knowledge, the questioning will move on to the supplemental nerve blocks that may be necessary. This will be preceded by the discussion of laryngeal innervation.

Direction the viva will take
You will be asked to describe the nerve supply to the larynx.

Sensory innervation
- The sensory innervation of the larynx is via the vagus (10th cranial nerve), which divides into the superior laryngeal nerve and the recurrent laryngeal nerve. The superior branch divides thereafter into internal and external laryngeal nerves.
- The internal laryngeal nerve innervates the inferior surface of the epiglottis and the supraglottic region as far as the mucous membrane above the vocal folds.
- The recurrent laryngeal nerve provides the sensory supply to the laryngeal mucosa below the vocal cords.

Motor innervation
- The recurrent laryngeal nerve supplies all the intrinsic muscles of the larynx, with the exception of the cricothyroid muscle. This is supplied from the external branch of the superior laryngeal nerve.
- The right recurrent laryngeal nerve leaves the vagus to loop beneath the subclavian artery, before ascending to the larynx in the groove between the oesophagus and the trachea.

- The left recurrent laryngeal nerve passes beneath the arch of the aorta and similarly ascends in the groove between oesophagus and trachea.

Direction the viva may take

You may be asked about the supplemental nerve blocks.

- **Glossopharyngeal nerve:** this provides sensory innervation to the oral pharynx, the supraglottic area, the base of tongue and the vallecula. It can be blocked by submucosal infiltration behind the tonsillar pillars.
- **Superior laryngeal nerve:** this can be anaesthetized by bilateral injections which can be performed either by walking off the greater cornua of the hyoid to penetrate the thyrohyoid membrane, or by walking off the superior alae of the thyroid cartilage.
- **Recurrent laryngeal nerve:** this nerve is usually blocked even if a 'spray as you go' technique has been used to anaesthetize the remainder of the airway. It is blocked via a transtracheal injection that is made through the cricothyroid membrane during inspiration. The inevitable cough distributes the solution (typically 4 ml of lignocaine 4%) more widely.

Further direction the viva may take

You may then be asked about the clinical consequences of injury to the laryngeal nerves.

- The external branch of the superior laryngeal nerve supplies the cricothyroid muscle, which tenses the vocal cords. Damage will be followed by hoarseness. If the injury is unilateral, this hoarseness will be temporary, because in time the other cricothyroid muscle will compensate. If it is bilateral the hoarseness will be permanent.
- The recurrent laryngeal nerve supplies all those muscles which control the opening and closing of the laryngeal inlet.
- Partial paralysis affects the abductor muscles more than the adductors and so with uni-lateral injury the corresponding vocal cord is paralysed. This also results in hoarseness.
- If both nerves are damaged then both cords oppose or even overlap each other in the midline. This leads to inspiratory stridor and has the potential to cause total respiratory obstruction.
- If one or both nerves are transected, the vocal cord(s) adopt the cadaveric position in which they lie partially abducted and through which airflow is much less compromised. Phonation may be reduced to a whisper.

The anatomy of the trachea and bronchi

Commentary

Anatomy of these areas is of self-evident importance both in anaesthesia and intensive care. It is possible that you may be given the opportunity to describe every bronchopulmonary segment but, because the terminology is cumbersome with considerable duplication, it is more likely, once you have demonstrated that you know the key points (such as the origin of the right upper lobe bronchus), that the viva will concentrate more on applied clinical aspects.

The viva

There are one or two ways in which clinical factors may introduce this question. One is pulmonary aspiration of gastric contents; another is the view obtained as a fibreoptic bronchoscope passes down the main conducting airways.

You may be asked whether you can predict which parts of the lung may be contaminated following an episode of aspiration.

- **Pulmonary aspiration of gastric contents:** the anatomy of the lobes and bronchopulmonary segments influences zonal contamination should pulmonary aspiration occur. If the patient is supine it is more likely that the apical segments of the lower lobes will be affected because of the direct posterior projection of the bronchus of the apical segment. If the patient is in the lateral position then aspiration is more likely to affect the upper lobes. If prone, the right middle lobe and lingula will be the site of the problem because of their downward and forward orientation, and if they are sitting, it will be the posterior or lateral basal segments of the lower lobes that are contaminated.

Alternatively, you may be asked the main structures that you see at bronchoscopy.

- **Fibreoptic bronchoscopy:** this is essentially a topic which needs visual aids, and so all that you will be required to do is give a brief description of the main structures that you see during bronchoscopy. Examiners will assume that most of your experience of the procedure will have been gained on intensive care and so your account will start beyond the endotracheal tube in the trachea. You will see first the trachea, the anterior wall, which is composed of complete cartilaginous bands, and the posterior wall, which is membranous. The carina separates the right and left main stem bronchi.
  — *Right side view:* the right main bronchus is wider than the left and is shorter at ~3 cm long. It is also angled more vertically than the left. Within ~2.5 cm of the bifurcation can be seen the right upper lobe bronchus. The right main then gives off the middle lobe bronchus, which is directed downwards and forwards. Just below the origin of the middle lobe bronchus and opposite to it is the bronchus of the apical segment of the lower lobe: beyond this the main stem of the lower lobe bronchus continues downwards.
  — *Left side view:* the left main bronchus is more obliquely placed and is about 5 cm in length. It gives off the left upper lobe bronchus near its termination at about 5 cm, which then divides into a superior division and a lingular bronchus. The anatomy of the left lower lobe bronchus is similar to the right.

You may then be asked to fill in some of the anatomical detail: this is likely to be limited to the upper airways, but should it include the bronchopulmonary segments then they are described below.

- **Trachea:** the trachea is a tube of cartilage with a membranous lining which is continuous inferiorly with the larynx. The trachea proper is 10–11 cm long, and extends downwards from the cricoid cartilage at the level of the sixth cervical vertebra, as far as the sixth thoracic vertebra (in full inspiration). It then divides into left and right main bronchi. Its diameter in the adult is around 20 mm. In the first year of life its diameter is 3 mm or less, and increases thereafter by about 1 mm per year of age until it attains adult dimensions.

— *Structure:* it comprises 16–20 C-shaped cartilages attached vertically by fibroelastic connective tissue, which helps explain the mobility of the structure. Through most of its course the trachea lies in the midline although at the bifurcation it is displaced slightly rightwards by the arch of the aorta. The posterior wall of the trachea is membranous.

— *Anterior relations:* in the upper part of the neck these are confined to skin and fascia, and to the isthmus of the thyroid overlying the second to fourth tracheal rings. In its lower cervical course the trachea is partly overlain by the sternohyoid and sternothyroid muscles, and by the jugular arch connecting the anterior jugular veins. In its thoracic course the manubrium sterni lies anteriorly, as do the remnants of the thymus, the inferior thyroid veins and the brachiocephalic artery.

— *Posterior relations:* the oesophagus lies posteriorly, and the recurrent laryngeal nerves run in grooves between the trachea and oesophagus.

— *Lateral relations:* in the upper neck the trachea is related to the lobes of the thyroid and to the carotid sheath. In its lower course it is related on the right to the lung and pleura, to the brachiocephalic artery and veins, to the azygos vein and to the superior vena cava. On the left it is related to the arch of the aorta and the left common carotid and subclavian arteries.

- **The right and left main bronchi:** the main bronchi are formed at about the level of T_5. The right is shorter (3 cm long), wider and angled more vertically than the left, which means that foreign bodies and tracheal tubes are more likely to enter its orifice than the left. The left main bronchus is more obliquely placed and is some 5 cm in length. Important relations on the right are the pulmonary artery which lies first below and then anterior to it, with the azygos vein above; on the left side the main bronchus lies below the arch of the aorta with the descending aorta behind and the left pulmonary artery lying in front. In children the angles of the bronchi at the carina are equal.

- **Bronchopulmonary segments – right lung:** within about 2.5 cm of the bifurcation the right main bronchus gives off the right upper lobe bronchus (which divides in turn within 1 cm into apical, anterior and posterior segments). It is this right upper lobe bronchus that is most at risk from inadvertent occlusion by a tracheal tube or a right-sided double-lumen endobronchial tube. The right main then gives off the middle lobe bronchus, which is directed downwards and forwards (before bifurcating into medial and lateral lobes). Just below the origin of the middle lobe bronchus, and opposite to it, is the bronchus of the apical segment of the lower lobe. This directs posteriorly, before dividing into superior, anterior basal and lateral basal segments. The medial, anterior, lateral, and posterior basal segments arise in due course from the main stem of the lower lobe bronchus, which continues in its downward direction.

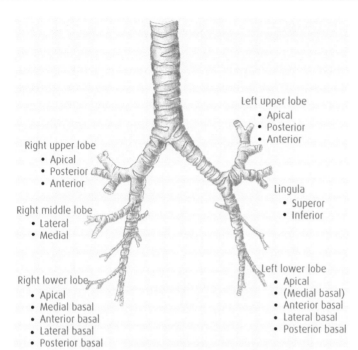

Fig. 2.5 The bronchopulmonary segments.

Left upper lobe
• Apical
• Posterior
• Anterior

Right upper lobe
• Apical
• Posterior
• Anterior

Right middle lobe
• Lateral
• Medial

Lingula
• Superor
• Inferior

Right lower lobe
• Apical
• Medial basal
• Anterior basal
• Lateral basal
• Posterior basal

Left lower lobe
• Apical
• (Medial basal)
• Anterior basal
• Lateral basal
• Posterior basal

- **Bronchopulmonary segments – left lung:** the longer left main bronchus gives off the left upper lobe bronchus after about 5 cm, and this then divides into a superior division from which arise apical, posterior and anterior segments of the upper lobe, and a lingular bronchus from which arise the superior and inferior lingular segments. The anatomy of the left lower lobe is similar to the right, in that the left lower lobe bronchus gives off superior, anterior basal, lateral basal and posterior basal segments. The medial basal bronchopulmonary segment usually arises in common with the anterior basal, however, which means technically that there are only four rather than five bronchopulmonary segments on the left (Figure 2.5).

Direction the viva may take

You may be asked about double-lumen tubes.

- **Double-lumen endobronchial tubes:** these are used when one lung needs to be isolated so that the other can be collapsed to allow surgery. Such procedures include pulmonary resection, oesophagogastrectomy, surgery of the thoracic aorta, anterior spinal fixation and thoracoscopic sympathectomy. A left-sided tube is almost always favoured because this avoids the risk of inadvertently occluding the origin of the right upper lobe bronchus. Problems with malpositioned tubes are an important cause of mortality and morbidity (page 138). A double-lumen tube is positioned correctly when the upper surface of the bronchial cuff lies immediately distal to the bifurcation of the carina. The position of the tube should be checked endoscopically.

You may be asked briefly about awake fibreoptic intubation.

- Indications include known difficult intubation; known or suspected difficult intubation in a patient with a full stomach; morbid obesity; and patients with cervical spine disease or injury. Details of technique vary, but all involve railroading a tube (oral or, more commonly, nasal) down over the fibrescope and into the anaesthetized airway. Local anaesthetic techniques for this procedure are described on page 37.

If you have been asked about pulmonary aspiration of gastric contents then you may also be asked about management.

- The cardinal sign will be otherwise unexplained desaturation. In a patient who has not received neuromuscular blockers this may be preceded by coughing which fails to settle as anaesthesia deepens. In a paralysed patient aspiration may be silent. Auscultation may reveal rhonchi and/or crepitations. Chest X-ray changes often occur early enough to support the diagnosis of significant aspiration, although they can be delayed for 6 hours or more. Management is essentially expectant. If a patient does not need supplemental oxygen to maintain a normal SpO_2 after 2 hours then it is unlikely that there will be significant sequelae. (Some anaesthetists prefer to wait 4–6 hours before making that judgement.) Should the patient remain oxygen-dependent then he or she will need supportive therapy which in severe cases may include intubation and ventilation. There is no evidence of any benefit from the administration of prophylactic antibiotics or steroids.

Surface anatomy of the neck (percutaneous tracheostomy and cricothyroidotomy)

Commentary

If these procedures are performed incorrectly the results can be disastrous. The applied anatomy is not complex but you should give a simple authoritative account of the techniques, particularly in relation to the potentially life-saving manoeuvre of cricothyroidotomy. If the techniques that you describe put the patient at risk then you cannot but fail this question.

The viva

This question is specific, but the examiner, mindful of the need to emphasize its clinical relevance, may preface the request to describe the surface anatomy of the neck by explaining that the questioning will in due course move on to the surgical airway.

It does not matter particularly how you approach the answer; one way is to outline the anatomy from above downwards.

- The hyoid bone lies at the level of the third cervical vertebra (C_3). Lying just above and behind is the epiglottis.
- The bifurcation of the common carotid artery is at the level of the fourth cervical vertebra (C_4), slightly above the notch of the thyroid cartilage.
- The larynx lies opposite the fourth, fifth and sixth cervical vertebrae ($C_{4,5,6}$).
- The cricoid cartilage is at the level of the sixth cervical vertebra (C_6).
- The trachea extends from the sixth cervical vertebra (C_6) down as far as the fifth or sixth thoracic vertebra ($T_{5,6}$) at end-inspiration.
- The suprasternal notch is located at the level of the second and third thoracic vertebrae ($T_{2,3}$).

Direction the viva may take

You may be asked further about the anatomy relevant to the two clinical techniques (of percutaneous tracheostomy and cricothyroidotomy), which have different indications but broadly similar complications.

- The trachea comprises 16–20 C-shaped cartilages, which lie anteriorly in the neck covered by skin and the superficial and deep fascial layers. The second, third and fourth rings are covered by the isthmus of the thyroid. The great vessels of the neck lie laterally, and so identification of the midline is crucial.
- The cricothyroid membrane spans the inferior border of the thyroid cartilage and the superior border of the cricoid cartilage, and immediately overlies the subglottic region of the larynx. It is covered anteriorly by skin and by superficial and deep fascia. Immediately lateral are the sternocleidomastoid muscle, the sternothyroid and the sternohyoid muscles and the carotid sheath.

Percutaneous tracheostomy

- This is an elective, not an emergency procedure, which in the context of intensive care has become a well established alternative to definitive surgical tracheostomy. Its indications are the same as for formal tracheostomy in the critically ill: typically to simplify airway management in a patient who otherwise would face the problems of long-term tracheal intubation.
- Different techniques have been described (by Ciaglia, by Griggs and by Fantoni, for example). Most are variations on a theme (dilatation over a guidewire), but describe the one with which you are most familiar.
- A typical technique is described as follows.
    — Guided by the surface anatomy as described above, a skin incision is made to allow a needle and guidewire to be placed through the fibroelastic tissue that joins the tracheal rings.
    — The isthmus of the thyroid gland covers the second to fourth tracheal rings. A higher approach through the subcricoid membrane or between the first and second tracheal rings does avoid the thyroid isthmus, but is associated with a greater incidence of tracheal stenosis. It is for this reason that

many intensivists now prefer a low approach, below the second or even third ring.

— The diameter of the hole is enlarged with progressively larger dilators to the point at which it will accept a definitive tracheostomy tube. An alternative is the use of a single tapered dilator.

— It is usual for a second anaesthetist to monitor this procedure from within the trachea by using a fibreoptic bronchoscope. The posterior wall of the trachea may be so ragged and friable that it can easily be perforated.

Further directions the viva could take

You may be asked to list the complications.

- Haemorrhage (immediate or delayed); the creation of false passage; tracheal or oesophageal perforation; barotrauma; subcutaneous emphysema; failure and accidental decannulation.
- Subglottic stenosis is a cause of serious morbidity: it is more common after cricothyroidotomy than after percutaneous tracheostomy.

You may be asked to compare percutaneous tracheostomy with cricothyroidotomy.

- Both techniques bypass the normal translaryngeal route to secure the airway, but the circumstances and urgency of their use differ considerably. Percutaneous tracheostomy is an elective procedure, whereas cricothyroidotomy is an emergency procedure which is usually invoked only when all other attempts to secure a definitive airway have failed and when critical hypoxia is imminent.
- The cricothyroid membrane is used for emergency access because it is readily identifiable and because it is relatively avascular.
- The patient is positioned with the neck extended to allow identification of the membrane. After stabilization of the overlying skin, which can be lax, a small vertical incision in the skin is followed by a transverse incision in the membrane. A spreader or scalpel handle is used to open the airway, after which an appropriate tube can be inserted under direct vision. The purpose-made devices typically have an internal diameter of 4 mm.

The stellate ganglion

Commentary

Stellate ganglion block is a common procedure in the chronic pain clinic, is simple to perform, and has significant potential complications. You may well not have carried out this block yourself but, as one of several procedures in the neck undertaken by anaesthetists (others include interscalene block, deep cervical plexus block and internal jugular cannulation), its anatomy is of some relevance.

The viva

You may first be asked about indications for the block, and the clinical part of the viva may concentrate on stellate ganglion block following inadvertent intra-arterial injection, this being one of the classic anaesthetic indications. Very few of the others listed are likely to lie within your current experience.

- You could start by commenting that the evidence base for the therapeutic use of stellate ganglion blocks is not strong, but the technique has a long tradition of use in the management of chronic pain.
- **Indications:** these include any condition requiring sympathetic block of the head, neck and upper limb.
  — *Neuropathic pain conditions:* complex regional pain syndromes (CRPS) types I and II, post-herpetic neuralgia of head and neck, shoulder–hand syndrome (following CVA or ischaemia), phantom limb pain, pain associated with upper limb denervation. There is evidence from at least one controlled study which suggests that early stellate ganglion block may prevent the progression of CRPS in some patients.
  — *Ischaemic conditions:* thrombosis or microembolism, vasospastic disorders (e.g. Raynaud's disease), scleroderma, frostbite and inadvertent intra-arterial injection in the upper limb (pages 79–80).
  — *Angina pectoris:* severe refractory chest pain due to coronary ischaemia (page 50).
  — *Miscellaneous:* hyperhidrosis and treatment of pain associated with Paget's disease of bone.

You will then be asked to describe the relevant anatomy.

- The cervical sympathetic chain lies either side of the vertebral column in the fascial space: posterior lies the fascia over the prevertebral muscles; anterior is the carotid sheath.
- The area where the inferior cervical and the first thoracic ganglia meet, either in close proximity or fusion, is referred to as the stellate ganglion.
- The ganglion extends from the neck of the first rib, where its lower part is covered anteriorly by the dome of the pleura, to the transverse process of C_7 where the vertebral artery lies anterior. By the level of C_6 the vertebral artery has moved posteriorly into the foramen transversarium pending its ascent into the skull.
- Much of the sympathetic nerve supply to the head and neck as well as to the upper extremity synapses in or near the stellate ganglion. A successful block will be signified by ipsilateral Horner's syndrome (ptosis, miosis, enophthalmos and anhidrosis).
- Sympathetic pre-ganglionic fibres leave the cord from segments as widely separated as T_1–T_6 and, although many converge in or around the stellate ganglion, some may bypass it. For this reason, large volumes of local anaesthetic solution may be needed to fill the space in front of the prevertebral fascia down to T_4, but this will produce reliable sympathetic blockade of the head, neck and upper limb. It is more accurately described as a 'cervicothoracic block'.

Direction the viva may take

You may then be asked about a technique of stellate ganglion block, and finally about its complications.

- **Techniques:** two approaches are described: the anterior (sometimes called the 'paratracheal' anterior) approach and the paratracheal approach.
  - *Anterior approach:* the trachea and carotid pulse are gently retracted to allow identification of the most prominent cervical transverse process (the Chassaignac tubercle) at C_6, the level of the cricoid cartilage.
  - A lower approach to the ganglion's actual location at C_7 risks both pneumothorax and vertebral artery puncture.
  - The carotid sheath is moved laterally, and the trachea medially, before a $25-30 \, mm \times 23-25G$ needle is directed perpendicularly down on to the tubercle.
  - Once it has encountered bone the needle is withdrawn 4–5 mm. If this is not done there is a higher incidence of upper limb somatic blockade.
  - Local anaesthetic in low concentration and high volume (such as lignocaine 0.5% or bupivacaine $0.125\% \times 15-20 \, ml$) is injected.
  - *Paratracheal approach:* The needle insertion is two fingerbreadths lateral to the suprasternal notch and two fingerbreadths superior to the clavicle. This identifies the transverse process of C_7, immediately below Chassaignac's tubercle at C_6, at the level of the cricoid cartilage.
  - The sternocleidomastoid and carotid sheath are moved laterally before the needle is directed perpendicularly down on to the transverse process.
  - Once it has encountered bone the needle is withdrawn 0.5–1.0 cm.
  - Local anaesthetic in low concentration and high volume is injected as above.
  - This lower approach risks pneumothorax as well as vertebral artery puncture.
  - *Complications* include local trauma and haematoma (which may compress the airway if severe); recurrent laryngeal nerve block, which causes hoarseness; brachial plexus block, because via the anterior approach only a layer of fascia separates the plexus and the ganglion which is anterior to it; carotid or vertebral arterial puncture and possible intravascular injection (with the paratracheal lower approach); intrathecal injection; pneumothorax (if the approach is too low) and deep cervical plexus block (if the approach is too high).

Myocardial blood supply

Commentary

This is functional rather than practical anatomy. There is considerable overlap in the arterial supply to areas of the myocardium, and so it is not always possible to diagnose the site of coronary artery occlusion from ECG or echocardiographic changes. After you have been asked about the anatomy, which you may find easier to explain with the help of a diagram, the viva is likely to move on to the physiology of coronary perfusion.

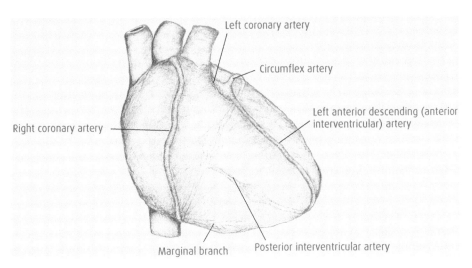

Left coronary artery

Circumflex artery

Left anterior descending (anterior interventricular) artery

Right coronary artery

Marginal branch

Posterior interventricular artery

Fig. 2.6 Coronary arterial supply.

The viva

You will be asked to describe the arterial supply and venous drainage of the heart.

- **Arterial supply:** the heart is supplied by the right and left coronary arteries; these originate from the ascending aorta (anterior and posterior aortic sinuses, located just above the cusps of the aortic valve) (Figure 2.6).
- **Right coronary artery:** this passes between the pulmonary trunk and the right atrial appendage to descend in the anterior atrioventricular groove.
- It gives off atrial and ventricular short branches to supply those structures.
- At the inferior border of the heart it effectively divides into the marginal branch which travels along the right ventricle towards the apex and the posterior interventricular artery which continues in the groove of the same name to anastomose with the circumflex artery (the corresponding branch of the left coronary artery). This anastomosis is variable.
- The right main coronary artery or its branches supply the right ventricle and right atrium, part of the interventricular septum, the sinoatrial node, SAN (in 65%), the bundle of His, the atrioventricular node, AVN (80%) and the conducting system (80%). It also supplies a small diaphragmatic part of the left ventricle.
- **Left coronary artery:** this is larger than the right and, after arising from the posterior aortic sinus, passes between the left atrial appendage and the pulmonary trunk.
- It divides shortly into the anterior interventricular (also known as the left anterior descending, LAD) artery, which passes down the interventricular groove giving off anterior ventricular branches, and into the circumflex artery. This continues in the atrioventricular groove to anastomose with the inferior interventricular artery as above.

- The left coronary artery or its branches supply the left ventricle and left atrium, part of the interventricular septum, the SAN (in 35%), the AVN (20%) and the conducting system (20%).
- The innermost part of the endocardium receives oxygen directly from the blood within the ventricle.
- **Venous drainage:** as much as a third of cardiac venous blood drains directly into the cardiac chambers via the venae cordis minimae (a network of small veins). The remainder is drained by larger veins which tend to accompany the coronary arteries.
- Most of the remaining venous blood drains into the right atrium via the coronary sinus, which is located to the left of the opening of the inferior vena cava, and which lies in the posterior atrioventricular groove.

This is probably all the information that will be required of you, but for completeness a fuller account of the venous drainage is summarized below.

- The main veins which drain into the sinus are: the *great cardiac vein*, which lies in the anterior interventricular groove (with the LAD); the *middle cardiac vein*, which lies in the inferior interventricular groove containing the anastomosis between the inferior interventricular and the circumflex arteries; the *small cardiac vein* accompanying the marginal branch of the right coronary artery; the *oblique vein* on the posterior surface of the left atrium; the *anterior cardiac vein*, which lies with the right coronary artery in the anterior atrioventricular groove and which drains directly into the right atrium.

Direction the viva may take
You may be asked about the physiology of coronary perfusion.

- At rest, about $250\,\text{ml}\,\text{min}^{-1}$, or 5%, of the cardiac output is supplied to the myocardium through the coronary arteries. This can increase fivefold during vigorous exercise.
- Flow is governed by the driving pressure. In the presence of a fixed coronary stenosis, this pressure gradient is crucial. In the absence of a stenotic lesion, the main variable that determines flow is the calibre of the blood vessels. Vasodilatation occurs mainly in response to the presence of local metabolites such as hydrogen ions, adenosine, potassium, phosphate, carbon dioxide and prostaglandins. Autonomic control of vascular tone is present but is a negligible influence in comparison.
- Myocardial tissue has a high oxygen extraction ratio (80%), which limits its capacity for anaerobic metabolism. Increased oxygen demand has to be met by an increase in coronary perfusion.
- During systole the subendocardial pressure in the left ventricle exceeds that in the outer part of the myocardium and so, in the main, arterial flow occurs through the arteries only in diastole. There is, however, some flow to the outer areas of the left ventricle throughout the cardiac cycle. In the right side of the heart, which is a lower pressure system, coronary perfusion persists throughout systole and diastole. At an average heart rate of 72 beats per minute, about 0.3 seconds will be spent in systole and 0.5 in diastole. High heart rates can compromise ventricular perfusion as well as ventricular filling.

Further direction the viva could take

You may be asked about the factors that determine the balance between myocardial oxygen supply and demand.

- **Supply:** coronary blood flow (as discussed above); O_2 content of blood (dependent on haemoglobin concentration and SpO_2); position of the oxygen–haemoglobin dissociation curve.
- **Demand:** systolic arterial pressure (afterload); left ventricular end-diastolic pressure (preload); myocardial contractility; heart rate.

Alternatively, you may be asked about the innervation of the heart and the implications for the transplanted heart (pages 49–50).

Myocardial innervation

Commentary

This sounds straightforward. The viva may include the broad aspects of transplant physiology which are increasingly well recognized given that there are more such patients presenting for non-cardiac surgery; however, just when you think that all is going well you may be asked about the origin of cardiac pain. This is a deceptively simple question because the neural basis of angina pectoris is more complex than it sounds, and most people have never given it much thought. This may even apply to the examiner who has been presented with the question to ask you, and so you perhaps need not fear that you will have to cover the topic in great detail.

The viva

You may be asked about the physiology of the transplanted heart.

- **Autonomic denervation:** the transplanted heart loses both sympathetic and parasympathetic efferent and afferent neurones. This leads to a (predictable) alteration in some aspects of cardiac physiology, including the absence of anginal pain.
- **Sympathetic denervation:** despite the lack of a direct neuronal supply, the heart still responds normally to circulating catecholamines. This humoral response is of relatively slow onset and takes some minutes to develop. The response to exogenous catecholamines is similarly delayed.
- **Parasympathetic denervation:** there may be some residual vagal activity associated with the vestigial recipient right atrium which is part of the anastomosis, but this does not extend to the donor atria. Vagal effects are absent and so drugs which usually have muscarinic actions do not cause bradycardia, and drugs which are vagolytic do not increase the heart rate. In normal individuals the resting heart rate is governed by vagal tone. In heart transplant patients, therefore the rate is higher, commonly around 100 beats per minute.

- **Starling mechanism:** the myocardial response to stress is maintained, with increases in contractility and cardiac output in response to any rise in left ventricular end-diastolic volume (LVEDV). It is important to avoid hypovolaemia in these patients.
- **Other considerations:** a discussion of anaesthetic problems is unlikely to feature at this stage, but is summarized briefly below for completeness. Such problems include: accelerated graft atherosclerosis owing to chronic rejection; absence of warning symptoms of angina; immunosuppression by drugs such as corticosteroids (with a wide range of side effects, from myopathy to hyperglycaemia), cyclosporin (with effects on renal and hepatic function) and azathioprine (myelosuppression).

Direction the viva will take

Following the introduction you will be asked in more detail about cardiac innervation.

- **Autonomic nervous system:** the innervation of the heart is predominantly autonomic. Efferent and afferent fibres originate from the cardiac plexuses, which are aggregations of autonomic nerves and ganglia. The superficial plexus lies below the arch of the aorta in front of the right pulmonary artery, and the deep plexus lies anterior to the bifurcation of the trachea and behind the arch of the aorta.
- **Parasympathetic supply:** this is from branches of the vagus nerves that enter the cardiac plexus. The right vagus innervates the SAN whereas the left vagus innervates the AVN. There can be some overlap. Vagal efferents supply atrial muscle, but innervate the ventricular myocardium only sparsely. Vagal stimulation vasoconstricts the coronary arterial circulation. These effects are mediated via muscarinic receptors.
- **Sympathetic supply:** the sympathetic fibres originate mainly from the upper thoracic spinal cord (segments T_2–T_4) and are distributed through the middle cervical and the stellate (cervicothoracic) ganglia as well as through the first four ganglia of the thoracic sympathetic chain. The fibres pass into the cardiac plexus and thence to the SAN and the cardiac muscle. Ventricular sympathetic innervation is denser than atrial. Sympathetic stimulation dilates coronary arteries via actions on beta-adrenoceptors.

Further direction the viva may take

You may then be asked about the origin of cardiac pain.

- The localization of somatic pain is usually precise, whereas visceral sensations are limited to discomfort (due, for example, to distension) and to pain. There are many fewer visceral sensory fibres than somatic sensory fibres in the dorsal roots, which helps to explain why visceral pain is poorly localized.
- How does cardiac pain originate? In a normal heart the oxygen supply can be increased six-to-eightfold in response to increased demand, such as during exertion. At the point at which demand exceeds supply there is an accumulation of lactate and other metabolites. Exercise is then limited by fatigue and dyspnoea, but not by cardiac pain. In a patient with coronary artery disease it is common for cardiac pain to precede fatigue. Why should this be so? A number of substances (which include lactate, potassium, adenosine, prostaglandins and bradykinins) are released from

ischaemic areas of the myocardium. It appears that these substances may sensitize sympathetic afferents, in particular those neurons which have a so-called acid-sensing sodium channel. Lactate increases the activity of these channels and enhances their excitability. This increased sensitization is not an acute phenomenon, because systemic lactic acidosis is not associated with chest pain.

- Pain is the only sensation that is evoked from the heart, but it too is more vaguely localized. Sympathetic afferents account for only around 2% of the total number of afferents to the upper thoracic cord. Stimulation of these afferents leads to excitation of spinothalamic tract cells (T_1–T_5) which also receive somatic input from overlying structures. This convergence onto a common pool of spinothalamic tract cells helps account for the classic nature of anginal pain which is frequently referred to the arm and chest. The convergence is on tracts with afferents from deep (muscle) rather than cutaneous (skin) structures. In addition, vagal afferents transmit nociceptive information to the spinothalamic tract at the level of C_1 and C_2 which explains referred pain in the neck and jaw. This vagal innervation is one of the reasons why not all cases of refractory angina can be treated successfully by sympathetic block.

- Sympathetic afferents from viscera such as the gallbladder and the oesophagus also converge on this pool of spinothalamic tracts; hence the similarity of symptoms that these structures can evoke.

- The above is a simplification which does not include other ascending spinal tracts that are involved, and does not entirely account for aspects such as the specific emotional components of cardiac pain. 'Angor animi', for example, which is a profound sense of impending death, is a sensation that is said to be unique to myocardial pain, but is one whose neural processing has not been elaborated.

Intercostal nerves

Commentary

This area of anatomy was of more direct relevance before thoracic epidural anaesthesia, paravertebral injection and intrapleural catheterization became common analgesic techniques. Intercostal nerve blocks were used to provide analgesia for subcostal surgical incisions and to treat the pain of fractured ribs. The topic, however, continues to be asked, but because the list of indications for intercostal block is shrinking, the viva will concentrate on the anatomy and on the distribution of injected drugs more than on clinical techniques of nerve blockade.

The viva

The subject may be introduced by a question about local anaesthetic techniques for managing thoracic pain.

- Analgesic options include thoracic epidural anaesthesia (effective, but bilateral in distribution with the generic disadvantages of epidural block); paravertebral block (effective, unilateral, but with potential complications of epidural spread and pneumothorax); and intrapleural block (simple but, according to at least some studies, less effective than the previous two methods). Arguably, intercostal nerve block is also less satisfactory, but none of the other techniques lend themselves as well to a discussion of anatomy.

You may be asked about the indications for intercostal nerve block.

- **Indications:** intercostal nerve block can provide effective analgesia for upwards of 12 hours. Historically, it was used for analgesia following subcostal and loin incisions (for gallbladder and renal surgery), after thoracotomy and to provide analgesia for fractured ribs. Only the last indication now applies, and here the technique has been superseded by intrapleural and epidural block. It has been used to alleviate the discomfort of herpes zoster. A block of T_{10}, T_{11} and T_{12} provides effective analgesia following appendicectomy, but it is rarely used for this purpose, possibly because in the UK relatively inexperienced trainees give the majority of anaesthetics for this operation.

You will be asked the anatomy of an intercostal nerve.

- The intercostal nerves are the ventral somatic rami of the spinal nerves from T_1 to T_{11}. T_{12} is a subcostal nerve which is not closely associated with its corresponding rib, and which in addition links with fibres from the first lumbar nerve. T_1, T_2 and, occasionally, T_3 are also atypical, in that some of their fibres join with fibres of the brachial plexus, as well as contributing to the formation of the intercostobrachial nerve.
- The typical intercostal nerve exits the intervertebral foramen to lie initially between the posterior intercostal membrane and the pleura. Thereafter, the nerve lies between the internal and the innermost (intercostalis intimis) intercostal muscles.
- Each nerve lies in the neurovascular bundle comprising the artery, vein and inferiorly the nerve, which runs in a groove beneath each rib. The overhanging external edge of the rib protects this bundle from direct trauma. The groove is also invested in the fascia of the external and internal intercostal muscles.
- The groove is well defined until it reaches the mid-axillary line, at which point the nerve divides.
- Motor filaments supply the intercostal, the transversus thoracis and the serratus posterior muscles. The lower intercostal nerves also supply motor fibres to the abdominal muscles.
- Sensory branches supply the overlying skin as well as supplying the parietal pleura and the costal part of the diaphragm.
- The first sensory branch arises as the posterior cutaneous branch, which supplies the skin and muscles of the paravertebral area.
- The second sensory branch arises as the lateral cutaneous branch after the division of the nerve at around the mid-axillary line. The terminal fibres of this branch supply the skin and subcutaneous tissue of much of the chest and abdominal wall.
- The third and final sensory branch arises as the anterior cutaneous branch which is the continuation of the main intercostal nerve, and which supplies the skin and subcutaneous tissue of the anterior chest and abdominal walls.

Direction the viva may take

You may be asked to describe a technique of intercostal block. You may never have seen this block performed, and it will come as no surprise to your examiners if you admit as much. Your account therefore may be theoretical, but it must be safe.

- The intercostal injection is usually made at the angle of the rib, before the nerve divides.
- The skin of the back is tensed gently in a cranial direction before a needle and syringe is advanced to encounter the lower surface of the appropriate rib. The skin tension is then released. This helps the needle to move to its correct position.
- The needle is then carefully 'walked off' the inferior surface, before being directed a further 2–3 mm inwards to pierce the fascia of the innermost intercostal muscle (the posterior intercostal membrane) and enter the subcostal groove.
- Following injection of 3 or 4 ml of solution, for example bupivacaine 0.25–0.5% with adrenaline, the needle is withdrawn to rest on the posterior surface of the rib. The next space can then be located in the same way without risking inadvertent injection in the same space. This can easily happen in individuals even of modest size, and is common in the obese.
- Complications include pneumothorax (incidence of less than 1%), respiratory embarrassment in patients with any diaphragmatic impairment, and systemic toxicity if a large number of nerves are blocked. The rich vascular supply to the area means that systemic absorption following intercostal block exceeds that from almost any other site.

Further direction the viva could take

You may be asked about the distribution of local anaesthetic following injection.

- Contrast studies have confirmed that local anaesthetic spreads not only along the rib but can also track medially as far as the sympathetic chain. It also extends to several dermatomes above and below the site of injection, probably via direct subpleural spread. The intercostal, subpleural and paravertebral spaces are all in anatomical continuity, and so it is not surprising that injection of sufficient volume may lead to spread throughout all three.

The diaphragm

Commentary

The diaphragm is an important anatomical area for anaesthetists and acts as a radiographic marker for other disease processes. A raised hemidiaphragm, for example, may indicate pulmonary or abdominal pathology, and gas under the diaphragm is pathognomonic of visceral perforation. So even though primary diaphragmatic problems are rare, the examiners will expect you to demonstrate knowledge of the anatomy that allows you to use it as an indicator for these other conditions. The diaphragm is a vital respiratory structure, but its physiological functions are unlikely to figure in any detail in this predominantly anatomical question. However, the viva may well be linked to questions about the phrenic nerve. Anatomically, the diaphragm was viewed by the ancient Greeks as a partition between body cavities (it derives from the words for 'across' and 'partition'). Philosophically, however, they believed it to be the organ of thinking, and so also called it the 'phren' (Greek for 'mind'). Hence the derivation of the word 'phrenic'. Here, as elsewhere, this etymological information is probably of more use in a pub quiz than in the final FRCA, but should you get as far as discussing it you will either be doing brilliantly well or will be the victim of a particularly eccentric examiner.

The viva

You may be asked first about the course of the phrenic nerve, where it might be blocked or damaged and what would be the effects of phrenic nerve palsy.

- The phrenic nerve arises from the anterior primary ramus, principally of C_4 but with contributions from C_3 and C_5. The nerve is formed from these roots at the upper lateral border of the scalenus anterior muscle, and then descends on the anterior surface of this muscle, behind the prevertebral fascia.
- At the root of the neck it runs in front of the subclavian artery and behind the subclavian vein to enter the thorax. Thereafter, the intrathoracic course of the right and left phrenic nerves is different.
- **Right:** on the right the nerve follows the great veins, passing lateral to the innominate vein, the superior vena cava (SVC), the pericardium overlying the right atrium and the supra-diaphragmatic part of the inferior vena cava (IVC). It penetrates the diaphragm close to the hiatus traversed by the IVC. Some fibres also pass directly through the hiatus.
- **Left:** the course of the left phrenic nerve is longer. After passing between the left subclavian and the left common carotid arteries the nerve crosses the arch of the aorta, descends anterior to the left hilum of the lung, and continues immediately lateral to the left ventricle before penetrating the diaphragm. On both sides the nerve lies medial to the mediastinal pleura.
- It is common for the phrenic nerve to be blocked secondarily by local anaesthetic techniques such as interscalene and deep cervical plexus blocks. It may be damaged during surgery, for example during radical neck dissection, and may also be affected by disease processes, typically metastatic malignant disease of the lung. There are also reports of phrenic nerve palsy complicating long-term central venous catheterization.
- **Phrenic nerve palsy:** this may be asymptomatic. During quiet breathing some 75% of respiratory function is diaphragmatic, although when the minute volume is high, around 60% of the tidal volume is provided by the accessory muscles. It may be found as an incidental finding on a plain chest X-ray which will show a raised hemidiaphragm. (There are other causes, which include pregnancy, ascites, obesity, intra-abdominal malignancy and pulmonary lobar collapse.) Fluoroscopy will reveal paradoxical upward movement during inspiration. The phrenic nerve

can be paced by stimuli applied where it lies on the scalenus anterior muscle in the neck.

- **Spinal cord injury:** cord lesions at the level of C_2 and C_3 cause respiratory tetraplegia. Injuries at C_4 and below permit some phrenic nerve function, but vital capacity is reduced to about 25% of normal. Damage below C_6 allows full diaphragmatic function.

Direction the viva will take

You will then be asked to describe the basic anatomy of the diaphragm itself.

- **Diaphragm:** the diaphragm is the dome-shaped muscular and fibrous partition which separates the abdominal from the thoracic viscera.
- **Vertebral part:** this part of the diaphragm originates from the right and left crura, which arise from the front of the vertebral bodies of L_1–L_3 and L_1–L_2, respectively, and from the arcuate ligaments. The median ligament is a fibrous band which links the crura; the medial ligament is a tendinous arch arising as a thickening of the fascia of the psoas major muscle; the lateral ligament arises as another thickening of fascia, in this case from the quadratus lumborum muscle.
- **Costal part:** this part of the diaphragm arises from the six lowest ribs and their costal cartilages.
- **Sternal part:** this part comprises two small attachments from the xiphisternum.
- **Central tendon:** the muscle fibres converge into the central tendon, which is a tough aponeurosis near the centre of the dome of the diaphragm and which is merged above with the connective tissue of the pericardium.
- **Foramina:** there are three important openings in the diaphragm. Through one foramen at the level of T_8 pass the IVC and some fibres of the right phrenic nerve. Through another aperture at the level of T_{10} pass the oesophagus and vagus nerves. Through the final opening at the level of T_{12} pass the aorta, the thoracic duct and the azygos vein.
- **Motor supply:** motor innervation is supplied solely by the phrenic nerve (mainly C_3, C_4 and C_5 as above) whose long thoracic course reflects the descent of the diaphragm during fetal development.
- **Sensory supply:** the central part of the diaphragm is innervated by the sensory afferents of the phrenic nerve, hence the tendency for subdiaphragmatic pain to be referred to the shoulder tip, which shares the sensory innervation of C_5. The peripheral area of the diaphragm is innervated by the lower intercostal nerves.

Further direction the viva may take

There are a number of miscellaneous areas of clinical relevance about which you could be asked.

- **Position on chest X-ray:** after forced expiration, the right cupola (which is higher than the left because of the upward pressure of the liver) is level anteriorly with the fourth costal cartilage, and level posteriorly with the eighth rib. During quiet respiration the diaphragm moves only about 1.5 cm but this excursion can increase to 10 cm or more with deep inspiration.

- **The cardio-oesophageal sphincter:** the fibres of the crura that surround the cardio-oesophageal junction exert a pinchcock effect on the oesophagus which contributes to the prevention of gastro-oesophageal reflux. Laxity of this oesophageal hiatus is associated with hiatus hernia in which the lower oesophagus and stomach slide into the chest, causing symptoms of dyspepsia and reflux. (This is a sliding hernia; the much less common rolling hernia occurs when the fundus of the stomach rolls up through the hiatus in front of the oesophagus which remains intra-abdominal. Patients have dyspepsia but no reflux.) You should be prepared to detail your management of anaesthesia in a patient with hiatus hernia. This would usually involve a precise clinical history seeking the symptoms and characteristics of oesophageal reflux which, if positive, would mandate rapid sequence induction following administration of agents to reduce gastric acidity.
- **Neuromuscular block:** the diaphragm is amongst the muscles most resistant to muscle relaxants. Postoperative respiration may therefore be adequate even though the patient subjectively may feel profoundly weak.
- **Diaphragmatic hernia:** these may be congenital, occurring in utero (the incidence is 1 in 4000 live births) and preventing the proper development of the lung, or traumatic. Surgical repair in the neonate requires tertiary paediatric centre expertise, specific details of which you will not be expected to know. Traumatic herniation may be associated with immediate symptoms requiring surgical repair; equally, there are cases in which the abnormality has been diagnosed years after an injury from which the patient has been asymptomatic.

The liver

Commentary

The liver is an organ of complex metabolic and biosynthetic importance, which means that the clinically orientated parts of the viva could follow one of several routes, examples of which include drug handling, protein synthesis and the anaesthetic implications of impaired liver function. Questions on its basic anatomy are likely to concentrate less on gross anatomy and more on its microstructure. This is not easy. The liver acinus is not a homogenous structure like the glomerulus of the kidney, and the traditional view that was based on the histological appearance of a hepatic lobule has been superseded by the concept of a functional unit. Different parts of the lobule appear to have not only a varied blood supply but also dissimilar metabolic functions. As you are unlikely to have enough time for a coherent discussion of this metabolic zonation, a simplified account of both the classical and functional anatomy is given below. Because it is complicated, most examiners will be content if you are able to describe the basic architecture, particularly if you can also convey that you know this to be an over-simplification. The oral will then move on to the clinical aspects which will be of more interest to both.

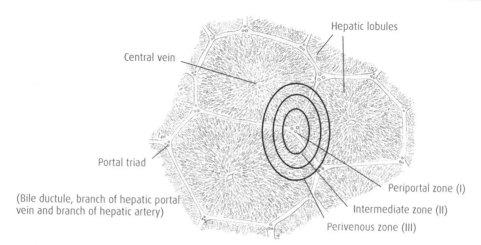

Hepatic lobules

Central vein

Portal triad

(Bile ductule, branch of hepatic portal vein and branch of hepatic artery)

Periportal zone (I)

Intermediate zone (II)

Perivenous zone (III)

Fig. 2.7 Microscopic anatomy of the liver.

The viva

As there is much clinical information that could be discussed, the examiner will probably concentrate on dispatching the anatomy first. You will be asked briefly about the gross anatomy of the liver and then in more detail about its functional microstructure.

- The liver is the largest organ *in* the body, although skin is actually the largest organ *of* the body. Its weight varies with factors such as gender and body habitus, but ranges from 1.0 to 2.5 kg.
- It is divided into right and left lobes, with the right accounting for about 85% of the mass of the whole. It lies directly beneath the diaphragm to fill the right hypochondrium, while its inferior relations include parts of much of the abdominal viscera (including the lesser curve of the stomach, the duodenum, the hepatic flexure of the colon and the right kidney and adrenal gland). It is covered by connective tissue which forms a capsule (Glisson's capsule).
- **Blood supply:** this totals about 1500 ml min^{-1} (range 1000–2000 ml min^{-1} depending on factors such as size) and is derived from two primary sources. These are the **hepatic artery**, which supplies about 30% of the total flow (500 ml min^{-1}), has an oxygen saturation of 98% and accounts for around 50% of total oxygen delivery; and the **portal vein**, which has an oxygen saturation of 60–75% (depending on gastrointestinal metabolic demand), supplies 70% of total flow (1000 ml min^{-1}) and accounts for the remaining 50% of oxygen delivery.
- **Traditional microscopic architecture (Figure 2.7):** the liver comprises numerous lobules, each approximately 1 mm in diameter and hexagonal in shape. Each lobule contains a central vein, which is a thin-walled venular tributary of the hepatic vein, and from which extend plate-like layers of hepatocytes one cell thick radiating to the borders of the lobule. Between these radiations are sinusoidal blood channels up to 12 μm wide which drain into the central vein and thence via collecting veins to the IVC. At each corner of the lobule is the **portal area** in which lie a branch of the hepatic portal vein, a branch of the hepatic artery, which drain into the sinusoids, and

a bile duct (strictly an interlobular bile ductule). These are the **portal triads** (although the portal areas do also contain lymphatics and nerves). The sinusoids are lined by endothelium whose cells include the Kupffer cells, which are mobile phagocytes (although they may have other metabolic functions), and Pitt cells, which are mobile lymphocytes that are active against tumour cells and infective pathogens. Hepatocytes themselves are large polyhedral cells measuring up to $30 \times 20\,\mu m$.

- **Functional anatomy – Rappaport's acinus (Figure 2.7):** this is a functional unit which consists of more than one lobule and whose central axis is a portal triad. Blood moves from this region towards the centrilobular veins, with a progressive decrease in oxygenation and metabolic activity. This drainage territory is divided into three concentric zones, which are separate functionally, if not anatomically. The **periportal zone (I)** has the highest oxygen saturation. It is also metabolically the most active, containing transaminases which mediate both protein anabolism and catabolism. The **intermediate zone (II)** has similar, but diminished functions to those not only of zone I but also of the **perivenous zone (III)**, which has the poorest oxygenation and which contains perivenous (centrilobular) hepatocytes. These nonetheless have high quantities of cytochromes P450 and are active in drug biotransformation. (You can see that this concept of metabolic zonation is more difficult to encapsulate anatomically, which is why both you and the examiner might find the traditional view somewhat easier to summarize.)

Direction the viva may take

You may be asked about aspects of liver function. Each could potentially include substantial detail but, as this is primarily a question about hepatic functional anatomy rather than liver function, you will be required to give only a relatively superficial overview.

- **Drug biotransformation:** the liver metabolizes drugs that reach it via the hepatic and the portal circulations. Phase I reactions, which involve oxidation, reduction and hydrolysis, are catabolic, and, while they render the drug more water-soluble, may create metabolites that are more toxic than the parent compound. Most, but not all phase I reactions involve the P450 mono-oxygenase system (page 374) and take place on the smooth endoplasmic reticulum within hepatocytes. Thiopental, for example, is oxidized, while pethidine is metabolized by ester hydrolysis. The P450 system does not degrade ethanol (alcohol), which is metabolized to acetaldehyde by the cytoplasmic enzyme alcohol dehydrogenase. Phase II reactions are anabolic (synthetic) and involve the formation of a conjugate which is more water-soluble than its precursor. A common example is the conjugation of morphine to 3- and 6-glucuronides.
- **Protein synthesis:** the liver produces plasma proteins, amongst the more important of which are albumin, prealbumin and some globulins $(\alpha_{1-2}, \beta$ but not $\gamma)$. It synthesizes coagulation factors I (fibrinogen), II (prothrombin), V, VII, IX, X and XI. It also synthesizes antithrombin, protein C and protein S. It produces purine and pyrimidine bases.
- **Carbohydrate metabolism:** the major processes are gluconeogenesis (glucose production from amino acids, lactate and glycerol), glycogenesis (formation of

glycogen from glucose) and the converse process of glycogenolysis (formation of glucose from glycogen breakdown).

- **Lipid metabolism:** the liver synthesizes cholesterol as well as high and low density lipoproteins. It also produces triglycerides and ketone bodies following partial oxidation of fatty acids.
- **Bile synthesis:** bile emulsifies fats in the gastrointestinal tract, and provides a means of eliminating drugs, toxins and other compounds. Hepatic breakdown of haemoglobin produces the bile pigments bilirubin and biliverdin.
- **Storage:** the liver is the major site of storage of a large number of compounds, including vitamins A, B_{12}, D, E and K, iron, copper and glycogen.
- **Immunological functions:** Kupffer and Pitt cells are mobile phagocytes that are active against pathogens and tumour cells.
- **Erythropoiesis:** until 32 weeks of gestational age the liver is the primary site of fetal red blood cell production.

You may be asked about the implications of anaesthesia in the jaundiced patient (pages 361–2).

- **Implications of jaundice:** these include impaired coagulation; renal failure (hepatorenal syndrome); altered drug metabolism owing to conversion of cytochrome P450 to the inactive P420; hypoproteinaemia may increase the proportion of free active drug; jaundice may be due to an infective disease (hepatitis A, B, C); bradyarrhythmias (owing to high concentrations of bile salts); inaccurate oxygen saturation monitoring (bilirubin absorption coefficient is similar to deoxygenated haemoglobin, and so SpO_2 will read artificially low).

The coeliac plexus

Commentary

You are unlikely to have had much, if any, direct experience of the coeliac plexus. Coeliac plexus block is no longer a procedure that can be undertaken blind without imaging, and its indications are limited to severe intractable pain. This question, however, remains a perennial favourite despite the fact that most examiners expect only theoretical knowledge. You will none the less need to know the anatomy reasonably well, because even the most sympathetic examiner has no choice but to pursue the topic. There is nowhere else to go and the 7 or 8 minutes otherwise will seem interminable.

The viva

You may be asked about the indications for coeliac plexus block.

- **Therapeutic block:** the plexus can be blocked in conjunction with intercostal nerves to provide analgesia for intra-abdominal surgery. This technique does not have many enthusiasts. More commonly it is used for the relief of malignant visceral pain, typically that due to carcinoma of the pancreas. Neurolytic blocks give good analgesia in up to 90% of patients, although the effect may only last for a number of months.

- **Non-malignant pain:** the commonest such condition is chronic pancreatitis. Many clinicians are reluctant to use coeliac plexus block in such patients both because of the risks of paraplegia (1–2 per 1000 owing to acute ischaemia at the watershed area of the cord) and because its effective duration is limited. Coeliac plexus block for non-malignant visceral pain is also generally less successful, with only around 60–70% of patients reporting good pain relief.
- **Diagnostic block:** coeliac plexus block using local anaesthetic alone can be used for diagnostic purposes, and for attempting to break a sympathetically mediated acute pain cycle.

You will be asked about the anatomy.

- It is the largest sympathetic plexus and lies anterior to the abdominal aorta where, as a dense network of nerve fibres, it surrounds the root of the coeliac artery at the level of L_1.
- It is a bilateral structure. There are two ganglia, right and left, which are closely related to the crura of the diaphragm.
- The plexus receives the greater splanchnic nerve (fibres from $T_5-T_{9\ or\ 10}$) and the lesser splanchnic nerve (fibres from $T_{9/10}$ or $T_{10/11}$).
- The plexus also receives some filaments bilaterally both from the vagus and the phrenic nerves.
- Superiorly lie the crura of the diaphragm; posteriorly is the abdominal aorta; laterally are the adrenal glands in the superior poles of left and right kidneys. The important anterior relation is the pancreas.

Direction the viva may take

You may then be asked how you might perform a block. Remember that the examiner's knowledge may be as theoretical as yours and that your collective experience may be small. You are unlikely to be picked up on small details as long as your overall account is plausible and safe. If your examiner does happen to work in chronic pain management they should not allow their specialist knowledge to influence the standard that is expected of you.

Technique of coeliac plexus block

- The patient lies prone.
- The spinous process of T_{12} forms the apex of a flattened triangle whose base is a line joining the 12th ribs, and which ends 7–8 cm from the midline.
- A 10–15 cm 20G needle (depending on the size of the patient) is directed medially and rostrally along the lines of this triangle, and towards the lateral border of the body of the first lumbar vertebra.
- When the needle encounters the vertebral body it is withdrawn almost to skin before redirection so that it can be walked off the anterolateral side of the vertebra to advance a further 2–3 cm.

- The diffuse nature of the para-aortic plexus means that 20–25 ml of local anaesthetic will be required on each side. Neurolytic agents should be injected only under X-ray control, after needle placement has been confirmed by contrast media.
- All neurolytic drugs lead to indiscriminate neural destruction. Alcohol (50–100%) is usually preferred to phenol (5–8%) for coeliac plexus block. It can be very painful on injection, but does not cause the vascular injury that is associated with phenol (which is a potential problem for a block such as this which is para-aortic). Transient intoxication may occur in the elderly.
- The duration of effective action may be limited to 1–6 months. The neuritis that can accompany the regeneration of nerves may be as severe as the original symptoms.

If there is time, the questions will include complications of the block.

- **Complications:** these include hypotension (it is a sympathetic block), anterior spinal artery syndrome (page 63), subarachnoid, epidural and intrapsoas injection, intravascular injection (the aorta is very accessible on the left, the inferior vena cava is less vulnerable on the right), retroperitoneal haemorrhage and visceral puncture. The kidney is the organ that is most vulnerable. The neurolytic agent may also spread unpredictably, causing paresis, paralysis and dysaesthesia.

Blood supply to the spinal cord

Commentary

This is another area of 'theoretical' anatomy. Its main clinical relevance lies in the potential for catastrophic neurological damage secondary to ischaemia. For most anaesthetists, happily, this is also theoretical, but it is of obvious importance for those involved in surgery of the thoracic aorta. Otherwise the required knowledge may perhaps allow you some day to astound colleagues as you alone correctly diagnose an anterior spinal artery syndrome.

The viva

You will be asked to describe the arterial blood supply to the cord. Alternatively, the questioning could be initiated by a discussion of some possible causes of ischaemia.

- The spinal cord is supplied by paired posterior arteries and a single anterior artery, together with a series of smaller feeder radicular arteries.
- The two posterior arteries arise from the posterior inferior cerebellar arteries. These descend to the posterior nerve roots, to which they lie medially, and give off penetrating vessels to the posterior white columns and the rest of the posterior grey columns.
- The anterior spinal artery is a single midline artery, which is formed between the pyramids of the medulla oblongata from terminal branches of the vertebral arteries.

It descends the cord in the midline in the anterior median fissure, giving off numerous circumferential vessels. The central branches of the artery supply up to two-thirds of the cross-sectional area of the cord.

- The anterior and two posterior arteries are fed by a variable number of smaller radicular arteries which approach the spinal cord along both ventral and dorsal nerve roots. These arteries, whose number may vary from about 25 to 40, arise from the spinal branches of the subclavian artery, the aorta and the iliac arteries inferiorly.
- In the cervical and upper thoracic regions the anterior spinal artery begins with contributions from the vertebrals, and then receives feeders from the subclavian, the thyrocostal and the costocervical arteries. From the level of T_4 down to T_9 the feeding branches of the intercostal arteries are relatively small.
- The three main arteries are also supplied by a few of the spinal branches of the vertebral, deep cervical, ascending cervical, posterior intercostal, lumbar and lateral sacral arteries. Only about six or seven of these make any significant contribution to the anterior artery, and a similar number supply the posterior arteries (but not at the same level). These feeding arteries terminate in a series of short lengths which anastomose across the midline from posterior to anterior. The posterior radicular arteries are larger than the anterior.
- The largest of the feeder arteries is the radicularis magna, or anterior radicular artery of Adamkiewicz. This originates from the aorta at a variable level, and supplies the low thoracic and lumbar regions of the cord. It enters on the left in 80% of subjects, through any one of the intervertebral foramina between T_8 and L_3. In a small number of patients (around 15%), the artery of Adamkiewicz originates high on the aorta, at the level of T_5, in which event the contribution of iliac tributaries to the lumbar cord enlarges. This renders the conus medullaris vulnerable should there be subsequent damage to this iliac supply, for example, by ligation during pelvic surgery.
- This anatomical arrangement ensures an adequate blood supply across three large and discrete areas of the cord: the cervical, the upper thoracic and the thoracolumbar. There is, however, a much poorer vertical anastomosis between the cervical, thoracic and lumbar areas, and at these watershed zones, particularly at T_4/T_5, the spinal cord is acutely vulnerable to ischaemia.

Direction the viva may take

You may be asked about the clinical situations in which cord damage may arise.

- This may occur following profound hypotension from any cause, including subarachnoid and extradural anaesthesia. Spinal cord ischaemic damage has also been associated specifically with hypotension secondary to coeliac plexus block.
- Injury may result from aortic surgery, particularly for repair of aneurysms of the thoracic aorta, although the incidence in elective procedures is now quoted as less than 5%. Risk factors, predictably, are those which worsen ischaemia: in particular the duration of aortic cross-clamp time, as well as the pre-morbid state of the patient's circulation, the patient's age, and the difficulty of the surgical procedure.

Further direction the viva could take

You may be asked how risks to the cord during aneurysm surgery can be minimized.

- Spinal cord function can be monitored using somatosensory evoked potentials (SSEPs).
- Non-pharmacological methods include hypothermia, the use of shunts and oxygenated bypass circuits, and CSF drainage. By analogy with cerebral perfusion pressure (CPP), the mean spinal arterial pressure (MAP) can be increased if CSF pressure is reduced. (CPP = MAP − [CVP + ICP], where CVP is central venous pressure and ICP is intracranial pressure.) Some surgeons have advocated reattachment of intercostal vessels, although others contend that the routine reimplantation of segmental vessels is not supported by evidence.
- Pharmacological interventions include intrathecal vasodilators such as papaverine, systemic calcium channel blockers, and the use of oxygen-derived free radical scavengers.

You may be asked about **anterior spinal artery syndrome.**

- This describes the situation in which critical ischaemia of the anterior part of the spinal cord leads to loss of the corticospinal and vestibulospinal tracts, which are motor; and the spinothalamic tracts, which subserve deep touch and pressure sensation. This results in a lesion that is primarily motor below the level of cord damage. Vibration sense, light touch and proprioception are mediated via the posterior columns and these remain undamaged.

The lumbar sympathetic chain

Commentary

The anatomy of this area is not detailed and so the viva is likely to move on quite quickly to clinical aspects of the subject. Lumbar sympathectomy is a procedure which is undertaken mainly by chronic pain specialists, and you may well not have seen it done. The same may apply to lumbar plexus (psoas compartment) block, which you may also be invited to discuss. If you are struggling for facts then do not guess, but instead fall back on the anatomy. If you are able to show that you could work out a safe theoretical approach by virtue of your anatomical knowledge then you are likely to pass, even though the practical details may be incomplete.

The viva

You may be asked for the indications for lumbar sympathectomy.

- **Indications:** the block is performed to improve impaired circulation of the lower limb, the commonest cause of which is peripheral vascular disease. It is also used to treat syndromes in which sympathetically maintained pain is a feature, such as the complex regional pain syndrome, and for phantom limb and other neuropathic pain. It has been used to alleviate renal colic, and to manage chronic urogenital pain.

You will be asked to describe the anatomy of the lumbar sympathetic chain.

- The sympathetic outflow originates in the hypothalamus, medulla and spinal cord as pre-ganglionic myelinated efferents. These exit the cord with the ventral nerve roots of the first thoracic nerve down to the second, third and, in some subjects, the fourth lumbar spinal nerves (T_1–L_{2-4}). These efferents pass via the white rami communicantes to synapse in the sympathetic ganglia of the paravertebral sympathetic trunk, which is closely related to the spinal column throughout its length.
- The lumbar part of the sympathetic trunk lies in a fascial plane on the anterolateral aspect of the vertebral bodies. Posterolaterally is the fascia of the sheath of psoas major, and anterolaterally is peritoneum. On the left side the anterior relation is the aorta, while on the right it is the IVC.

Direction the viva may follow

You may be asked how you would perform a lumbar sympathetic block.

- **Technique:** several techniques have been described. Choose the one with which you are familiar, but if you have never seen this procedure performed then you can cite the account which follows as the 'traditional approach'. The block should always be undertaken with the help of an image intensifier. With the patient in the lateral position and after infiltration of the skin, a 120-mm needle is inserted 8–10 cm from the midline at the lateral margin of the erector spinae muscle and at the level of the L_2 spinous process (the procedure is repeated at L_3 and L_4). The needle is then directed inward and medially at an angle of 45° towards the vertebral body. As soon as the needle encounters bone it is partly withdrawn prior to reinsertion at a steeper angle, which will allow the needle (with the bevel facing towards the vertebra) to slide past the vertebral body and through the psoas fascia to lie close to the sympathetic chain. After aspiration checks for blood (the aorta is on the left, the IVC on the right), a small volume of contrast medium is injected. Correct placement is indicated by localized linear spread along the vertebral column. If the needle is lying within the psoas compartment then the contrast will track away from the vertebral body. Local anaesthetic is then injected or, if a permanent block is sought, either absolute alcohol or a dilute solution of phenol (5%) can be used.
- **Complications:** these include puncture of the aorta or IVC, inadvertent subarachnoid injection, profound hypotension, genitofemoral nerve neuritis (occurring in 5–10% of patients and presenting as pain in the groin), injury to somatic nerves (1%) and perforation of the intervertebral disc. Some of these complications are associated with mechanical damage caused by the advancing needle, others by the substance that is injected. L_1 genitofemoral neuralgia, for example, is much more common after alcohol has been used. Ureteric strictures have also been reported following the use of alcohol and phenol.

Further direction the viva could take

You may be asked to contrast lumbar sympathetic block with lumbar plexus block.

- The lumbar plexus is formed from the anterior primary rami of the first four lumbar nerves, together with a small contribution from the 12th thoracic nerve. After emerging from the intervertebral foramina the nerves lie just within the substance of the psoas major muscle (and within its sheath). The nerves formed by the plexus include the femoral, obturator, iliohypogastric, ilioinguinal, genitofemoral and the lateral cutaneous nerve of the thigh. All except the obturator nerve emerge laterally in the plane between the psoas and quadratus lumborum. The obturator nerve issues medially before descending beneath the iliac vessels.
- **Lumbar plexus block:** this block (sometimes called psoas compartment block) can provide effective analgesia (as well as motor block) to much of the groin and upper leg. It should, therefore, offer a useful alternative to field block for inguinal herniorrhaphy, and to '3-in-1' blocks for proximal hip surgery (cannulated and dynamic hip screws). The analgesia afforded by the block is rarely dense enough to allow surgery without general anaesthesia, and nerves such as the femoral and obturator can as readily be blocked at more distal sites.
- **Technique:** various approaches have been described. With the patient in the lateral position with the side to be blocked uppermost, a needle is directed perpendicular to the skin to encounter the transverse process of L3. This site is chosen because the process is longer and wider than those of the other lumbar vertebrae. The needle is then walked off superiorly, penetrating first the fascia of quadratus lumborum and then that of the psoas sheath. Some anaesthetists use a nerve stimulator, although because the fibres of the plexus are separated and embedded within the body of the muscle this technique may not always succeed. An alternative is to use a Tuohy epidural needle with a loss-of-resistance device attached. The loss of resistance as the needle penetrates the sheath is not dissimilar to that which occurs when the epidural space is entered. The advantage of this approach is that an epidural catheter can be inserted to provide continuous analgesia. It also allows verification of placement, because an injection of contrast medium will outline the borders of the psoas compartment should the catheter be in the correct place. (Various catheter-over-needle sets are now available.) A single bolus injection may require 20–40 ml of local anaesthetic to achieve a satisfactory block.

Innervation of the inguinal region

Commentary

This in essence is a straightforward question about field block for inguinal hernia repair based on anatomical knowledge. If you provide reasonably comprehensive anatomical details it will prevent the viva moving away from the core topic into areas such as ultrasound guidance or local anaesthetic toxicity.

The viva

You will be asked to describe the nerve supply to the inguinal region.

- **Supply:** the skin over the lower abdomen is supplied by the first and second nerves of the lumbar plexus, L_1 and L_2, together with a contribution from the subcostal nerve, T_{12}.
- **Iliohypogastric nerve:** this arises from L_1, emerges from the lateral border of the psoas muscle, and passes obliquely behind the kidney to perforate the posterior part of the transversus abdominis muscle above the iliac crest. It lies then between transversus and the internal oblique where it divides. Its anterior cutaneous branch runs forward between those muscles before passing through the internal oblique about 2 cm medial to the anterior superior iliac spine. It pierces the aponeurosis of the external oblique muscle about 3 cm above the external inguinal ring and supplies sensation to suprapubic skin.
- **Ilioinguinal nerve:** this also arises from L_1, emerging from the lateral border of the psoas muscle and passing below the larger iliohypogastric nerve to perforate the posterior part of the transversus abdominis muscle near the anterior iliac crest. It lies below the internal oblique, before piercing it to traverse the inguinal canal accompanied by the spermatic cord. It exits the external inguinal ring to supply the skin of the upper thigh, the skin over the root of the penis or the mons pubis, and the skin of the scrotum or labia.
- **Genitofemoral nerve:** this arises from L_1 and L_2, emerging on the abdominal surface of the psoas muscle opposite the third or fourth lumbar vertebra. It runs down on the body of the psoas muscle, retroperitoneally, and divides above the inguinal ligament into genital and femoral branches. The genital branch enters the inguinal canal via the deep inguinal ring to supply the cremaster muscle and to send some fine terminal branches to innervate scrotal skin. (In women it accompanies the broad ligament and contributes to cutaneous sensation of the mons and labia.) The femoral branch passes behind the inguinal ligament to enter the femoral sheath, lateral to the artery, before perforating the sheath and fascia lata anteriorly to supply the skin over the upper femoral triangle.

Direction the viva may take

You will be asked how you would perform a field block for inguinal herniorrhaphy. There are various techniques described: choose the one with which you are most familiar.

- Reliable anaesthesia for inguinal hernia repair is not always easy to achieve, and if the operation is done with the patient awake it is common for surgeons to infiltrate considerable volumes of supplemental local anaesthetic. Field block, however, is useful for postoperative analgesia.
- All three nerves need to be blocked, and subsequent infiltration may also be required over the skin incision itself, depending on its extent, and at the internal ring.
- A short bevelled needle is advanced via a point approximately 2 cm medial and 2 cm caudal to the anterior superior iliac spine. This blunter needle will better appreciate the resistance offered by the external oblique aponeurosis, which is penetrated often with a definite click. Injection of around 5 ml of local anaesthetic should be sufficient to block the iliohypogastric nerve at this point. If the needle is then

advanced through the internal oblique muscle for about 1–2 cm the same volume should block the ilioinguinal nerve which at this point lies below the muscle. The genitofemoral nerve is approached via an injection made from the pubic tubercle and extending fanwise from the midline to the external inguinal ring.

- Alternative techniques include the fanwise injection of large volume low concentration solutions in and between the oblique muscles (plus genitofemoral nerve block as above), lumbar plexus and lumbar paravertebral blocks. These latter two techniques are used infrequently.
- Ultrasound-guided block of the ilioinguinal nerve is becoming more commonplace, the technique allowing clear identification of the nerve between the transversus abdominis and the internal oblique muscles.

Further direction the viva could take
You may be asked about the use of ultrasound (page 337) or local anaesthetic toxicity (page 220).

The brachial plexus

Commentary
An understanding of the anatomy of the brachial plexus is the key to successful regional anaesthesia of the upper limb. The anatomy is detailed but is not so complex that it cannot be incorporated into a 7 or 8-minute viva question. It is a clinically important area of anatomy and is asked frequently. It is worth learning a schematic diagram of the plexus because it makes it much easier to explain it to the examiners. As it is a core topic of obvious clinical relevance, it is likely that the pure anatomy part of the question will precede discussion of its clinical aspects.

The viva
You will be asked about the formation of the brachial plexus (Figure 2.8).

- The plexus forms in the neck from the anterior primary rami of C_5, C_6, C_7, C_8 and T_1.
- These five roots merge in the posterior triangle of the neck to form three trunks.
- C_5 and C_6 form the upper trunk, C_7 the middle trunk (above the subclavian artery), and C_8 and T_1 form the lower trunk (posterior to the subclavian artery).
- At the lateral border of the first rib the three trunks each divide into anterior and posterior divisions.
- The three posterior divisions form the posterior cord (described according to its relationship with the axillary artery), from which derives the radial nerve (also the axillary, thoracodorsal and upper and lower subscapular nerves).
- The anterior divisions of the upper and middle trunks form the lateral cord, from which derive the median nerve (lateral head) and the musculocutaneous nerve (also the lateral pectoral nerve).

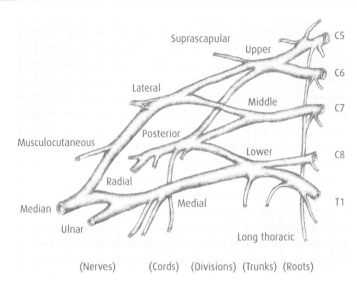

Fig. 2.8 The brachial plexus.

(Nerves)   (Cords)   (Divisions) (Trunks) (Roots)

- The anterior division of the lower trunk continues as the medial cord, from which derive the ulnar nerve and the median nerve (medial head) (also the medial cutaneous nerves of arm and forearm and the medial pectoral nerve).

Direction the viva may take
You will be asked about brachial plexus block. It is probable that you will be asked to describe an approach of your choosing. If possible, choose a block that you have performed.

- **Interscalene block.**
    — Interscalene local anaesthesia blocks the anterior primary rami of the nerves of C_5–C_8 and T_1 before they merge in the posterior triangle to form the trunks of the brachial plexus.
    — The cervical nerves leave the intervertebral foramina, and pass caudad and laterally between the scalenus anterior and the scalenus medius muscles. The nerves are enclosed within a fascial compartment which comprises the posterior fascia of the anterior scalene muscle and the anterior fascia of the middle scalene muscle.
    — The patient should lie supine with the head turned slightly away from the side of injection and with the arm by the side (gently pulled down if necessary to depress the shoulder).
    — After standard aseptic preparation, the interscalene groove between scalenus anterior and medius should be identified at the level of the cricoid cartilage (C_6).
    — If the awake patient is asked to lift the head off the pillow (which tenses the sternocleidomastoid muscles) or to give a sniff, the groove becomes more evident. In the anaesthetized patient, identification is helped by the fact that in more than 90% of subjects the external jugular vein overlies the groove at this level.

— It has been usual practice to identify the plexus using a peripheral nerve stimulator alone, but ultrasound-guided location is likely to become commonplace.

— The groove and the roots beyond are superficial and in most cases a stimulating needle no longer than 30 mm is needed. The needle should be held perpendicular to the skin in all planes as it is directed medially, posteriorly and caudally (inwards, backwards and downwards) towards the transverse process of C_6 (Chassaignac's tubercle). This is the approach as described by Winnie. An alternative is Meier's approach, in which the needle is directed caudad down the interscalene groove towards the subclavian artery. You will not be expected to discuss these in any further detail.

— Once muscle stimulation is apparent in the required distribution (usually shoulder movements mediated by $C_{5,6}$), 20–40 ml of solution may be injected after aspiration and with all due precautions. In common with most plexus blocks into fascial compartments, large volumes of appropriately dilute solutions may be needed to obtain adequate analgesia of all the nerves involved.

— Interscalene block is particularly useful for shoulder surgery. It can be used to provide analgesia for more distal structures in the upper limb, but it does not provide reliable block of C_8 and T_1, and so ulnar sparing is frequent (some reports quote 30–40%).

— Successful analgesia is almost invariably associated with block of the phrenic nerve which lies on scalenus anterior. The block should be used cautiously in patients with respiratory disease because it may reduce the functional residual capacity by up to 30%. Bilateral blocks should not be performed.

— *Complications:* these include intravascular injection (particularly into the vertebral artery), central spread via inadvertent dural puncture leading to a total spinal, phrenic nerve palsy (90%), Horner's syndrome (cervical sympathetic block, which is usually innocuous) (20%), vagal and recurrent laryngeal nerve block which may cause hoarseness (15%), but is usually benign, and pneumothorax (rare). (There are also generic complications such as systemic toxicity and neurapraxia.)

- **Supraclavicular block.**
   — This block provides analgesia for most of the upper limb. The three trunks are in close arrangement and the block is reliable. It can also be used for shoulder surgery, although the interscalene approach is usually preferred.
   — The three trunks lie on the first rib, between the insertion of the scalenus anterior and scalenus medius muscles, and immediately posterior to the subclavian artery (the pulsations of which can provide a landmark).
   — The trunks cross the rib at about the midpoint of the clavicle.
   — A number of approaches have been described: if you are familiar with one of them then explain it. In essence, the aim of the technique is to direct the needle down on to the first rib, and to contact the brachial plexus where it lies cephaloposterior to the subclavian artery.
   — Once muscle stimulation is apparent in the appropriate distribution, 20–40 ml of appropriate local anaesthetic solution (such as levobupivacaine 0.25–0.5%) may be injected after aspiration and with the usual precautions. If localization is accurate, then the smaller volumes will be effective.

— *Complications:* these include pneumothorax (the incidence may be 0.5–1.0% even in experienced hands, and may take up to 24 hours to develop), intravascular injection or puncture (subclavian artery or vein), phrenic nerve palsy (in 40–60%), Horner's syndrome in 70–90% (cervical sympathetic block) and neuritis (plus generic complications as above).

- **Subclavian perivascular or vertical infraclavicular block.** (several variations have been described.)
  — In effect this is an approach to the axillary sheath from a proximal direction, although the block provides analgesia similar to that offered by the supraclavicular approach. The subclavian perivascular block is actually made through a needle inserted above the clavicle. Unlike the other techniques, these alone reliably block the intercostobrachial nerve. These blocks are not that widely used in the UK and unfamiliarity with their details will not disadvantage you.

- **Axillary block.**
  — This has fewer complications than other approaches, is generally effective and is a popular technique.
  — The block provides good analgesia for surgery below the elbow. The musculocutaneous nerve may leave the axillary sheath proximal to the site of injection, in which event supplemental analgesia may be needed by blocking the nerve between brachioradialis and the lateral epicondyle at the elbow. This nerve innervates a substantial part of the radial side of the forearm, and so local anaesthetic sparing of this area is not purely academic.
  — The arm is abducted to 90° (hyperabduction may abolish the arterial pulsation). The advancing needle is directed at an angle of about 45° to the skin as far proximally as possible. In practice, this often means injecting at the lateral border of pectoralis major.
  — Once a twitch is elicited, the entire volume of local anaesthetic solution can be injected (after aspiration). It takes just over 40 ml to fill the axillary sheath as far as the coracoid process in adults, and, in theory, complete block of all three cords will follow circumferential spread round the sheath. Some anaesthetists prefer to identify the major nerves of the upper limb separately, and block each one in turn.
  — An alternative approach uses axillary arterial puncture as an end point. Following transfixion of the vessel, the needle is either advanced or withdrawn until aspiration is negative. The widespread use of nerve stimulators has made this technique less respectable than once it was.
  — Axillary brachial plexus block does not provide dense analgesia of the upper arm and does not block the intercostobrachial nerve (which arises from T_2 and T_3 and supplies the skin of the posterior upper arm). Patients may therefore be unable to tolerate the arterial tourniquet.
  — Cadaver studies have suggested that the connective tissue of the sheath can form septa between the parts of the plexus, effectively forming a fascial compartment for each nerve and thus limiting the circumferential, but not the longitudinal, spread of injected local anaesthetic. This may explain patchy and incomplete blocks (while providing a useful excuse for their failure).

Further direction the viva could take

It is important that you understand the indications for these different approaches (for instance, interscalene block for shoulder surgery, axillary block for a fasciectomy involving the fifth finger) and that you are aware of their limitations and complications. You may be asked therefore to compare and contrast some of the blocks.

The ulnar nerve

Commentary

You may well not get a full question on this single nerve: there are few indications for isolated ulnar block and so it might be linked to a discussion of the radial and median nerves. Other clinical aspects could include its vulnerability to damage during general anaesthesia and the clinical features of injury.

The viva

The questioning may start with the indications for ulnar nerve block.

- Ulnar nerve block provides analgesia for procedures on the medial (ulnar) side of the hand and forearm. The nerve supplies sensation to a relatively small area. Digital nerve blocks are an easy and reliable method of providing anaesthesia for finger surgery, and so ulnar block is usually reserved for more proximal operations such as palmar fasciectomy. It would be used in isolation only for disease that was restricted to the fifth finger and so is commonly performed jointly with blocks of the other major nerves of the arm.

You will be asked about the anatomy of the ulnar nerve.

- The ulnar nerve arises from the brachial plexus (page 67). The anterior division of the lower trunk continues as the medial cord, from which derives the ulnar nerve. Its fibres originate mainly from C_8 and T_1, although it may also receive a contribution from C_7.
- It passes through the extensor compartment of the upper arm, lying medial to the axillary and brachial arteries. It then continues medially on the anterior aspect of the medial head of triceps to pass beneath the medial epicondyle of the humerus, where it lies in the ulnar groove.
- It enters the forearm between the two heads of flexor carpi ulnaris. In the upper part of the forearm it lies deep to this muscle and separated from the ulnar artery. In the distal forearm it lies lateral to flexor carpi ulnaris and near to the medial side of the artery.
- About 5 cm above the wrist it gives off a dorsal branch before continuing into the hand lateral to the pisiform bone and above the flexor retinaculum.
- The ulnar nerve provides the motor supply to flexor carpi ulnaris, to the medial part of flexor digitorum profundus, and to the hypothenar muscles. It also

supplies all the small muscles of the hand apart from the lateral two lumbricals and the three muscles of the thenar eminence (abductor pollicis brevis, opponens pollicis and part of flexor pollicis brevis). It innervates the deep head of flexor pollicis.

- It supplies sensation to the elbow joint but gives off no branches in the upper arm. It supplies the skin over the hypothenar eminence and over the fifth finger as well as over the medial part of the fourth finger.

Direction the viva may take

You may be asked to describe a technique of ulnar nerve blockade. It can be blocked at various sites.

- **At the brachial plexus:** see page 67.
- **At mid-humeral level:** a line is drawn between the upper border of pectoralis major in the axilla and the mid-point of the flexor crease of the elbow. A parallel line is drawn along the middle of the humerus about 1 cm medial to it and, via a single injection point at this mid-point, all three major nerves of the forearm can be reached with a 50-mm stimulator needle. The ulnar nerve is below and medial to the brachial artery and superficial to the triceps muscle.
- **At the elbow:** the nerve can be blocked with about 5 ml of solution injected 2–3 cm proximal to the ulnar groove. Injection into the actual fibrous sheath at the elbow is said to be associated with a high incidence of residual neuritis.
- **At the wrist:** the nerve lies beneath the tendon of flexor carpi ulnaris, proximal to the pisiform bone, and medial and deep to the ulnar artery. An approach from the ulnar side of the tendon (3–5 ml of solution injected at a depth of around 1.5 cm) is less likely to encounter the artery, and will also block the cutaneous branches.

Further direction the viva could take

You may be asked about the potential for ulnar nerve damage and its clinical signs.

- **Damage:** even when the arm is lying in the neutral position by the side of the anaesthetized patient it is vulnerable to pressure, either from arm supports or from the table. It has become routine practice to protect the elbow with padding, and it has also become routine to blame anaesthesia for any ulnar nerve damage. This is despite the fact that ulnar nerve palsy has been reported even when every precaution has been taken. The nerve is also vulnerable to stretch and so the upper arm should not be displaced posteriorly, nor abducted to greater than 90°.
- **Symptoms and signs of injury:** apart from the sensory loss and paraesthesia of which the patient will complain, ulnar nerve injury is associated with the classic *main en griffe*, or claw hand. This is because the extensors of the fingers and the long flexors of the hand act unopposed. If the nerve is transected at the elbow the clawing is less marked. This so-called 'ulnar paradox' occurs because the flexor digitorum profundus is also paralysed.

The radial nerve

Commentary

The radial nerve is another of the three main nerves of the upper limb, and comprises another well defined area of anatomy. Upper limb surgery and trauma is common, and radial nerve block is a reliable means of producing useful analgesia. The nerve has a relatively large number of terminal branches whose detailed anatomy is beyond the scope of this viva, but you will need to know the effects of blocking the radial nerve proximal to its main divisions. Again, you may find that the viva incorporates the other two main nerves of the upper limb.

The viva

You may be asked about the indications for radial nerve blockade.

- Its main use is in conjunction with other blocks to provide analgesia for procedures on the lateral, radial side of the hand and forearm. Digital nerve blocks provide reliable anaesthesia for finger surgery, but radial block can be used for procedures on the base of the thumb and, in combination with musculocutaneous block, to allow the creation of forearm arteriovenous fistulas for dialysis.

You will be asked about the anatomy of the radial nerve.

- The radial nerve arises from the brachial plexus. The posterior divisions from each of the three trunks form the posterior cord (described according to its relationship with the axillary artery), from which derives the radial nerve. Its fibres therefore originate from C_5, C_6, C_7, C_8 and T_1, and it is the largest branch of the brachial plexus.
- The radial nerve descends beneath the axillary artery and passes between the long and medial heads of the triceps muscle into the posterior compartment of the arm. It then passes obliquely behind the humerus where it lies in a shallow spiral groove.
- In the lower third of the humerus the radial nerve enters the anterior compartment of the upper arm, descending into the forearm between brachialis medially and brachioradialis laterally. At the lateral epicondyle of the humerus it divides into its terminal deep and superficial branches.
- It is motor in the upper arm to triceps, in the lower arm to brachialis, brachioradialis, and to the extensor muscles of the wrist and hand.
- The area of sensory innervation that is of particular anaesthetic relevance includes much of the dorsum of the hand and the radial side of the forearm. (The ulnar nerve supplies the skin over the distal phalanges, the fifth finger and medial side of the fourth finger, and over the fifth and fourth metacarpals.) The radial nerve also supplies cutaneous sensation to the posterior aspect of the forearm and to the skin over the dorsal base of the thumb. (The musculocutaneous nerve supplies much of the radial surface of the forearm.)

Direction the viva may take

You may be asked to describe a technique of radial nerve blockade. It can be blocked at various sites.

- **At the brachial plexus:** see page 67.
- **At mid-humeral level:** see page 72. Via the single injection point at this mid-point the nerve can be located below and medial to the brachial artery where it lies on the posterior surface of the humerus in the spiral groove.
- **At the elbow:** the nerve can be blocked as it traverses the anterior aspect of the lateral epicondyle of the humerus. The needle is inserted some 2 cm lateral to the biceps tendon and directed towards the bone. Up to 10 ml of solution can be injected in a fanwise direction as the needle is withdrawn. The musculocutaneous nerve can also be blocked at the elbow between the biceps and brachioradialis muscles.
- **At the wrist:** nerve block at the wrist is effectively a superficial field block of the terminal sensory branches. Local anaesthetic solution can be injected along the lateral border of the radial artery, extending dorsally to include the area delineated by the extensor tendons of the thumb.

Further direction the viva could take

You may be asked about the potential for radial nerve damage and its clinical signs.

- **Damage:** the radial nerve is subject to various types of injury and may be damaged by compression against the upper humerus, as in the so-called 'Saturday night' or 'crutch' palsy. The pressure exerted by an arterial tourniquet can also damage the nerve by the same mechanism. Its close relation to the humerus makes it vulnerable to damage in mid-humeral fractures, and the posterior interosseous branch may be traumatized in injuries to the head of the radius.
- **Symptoms and signs of injury:** overlap of innervation means that sensory loss and paraesthesia may be confined to a relatively small area on the dorsum of the hand. Otherwise, radial nerve injury is typically associated with wrist drop due to paralysis of the extensor muscles. If the damage to the nerve has occurred below the elbow then the functional preservation of extensor carpi radialis longus will minimize this effect.

The median nerve

Commentary

This is the third of the main nerves of the upper limb, and is another well defined area of anatomy. As with the questions on the ulnar and radial nerves, you will be expected to outline the anatomy and to discuss the relevant local anaesthetic blocks. The viva is likely to include questions on the other nerves of the upper limb.

The viva

You may be asked about the indications for median nerve blockade.

- Its main use is the provision of analgesia for procedures on the radial palm. The fingers and distal thumb can readily be anaesthetized using digital nerve blocks, but median nerve block is useful for procedures such as carpal tunnel release and palmar fasciectomy.

You will be asked about the anatomy of the median nerve.

- The median nerve arises from the brachial plexus. The anterior divisions of the upper and middle trunks form the lateral cord, from which derives the lateral head of the median nerve.
- The anterior division of the lower trunk continues as the medial cord, from which derives the medial head of the median nerve. Its fibres originate, therefore, from C_5, C_6, C_7, C_8 and T_1.
- The nerve passes into the arm lying lateral to the brachial artery which it then crosses to descend on its medial side to the antecubital fossa, where it is protected by the bicipital aponeurosis.
- It passes down into the forearm between the bellies of the deep and superficial flexors of the fingers (flexor digitorum profundus and superficialis) and at the wrist lies lateral to or just beneath the tendon of palmaris longus, and medial to flexor carpi radialis.
- It enters the hand beneath the flexor retinaculum before dividing into a leash of terminal branches.
- It is motor in the forearm to several of the superficial flexors (excluding flexor carpi ulnaris) and in the hand to muscles of the thenar eminence: abductor pollicis brevis, part of flexor pollicis brevis, and the opponens pollicis. Its anterior interosseous branch also supplies flexor pollicis longus, pronator quadratus and part of flexor digitorum profundus.
- The cutaneous innervation extends to the radial aspect of the palm, and the palmar surface of the radial 3½ digits, together with their dorsal tips as far as the first interphalangeal joint.

Direction the viva may take

You may be asked to describe a technique of median nerve blockade. It can be blocked at various sites.

- **At the brachial plexus:** see page 67.
- **At mid-humeral level:** see page 72. Via the single injection point at the mid-point, the nerve lies above the brachial artery with which it runs parallel.
- **At the elbow:** the nerve can be blocked immediately medial to the brachial artery as it crosses the intercondylar line. The needle is directed perpendicularly and should find the nerve within 1–2 cm.
- **At the wrist:** the nerve lies in the midline on the radial border of the palmaris longus tendon. The needle is directed perpendicularly some 2 cm proximal to the distal flexor crease of the wrist. The nerve is superficial and lies beneath the deep fascia at a depth of 1cm or less.

Further direction the viva could take

You may be asked about the potential for median nerve damage and its clinical signs.

- **Damage:** the median nerve is most vulnerable to trauma at the wrist, although it can be injured in supracondylar humeral fractures and following injury to the distal radius. The commonest lesion occurs as a result of compression of the nerve in the carpal tunnel.
- **Symptoms and signs of injury:** trauma at the wrist will paralyse the thenar muscles and cause significant sensory loss. More proximal injury leads to weak wrist flexion, loss of pronation, and loss of flexion of the thumb, index and middle finger. Atrophic changes and wasting of the thenar eminence flatten the contours of the hand.

The antecubital fossa

Commentary

In common with the femoral triangle, the anatomy of the antecubital fossa is straightforward, and it too lends itself readily to simple diagrams which are worth practising. Alternatively, you may find yourself automatically demonstrating on your own arm: this can be an effective technique which may make the anatomy easier to learn. Questioning may extend to practical clinical matters such as inadvertent intra-arterial injection, nerve blocks at the elbow and the insertion of long lines. Non-medical personnel who undergo training in venepuncture and cannulation are required to learn the detailed anatomy of this area, and so the FRCA examiners will expect at least as much.

The viva

You will be asked to describe the anatomy (Figure 2.9).

- The antecubital, or cubital, fossa is a triangular intermuscular depression on the anterior surface of the elbow joint.
- The base of the triangle is formed by the line which joins the medial and lateral epicondyles of the humerus.
- The lateral side of the triangle is formed by the medial edge of the brachioradialis muscle, while the medial side is formed by the lateral border of the pronator teres.
- The floor consists of the brachialis and supinator muscles.
- The roof (from above down) comprises skin, subcutaneous tissue and the deep fascia, which includes the bicipital aponeurosis.
- Within the fossa lie the tendon of the biceps muscle and the terminal part of the brachial artery, which lies in the centre of the fossa prior to its division into the radial and ulnar arteries opposite the neck of the radius. It also contains the associated veins and the median and radial nerves.

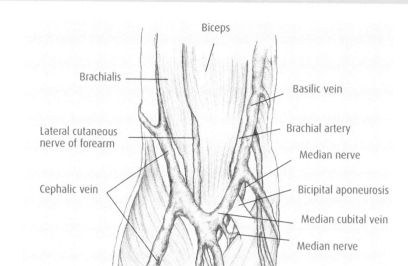

Fig. 2.9 The antecubital fossa.

- The anatomy of the superficial veins varies greatly, but that of a typical subject can be described as follows.
  - *Cephalic vein:* this drains the radial side of the forearm, and ascends over the lateral side of the fossa to lie in a groove along the lateral edge of the biceps. At the lower border of pectoralis major it moves deeper to lie between pectoralis major and deltoid before penetrating the clavipectoral fascia to join the axillary vein.
  - *Basilic vein:* this drains the ulnar side of the forearm and rises along the medial border of biceps to pierce the deep fascia in the middle upper arm before going on to form the axillary vein.
  - *Median cubital vein:* this originates from the cephalic vein distal to the lateral epicondyle, and then runs upwards and medially across the antecubital fossa to join the basilic vein above the elbow.

Direction the viva may take
You are likely to be asked about the clinical relevance of the anatomy.

- The antecubital fossa is the commonest site for venepuncture as well as being a site for venous cannulation. One potential hazard is inadvertent puncture or injection into the brachial artery. The danger of this happening is lessened by the presence of the bicipital aponeurosis, which is an extension of the medial lower border of the muscle and tendon of biceps. It passes downwards and medially to merge with the deep fascia at the origin of the forearm flexor muscles, separating as it does so the brachial artery from the median cubital vein. (This is the reason why historically it was known as the 'grâce à Dieu' fascia.)

- The lateral cutaneous nerve of the forearm crosses the fascia of the roof of the fossa and, although it lies deep to the cephalic vein, may still be vulnerable to damage from a needle or cannula.
- Long lines can be inserted via the antecubital veins, which offer a safer route to the central veins. Although cannulation at the elbow may be simple, the acute curve at the clavipectoral fascia may prevent a long venous catheter from gaining access to the central venous circulation. The length of the catheter precludes the rapid infusion of fluid.

Further direction the viva could take

You may be asked how you would recognize and manage inadvertent intra-arterial injection, and about nerve blocks at this site.

- Inadvertent intra-arterial injection is detailed on pages 79–80. An anomalous ulnar artery which lies superficially just below the median cubital vein is present in 2% of the population, and so it is not only accidental injection into the brachial artery of which anaesthetists must be aware.
- Nerve blocks at the elbow are described on pages 72, 74 and 75.

Arterial supply of the hand

Commentary

This is a straightforward area of anatomy. The topic is not large and so you may exhaust it quickly. The questioning may include topics such as the modified Allen test, the indications for direct intra-arterial blood pressure monitoring and problems associated with intra-arterial injection.

The viva

You may be asked about the indications for direct intra-arterial monitoring.

- **Indications:** intra-arterial monitoring gives beat-to-beat information about the blood pressure, which is particularly useful in patients with actual or potential cardiovascular instability. Many anaesthetists would also regard its use as mandatory whenever intravenous vasoactive drugs are used to manipulate the blood pressure. It is useful in patients in whom regular arterial blood gas analysis is indicated, and it is used routinely in the critically ill. It may also be indicated in patients in whom anatomical factors such as morbid obesity make it impossible to measure blood pressure by any other means.

This will lead on to a discussion of the modified Allen test for arterial patency.

- **Modified Allen test:** both the radial and ulnar arteries can be cannulated to allow direct intra-arterial measurement of blood pressure, but anaesthetists prefer reassurance that the circulation of the hand will not be jeopardized. The traditional method for assessing the adequacy of radial or ulnar arterial flow is the modified Allen test. After compression of both arteries at the wrist, the patient is asked to blanch the palm by clenching and then opening the hand. On releasing the compression of one or other of the arteries, depending on which is chosen as the site of cannulation, the palm should reperfuse, demonstrating thereby the adequacy of flow. Seven seconds or less is considered normal; longer than fifteen seconds is abnormal. Although the test continues to be used widely, it has a poor predictive value. Ischaemic complications have been reported following a normal Allen test and vice versa.

Direction the viva will take

You will be asked the basic anatomy of the arterial supply. The hand is supplied by the radial and ulnar arteries.

- **Radial artery:** in the distal forearm the radial artery lies between the flexor carpi radialis and brachioradialis. The tendons of these muscles comprise the landmarks between which the artery is palpated at the wrist.
  — Beyond the radial pulse the artery supplies a branch which contributes to the superficial palmar arch.
  — The main arterial branch continues over the scaphoid and beneath the extensor and abductor tendons of the thumb (extensor pollicis longus and brevis, and abductor pollicis longus), and passes between the first and second metacarpal bones to contribute to the deep palmar arch.
- **Ulnar artery:** in the distal forearm the ulnar artery lies superficially between the tendons of flexor carpi ulnaris and flexor digitorum superficialis.
  — It crosses beneath the flexor retinaculum to complete the superficial palmar arch. The ulnar arterial component is much more significant than the radial.
  — The deep branch enters the palm where it forms an anastomosis with the radial artery to complete the deep palmar arch.
  — The superficial palmar arch then gives off further branches including dorsal metacarpal and dorsal digital arteries. The deep palmar arch similarly branches, to form palmar metacarpal and palmar digital arteries.

Further direction the viva could take

You may be asked about inadvertent intra-arterial injection. Further discussion of direct arterial pressure measurement will only feature if you have exhausted the topic.

- **Intra-arterial injection:** this may occur when an intra-arterial catheter is mistaken for a venous cannula. Drugs that have been so injected include phenytoin, benzodiazepines, anaesthetic induction agents and antibiotics. In the awake patient severe pain in the hand is a cardinal feature. In the anaesthetized or sedated patient there may be ischaemic colour changes in the distal limb which, because of arterial spasm, may be pale, mottled or cyanosed. Thrombosis may follow. The degree of damage depends on the substance injected. Thiopental causes substantial damage because at body pH it precipitates into crystals which occlude small arterial vessels and provoke intense vasospasm mediated via local noradrenaline release. In contrast, propofol seems relatively innocuous. Any such injection should be treated as for the worst-case scenario, because clinical experience of intra-arterial injection of many drugs is limited.

- **Management:** after the injection of heparin 500–1000 units to reduce the risk of thrombosis, warm NaCl 0.9% can be given to dilute the substance. Arterial spasm can be treated with papaverine 40–80 mg, prostacyclin at a rate of $1\,\mu g\,min^{-1}$, tolazoline (which is a noradrenaline antagonist) and phenoxybenzamine (which is an α_1-antagonist). Sound though the recommendation may be, these drugs might well not be immediately available, and this advice may be impractical. Dexamethasone 8 mg given immediately may reduce arterial oedema. Perfusion can be enhanced by sympatholysis, either by a stellate ganglion block (which is quick to perform) or via a brachial plexus block using a catheter technique to provide analgesia and a continuous block. Maintenance anticoagulation is recommended for up to 14 days, and hyperbaric oxygen has also been suggested as a means of minimizing final ischaemic damage.
- **Intra-arterial monitoring:** see page 319.

Anatomy relevant to subarachnoid (spinal) anaesthesia

Commentary
Every candidate for this exam will have performed spinal anaesthesia. It is the default technique for obstetric anaesthesia and is regaining popularity elsewhere. Along with epidural analgesia it is a central area of anaesthetic practice. Ignorance of its main aspects can potentially put patients at grave harm, and so you will be expected to demonstrate that your knowledge is sound.

The viva
You may be asked first to describe the basic anatomy. Just as with the epidural space this is an area of such obvious clinical importance that the examiner will not feel the need to introduce it in any other way.

- The subarachnoid space is defined by its relation to the arachnoid mater, which is one of the three meningeal layers.
- **Meningeal layers:** there is continuity between the cranial and spinal meninges. The spinal subarachnoid space communicates freely with the ventricular system of the brain.

- **Dura mater:** this is the strongest of the meningeal coverings and consists of fibroelastic connective tissue. The cranial dura has two layers: an outer endosteal layer which lines the skull, and a meningeal layer which invests the brain. These two layers are closely applied, except where they separate to accommodate the large venous sinuses. At the spinal level, the endosteal layer continues down the vertebral canal as a lining of periosteum. The inner layer continues downwards as the spinal dura. The width of the dura varies with the spinal level: in the lumbar region it is between 0.3 and 0.5 mm thick, and it becomes progressively thicker towards the cervical region where it can be three times as large. The spinal dura also provides a cuff for nerve roots, which thins as each nerve approaches the intervertebral foramen. In some subjects this cuff is a more substantial structure, containing CSF which does not communicate with intrathecal CSF. These structures are known as Tarlov's cysts and may (rarely) explain the apparently impeccable spinal which then completely fails to work.
- **Arachnoid mater:** this is a fine non-vascular membrane, which is closely applied to the dura. The subdural space between these two layers is a potential capillary space, containing a small amount of lubricant serous fluid. It is widest in the cervical region, and laterally, adjacent to the nerve roots themselves.
- **Pia mater:** this is a fine vascular membrane which invests the spinal cord. Its lateral projections form the denticulate ligament, which attaches to the dura and support the cord. The filum terminale is the terminal extension of the pia mater which runs from the end of the spinal cord to attach to coccygeal periosteum. It is not purely vestigial: it stabilizes and anchors the cord within the CSF, and tethers the dura within the lower part of the epidural space. The filum contains neither neural tissue nor CSF.
- **Subarachnoid space:** this contains CSF, and the anterior and posterior roots of the 31 pairs of spinal nerves. The subarachnoid space extends laterally as far as the dorsal root ganglion.
- **CSF:** this is an ultrafiltrate of plasma, which is found in the spinal and cranial subarachnoid spaces and within the cerebral ventricles. It is formed by secretion and ultrafiltration from the choroid arterial plexus in the lateral third ventricles and the fourth ventricle. Its rate of production is constant at around $0.4 \, ml \, min^{-1}$ (575 ml per day). Its specific gravity at body temperature ranges from 1.003 to 1.009 (mean 1.006). The total volume in adults is between 120 and 150 ml, 25–35 ml of which is found in the spinal subarachnoid space and most of which is distal to the cord in the area of the cauda equina. The PCO_2 is higher than that of blood, and the pH of CSF is slightly below arterial pH at 7.32. Electrolyte concentrations are similar (but not identical) to plasma. The protein concentration is less, but levels are not uniform and demonstrate a gradient between the ventricles, where the concentration is low, and the lumbar region where they are highest. The mean protein concentration is $23–28 \, mg \, dl^{-1}$.
- The adult spine has a number of natural curves, the high points of which (in the supine position) are the fifth cervical (C_5) and the second or third lumbar ($L_{2/3}$) vertebrae, and the low points of which are the fifth and sixth thoracic ($T_{5/6}$) and the second sacral (S_2) vertebrae. This has relevance for the spread of intrathecal hyperbaric solutions.

Direction the viva may take

You may be asked what surface landmarks govern your approach to a particular vertebral level.

- The spinal cord in the adult ends at the level of the intervertebral disc at L_1/L_2. There is some variation and in up to 10% of subjects the cord may end as high as T_{12}/L_1 or as low as L_2/L_3. (In the neonate the cord ends at the lower border of L_3.) It is important to identify the vertebral level as accurately as you are able.
- A line drawn between the highest points of the iliac crests (the intercristal or Touffier's line) passes across either the spinous process of L_4 or the L_4/L_5 interspace. (Some textbooks say L_3/L_4.) This is the technique that is most commonly used by anaesthetists. It can be difficult to identify this point clinically, which is why neurosurgeons operating on the back identify the level radiologically prior to operation. Anaesthetists must be aware of this potential for inaccuracy, because a spinal needle which is advanced too high or without finesse risks penetrating the conus medullaris with permanent neurological deficit.
- The lowest rib (which is palpable only in very thin subjects) is at the level of T_{12}.
- The first spinous process which is clearly palpable is C_7, which is the vertebra prominens (although the spinous process of T_1 below it is actually more prominent still).
- The inferior angle of the scapula in the neutral position is at the level of T_7 or T_8.

Further direction the viva could take

There are various ways in which a viva on spinal anaesthesia may develop. You may be asked about complications, but this is relatively straightforward, and so it is more likely that you will be asked the factors that influence intrathecal spread.

- **Drug dose:** the prime determinant of spread is the mass of drug. The greater the amount of drug, the higher and more prolonged the block. The volume is of less importance: it has been demonstrated in obstetric anaesthesia, for example, that the injection of bupivacaine 15 mg in 15 ml (0.1%) will achieve a block of similar height to that obtained after injection of bupivacaine 15 mg in 3 ml (0.5%).
- **Level of injection:** in the supine patient with a normal spine the maximum height of the lumbar lordosis is at L_2/L_3. Less local anaesthetic will move rostrally if the injection is made below that level. In practice the final block height is similar but it may take longer to achieve.
- **Baricity of drug:** this is another important determinant. Plain solutions of local anaesthetic are approximately isobaric relative to CSF at room temperature (mean CSF specific density is 1.006). At body temperature they become slightly hypobaric. Hyperbaric ('heavy') solutions are made so by the addition of glucose. 'Heavy' bupivacaine contains glucose 8% (which is much more than the 0.8% which would render the solution hyperbaric). In the supine patient with a normal spine, hyperbaric solutions tend to pool in the thoracic kyphosis at $T_{5/6}$, and produce blocks which are generally higher but which are claimed to be more predictable than those produced by isobaric solutions. Solutions which pool in the lumbosacral area may have a relatively enhanced effect because the nerves of the cauda equina have a

large surface area and only a thin layer of pia mater. This appears to increase their sensitivity to local anaesthetic.

- **Patient position:** this is linked to baricity. If the patient is in the decubitus position, the curves of the spine have no influence. Trendelenberg positioning will clearly increase the rostral spread of a hyperbaric solution.
- **Patient height:** there may be reduced cephalad spread in taller subjects: the relationship is not reliable enough to allow any prediction.
- **Patient age:** there may be increased cephalad spread with advancing age, although again the block height cannot reliably be predicted.
- **Pregnancy:** term pregnancy is said to be associated with greater block height, which is made higher still with multiple pregnancy. The mechanism may relate to the relatively smaller volume of the dural sheath because of encroachment in the epidural space by the engorged venous plexus.
- **Speed and direction of injection:** forceful injection shortens the onset time but does not usually influence the final height of block. There are some data to suggest that if the side hole of a pencil point needle is directed rostrally, then block height may be increased.
- **Barbotage, weight of patient, gender of patient, adjuvant drugs, vasoconstrictors:** none of these factors has any significant effect on block height.

The extradural (epidural) space

Commentary

This is another key subject for anaesthetists. In many hospitals the numbers of epidurals that are now inserted for surgical analgesia matches those that are given to relieve the pain of labour. Detailed knowledge will be expected: you will be required to demonstrate a good three-dimensional grasp of the anatomy as well as being aware of all the material complications and their management.

The viva

You may be asked first to describe the relevant anatomy.

- The extradural (epidural) space is the area surrounding the dural sheath as it lies within the vertebral canal.
- It extends from the foramen magnum superiorly (where the dura is fused to the skull) to the sacral hiatus inferiorly. (This means that extradural local anaesthetic cannot under normal circumstances spread intracranially. So, in contrast to a 'total spinal', a patient with a high cervical block may stop breathing but will not be unconscious. There may be some intracranial diffusion of local anaesthetic, but this is unlikely to be significant.)
- The space is traversed by the dural sheath, whose thickness in the lumbar region is about 0.3–0.5 mm, and which comprises the membranes of the dura and arachnoid

maters, the subarachnoid space containing CSF, the spinal nerves of the cauda equina and the filum terminale. The filum terminale is an extension of the pia mater, which runs from the conus medullaris to the coccyx, effectively acting to stabilize the cord. It contains neither neural tissue nor CSF.

- Anteriorly, the epidural space is bounded by the bodies of the vertebrae and by the intervertebral discs, over which lies the posterior longitudinal ligament. The anterior dura mater and the posterior longitudinal ligament are so closely apposed that effectively there is no anterior space.
- Laterally, the epidural space is bounded by the pedicles and the intervertebral foramina.
- Posteriorly, it is bounded by the laminae of the neural arches.
- **Ligamenta flava:** these are not continuous. At each level there are two ligaments which meet in the midline and which connect the laminae of adjacent vertebrae. Each ligament extends from the lower part of the anterior surface of the lamina above to the posterior surface of, and upper margin of, the lamina below. Their fibres run in a perpendicular direction, but when viewed in the sagittal plane the ligaments are triangular in shape, with the apex of the triangle formed at the upper lamina. This explains why the ligamenta flava in different (or even the same) patients can appear to vary in thickness. The ligaments contain yellow elastic connective tissue: hence the name ('flavus' = 'yellow' in Latin).
- At the level of a typical lumbar vertebra, for example L_3, the space contains the spinal nerves, each of which is invested with a cuff of dura, with loosely packed fat, areolar connective tissue, lymphatics and blood vessels. These vessels include the rich valveless vertebral venous plexus of Batson. (The lack of valves means that they will engorge as intra-abdominal pressure increases, for example during a contraction in labour.)
- The depth of the posterior epidural space (between the ligamenta flava and the dura) varies with the vertebral level. In the mid-cervical region it is only 1.0–1.5 mm wide, and at T_6 it is deeper, at around 2.5–3.0 mm. The greatest depth is at the L_2 interspace in men, in whom this is 5.0–6.0 mm.

Direction the viva may take

You may be asked to discuss the complications of epidural anaesthesia. The list is long, and so once you have volunteered as many as you can recall, it is probable that the viva will concentrate on the recognition and management of only one or two.

Complications associated with the procedure

- These include inadvertent dural puncture and subsequent post-dural puncture headache (PDPH) (incidence of 0.5%); failure (1%); unilateral or patchy block (5–10%); inadvertent subdural block (0.1%); intravascular injection; retention of a fragment of needle or catheter; epidural haematoma. The risk of permanent neurological sequelae is very small. The incidence is quoted at 1 in 10 000 epidurals, but many of these complications are relatively minor, comprising, for example, little more than a patch of residual numbness. There is no evidence that routine epidurals lead to chronic back pain.

Complications associated with drugs that are injected

- These include hypotension owing to sympathetic block; a total spinal or high spinal block; evidence of systemic toxicity of local anaesthetic; urinary retention; pruritus, nausea and vomiting (usually associated with extradural opiate); respiratory depression. There are many case reports of accidental injection of the wrong solution. Many substances have been administered in this way, including various antibiotics, solutions of total parenteral nutrition (which provided good quality analgesia) and thiopental. The influence of obstetric epidurals on instrumental and operative delivery rates remains disputed.

Further direction the viva could take

You may be asked about your diagnosis and management of some of the more common or more complex complications.

PDPH

- **Diagnosis:** the incidence of inadvertent dural puncture should not exceed 0.5%, and the incidence is usually quoted at between 0.5% and 1.0%. The incidence of PDPH is highest in obstetric patients, over 80% of whom will develop symptoms. These are probably caused by traction on intracranial pain-sensitive structures such as the tentorium and blood vessels. The headache results from the failure of the choroid plexus to produce sufficient CSF to compensate for the loss through the breach in the dura. The onset is variable, with the headache commonly starting after about 12–24 hours. It can occur earlier or later. The headache may be frontal or occipital rather than global, but typically it is postural and relieved by recumbency or abdominal pressure. It may also be associated with photophobia, visual disturbance, neck and shoulder stiffness, and tinnitus. If the patient also complains of anorexia, nausea and vomiting, this is an indication that there is significant sagging of intracranial contents, with pressure on the brain stem at the foramen magnum. The patient may feel systemically unwell. The presentation is not always typical.
- **Management of severe PDPH:** assuming the failure of initial conservative treatment, advising recumbence when headache supervenes and simple analgesia, management may move on to other treatments. Cerebral vasoconstrictors such as caffeine and sumatriptan may improve symptoms, but they will not address the cause. Patients are instructed frequently to overhydrate. This has no influence on CSF production. The only agents which may increase it are corticosteroids. ACTH analogues such as tetracosactrin (Synacthen) are used by some anaesthetists, but their benefits are anecdotal. The only technique that is likely to provide immediate relief is an extradural blood patch (EBP). This will abolish symptoms in almost all patients but in at least 30% of mothers the procedure will need to be repeated. EBP has been associated with the development of chronic low back pain, and this risk must be weighed against those of persistent long-term headache or of neurological disaster (such as subdural haemorrhage) which has been reported in PDPH left neglected.

Inadvertent subdural block

- A catheter or needle may deposit solution in the subdural space between the dura and arachnoid mater. Radiologists maintain that during myelography there is a 1% incidence of subdural injection. It is much less commonly diagnosed in clinical anaesthesia. Some authorities cite an incidence of 1 in 1000.
- Subdural block is often patchy; it may be extensive and unilateral, may extend very high (the subdural space extends into the cranium), and it often spares the sacral roots. The dura and arachnoid are more densely adherent to each other anteriorly, and so there may be a relative sparing of motor fibres. Sympathetic block may be minimal and analgesia may be delayed. Horner's syndrome may be apparent.
- The use of a multi-holed catheter may further confuse the picture, because it is theoretically possible for the catheter to lie partly within the epidural and partly within the subdural space. Slow injection will favour emergence of the solution from the proximal epidural holes: more vigorous injection will favour dispersal through the distal subdural hole.

High block or total spinal

- Examiners may address a question about total spinal anaesthesia by asking you to describe what happens as the block ascends. A high block or developing total spinal is characterized by the development of paraesthesia and weakness of the upper limbs, respiratory embarrassment owing to intercostal paralysis, a weak voice and cough, and sensory loss over the skin of the neck and eventually the jaw. If the block is a total spinal then apnoea and unconsciousness will supervene. Pupils dilate. It is always said that a high sympathetic block will lead to hypotension and bradycardia because of local anaesthetic effects on the cardiac accelerator fibres (T_1–T_4). In practice, the cardiovascular changes are by no means always so predictable. High blocks regress quickly, whereas it might be some hours before a total spinal has worn off to the point at which comfortable respiration will be possible. Until this happens, anaesthesia must be maintained to prevent awareness.

The sacrum

Commentary

Caudal (sacral extradural) anaesthesia is a popular technique, particularly in children, in whom it can provide analgesia similar to that provided by a low lumbar epidural. In contrast to other neuraxial blocks it requires no equipment other than a needle, syringe and/or intravenous cannula, and is simple to perform. This is a core area of anatomy applied to anaesthetic practice.

The viva

You will be asked to describe the basic anatomy. (You will not be asked the origin of the name, but its etymological origin does add a certain poetry to the bare anatomical facts.)

- The sacrum was believed by the ancients to be the site of the soul, the bone which was the last to decompose, and thus the one around which the new body would form. Hence it was called the 'sacred bone'.
- It is a triangular-shaped bone that articulates superiorly with the fifth lumbar vertebra, inferiorly with the coccyx and laterally with the ilia.
- The dorsal roof comprises the fused laminae of the five sacral vertebrae and is convex dorsally (the curve is variable between sexes and races).
- In the midline there is a median crest, which represents the sacral spinous processes.
- Lateral to this is the intermediate sacral crest with a row of four tubercles, which represent the articular processes. The S_5 processes are remnants only and form the cornua, which are the main landmarks for identifying the sacral hiatus.
- At S_5 this failure of development of the spinous processes and laminae results in a hiatus in the roof of the canal. It is this sacral hiatus which allows access to the extradural space. It is covered by the sacrococcygeal membrane.
- Along the lateral border are anterior and posterior foramina which are the sacral equivalent of intervertebral foramina of higher levels, and through which the sacral nerve roots pass.
- In addition to the dura superiorly, the canal contains areolar connective tissue, fat, the sacral nerves, lymphatics, the filum terminale (which is an extension of the pia mater originating from the conus medullaris at the end of the spinal cord and which extends to the coccyx), and a rich venous plexus.

Direction the viva may take

You may be asked how you would perform a caudal block.

- Access to the canal is via the sacral hiatus at the level of the fifth sacral vertebra through the sacrococcygeal membrane. In up to 7% of subjects, fusion has taken place and so access is impossible. (Some authorities believe this to be an overestimate.)
- **Identification:** there are several ways of identifying the hiatus
  — The sacral hiatus is at the apex of an equilateral triangle completed by the posterior superior iliac spines.
  — If the tip of the index finger palpates the coccyx, the mid-point of the middle interphalangeal joint of the finger identifies the hiatus (in an 'average' adult).
  — With the hips flexed at 90°, a line extended along the mid-point of the thigh will end at the hiatus.
  — Palpation of the midline sacral crest caudally until the cornua are identified is useful only in lean subjects in whom the anatomy is not obscured by a sacral fat pad.
- **Drug doses:** in adults, a typical dose would be levobupivacaine 0.5% × 20 ml. In children, various formulae have been elaborated to achieve blocks of adequate height. A commonly used regimen is that described by Armitage in 1979: 0.5 ml kg^{-1} of (levo)bupivacaine 0.25% for sacral block (circumcision, hypospadias,

Armitage EN. (1979). Caudal block in children. *Anaesthesia*, **34**, 396.

anal procedures), $1.0\,\mathrm{ml\,kg^{-1}}$ for low thoracic block (for inguinal herniotomy) and $1.25\,\mathrm{ml\,kg^{-1}}$ for higher thoracic block up to T_8 (for orchidopexy). The addition of clonidine $2.0\,\mu\mathrm{g\,kg^{-1}}$ will double the duration of effective analgesia, while ketamine $0.5\,\mathrm{mg\,kg^{-1}}$ (preservative-free) will increase it by four times.

- The 'whoosh' and 'swoosh' tests have been described as methods of verifying accurate needle placement. In the 'whoosh' test a small volume of air (2 ml) is injected while the anaesthetist listens with a stethoscope over the lumbar spine. Some first deposit a small volume of fluid in the space; correct needle placement is confirmed by definite crepitus. The injection of air into the extradural space has well recognized disadvantages: the subsequent block may be patchy, and venous air embolism has been reported. The 'swoosh' test is similar in principle, except that auscultation is performed as the local anaesthetic itself is being injected.

Further direction the viva could take

You may then be asked about differences between children and adults, both in the performance of the blocks and in the way that they behave.

- **Anatomical differences:** the dura mater usually ends at the level of S_2 in adults (although it can descend to within about 5 cm of the hiatus in some subjects). At birth the dura is as low as S_4, but by around 2 years of age it ascends to adult levels.
- The sacral hiatus is easier to locate in children because it is not overlain by the sacral fat pad that later develops in adults.
- **Physiological differences:** the spread of solution in the sacral extradural space is influenced in adults by total volume, speed of injection and posture (one study has reported that higher levels are reached if the patient is 15° head up).
- There is good correlation in children between spread of a given dose and age. There is poor correlation between spread and weight and/or height.
- The sacral extradural space in children offers lower resistance to longitudinal spread than the adult. Epidural fat in children has a loose and wide-meshed texture, whereas in adults it becomes more densely packed and fibrous. There is less fibrous connective tissue in the sacral epidural space than in adults and this combination of factors means that local anaesthetic spread is greater.
- In children it is possible to direct a 20G 51-mm cannula rostrally to escape the sacral space altogether and allow what is in effect a lower lumbar epidural block. Generous volumes can be employed, therefore, if a high block is required. High blocks are much more difficult to achieve in adults. Hypodermic needles should not be used to perform caudal blocks in children; a cannula sized 20G or smaller should be used.
- Complications such as intrathecal injection are more likely in children less than 2 years of age. Otherwise, the incidence both of intrathecal and intravascular injection does not differ from that seen in adults.
- **Sympathetic effects:** children up to and beyond the age of 6 years show cardiovascular stability in the face of blocks that would cause sympathetic blockade and hypotension in adults. This is probably due to delay in the maturation of the autonomic nervous system.

You may also at any stage be asked about complications of the block.

- **Complications:** these include failure; intravascular injection (false negative aspiration may occur in 10% or more of cases, as negative pressure collapses the vein); intraosseous injection in young children; bowel perforation; dural and subdural puncture (which is characterized by an extensive, patchy block of slow onset). In obstetric practice the fetal head is vulnerable to an inaccurately placed needle. There are also the potential complications associated with the particular drugs injected (local anaesthetics, opiates, clonidine, ketamine).

The femoral triangle

Commentary
The anatomy of the femoral triangle is straightforward. It lends itself readily to simple diagrams: the first being the triangle itself, the second a transverse view to demonstrate that you realize that the femoral nerve lies in a fascial compartment quite separate from the femoral sheath. The question may then move on to the structures of significance to the anaesthetist, namely the femoral nerve, the femoral vein and the femoral artery. There is not a large amount of detail to cover.

The viva
You may be asked about the structures within the triangle that are of relevance to anaesthetists.

- **Femoral vein:** this is useful for central venous access (if other sites are unsuitable) and for siting large-bore cannulae for haemodiafiltration. It is the central vein of choice in infants and young children. It is also the site of access for insertion of vena caval filters. Access to the femoral vein is not always easy: it is commonly overlaid by the superficial femoral artery and its anatomy can be variable. The route is used commonly in children but is more of a last resort in adults in whom the subclavian veins are usually a better alternative.
- **Femoral artery:** this is used for arterial sampling and monitoring (again if other sites are unsuitable). The artery also provides access for angiography and for the insertion of intra-aortic balloon pump catheters.
- **Femoral nerve:** this can readily be blocked in this site.

You will then be asked to describe the anatomy (Figure 2.10).

- The triangle is bounded superiorly by the inguinal ligament (which curves from the anterior superior iliac spine to the pubic tubercle).
- Its lateral border is formed by the sartorius. (This is 'the tailor's muscle' which runs across the thigh from its origin at the anterior superior iliac spine to the medial side of the upper tibia, and is the longest muscle in the body.)

- Its medial border is formed by the adductor longus muscle (whose insertion is at the superior ramus of the pubis and which has a linear attachment to the linea aspera on the posterior aspect of the femur).
- Its roof is formed by areolar tissue, fascia lata, subcutaneous tissue and skin.
- Its floor is a trough comprised of the iliacus, psoas and pectineus muscles.
- Within the triangle lie the femoral canal, containing lymphatics, and immediately lateral to it, the femoral sheath, containing the femoral vein (medial) and femoral artery (lateral).
- Outside the femoral sheath and lying lateral to it is the femoral nerve. The nerve is invested in the fascia of the iliacus muscle (fascia iliaca), which separates it from the femoral sheath. Above this is the fascia of the tensor fascia lata muscle. The distance by which it is separated is variable. It may bear a close relation to the pulsation of the femoral artery or may be 1–2 cm or more lateral to it. It can also be separated from the femoral sheath by a small part of the psoas muscle.

Direction the viva may take

You may then be asked about the indications for, and a technique of, femoral nerve block.

- **Indications:** these include analgesia for fractured shaft of femur, perioperative analgesia for knee surgery and perioperative analgesia for hip surgery (usually as part of a '3-in-1' block). **Technique:** see page 92.

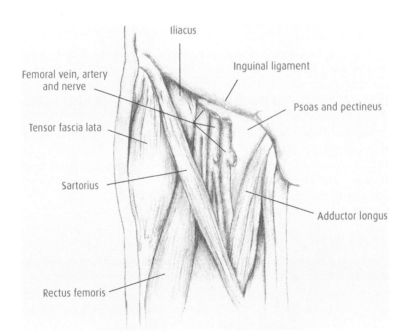

Fig. 2.10 The femoral triangle.

The femoral nerve

Commentary

The applied anatomy of the femoral nerve is not straightforward because it can be variable. Peripheral femoral nerve block is popular and useful, and so this is an important area of anatomical information. Take heart from the fact that this popularity is relatively recent, and so, unless your examiners have an interest in anaesthesia for orthopaedic surgery, their experience of this block may be less than yours.

The viva

You will be asked first to describe the anatomy.

- The femoral nerve originates from the anterior primary rami of L_2, L_3 and L_4 and enters the anterior thigh beneath the inguinal ligament (which runs from the anterior superior iliac spine to the pubic tubercle).
- The femoral sheath is formed from an extension of the extraperitoneal fascia and contains the femoral vein (medially) and artery (laterally). It does not contain the femoral nerve.
- The nerve is invested in the fascia of the iliacus muscle (fascia iliaca), which separates it from the femoral sheath. Above this is the fascia lata (see Figure 2.11).
- The distance by which it is separated from the vessel is variable. It may bear a close relation to the pulsation of the femoral artery or may be 1–2 cm or even more lateral to it. It can be separated from the femoral sheath by a part of the psoas muscle, and can also lie posterior to the artery.

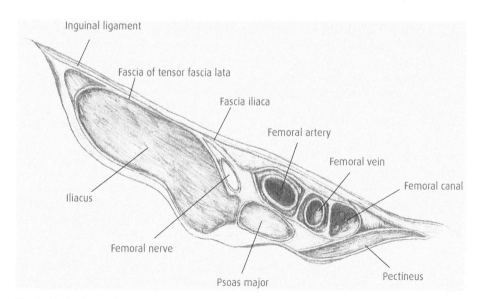

Fig. 2.11 The femoral nerve.

- The nerve usually starts to divide into its terminal branches at the base of the femoral triangle. In some subjects this division can start above the inguinal ligament.
- It divides into a leash of nerves which supply the muscles of the thigh. One of the main divisions continues as the saphenous nerve, which passes medially across the knee to provide sensory innervation as far as the medial aspect of the ankle and rear foot.

Direction the viva may take

The second part of the question is likely to be about femoral nerve, 3-in-1 and fascia iliaca blocks. It may touch briefly on the use of peripheral nerve stimulators (page 340).

- It is common for anaesthetists to assume that it is straightforward to perform a femoral nerve block and that the 3-in-1 block provides useful analgesia for hip surgery. Neither is necessarily true: the anatomy of the femoral nerve is variable and the benefits of '3-in-1' block are inconsistent.
- **Supply:** the nerve supplies the shaft of the femur, the muscles and skin of the anterior thigh as far as the knee, and via the saphenous nerve, the medial side of the lower leg as far as an area surrounding the medial malleolus.
- **Indications:** these include the provision of analgesia for fractured shaft of femur (which is usually very effective, particularly if an indwelling catheter technique is used), perioperative analgesia for knee surgery, and perioperative analgesia for hip surgery (usually as part of a 3-in-1 block).
- **3-in-1 block:** this describes a single injection, which aims to block the **femoral** nerve, the **obturator** nerve and the **lateral cutaneous** nerve of the thigh. A larger volume of local anaesthetic is used, and during injection firm distal pressure is applied. In theory this spreads the local anaesthetic rostrally back up into the psoas compartment so that all three nerves are blocked. The obturator nerve supplies the adductor muscles of the hip, part of the hip joint, skin on the medial side of the thigh, and part of the knee joint. The lateral cutaneous nerve supplies skin over the anterolateral thigh as far as the knee, and the over the lateral thigh from the greater trochanter down to the level of the mid-thigh. These nerves can also be blocked within the psoas compartment itself (page 65).
- **Efficacy:** 3-in-1 block can be effective for cannulated hip screws and sometimes for dynamic hip screws, but, as its anatomy demonstrates, in many cases it will not provide reliable analgesia for cutaneous sensation above the level of the greater trochanter, which is the site of incision for much hip surgery. It has been described, perhaps unfairly, as 'a nerve block in search of an operation'.
- **Fascia iliaca block:** this is an alternative to the standard 3-in-1 block, but which also blocks the femoral, lateral cutaneous and obturator nerves. Local anaesthetic is injected behind the fascia iliaca at the junction of the lateral with the two medial thirds of the inguinal ligament, and is directed upwards by the application of distal pressure. A short-bevelled needle allows identification of the two fascial layers (producing 'clicks' as it passes through tensor fascia lata and fascia iliaca), and it is not necessary to seek a motor response using a nerve stimulator. The fascial layers of the iliacus muscle form a potential space in which are found the three nerves. Some studies have claimed that fascia iliaca block provides better analgesia than either femoral or 3-in-1 blocks, but, given the anatomy it is hard to see why this should be so. In essence, it is a different mode of detection rather than a different nerve block.

- **Technique of femoral and 3-in-1 nerve block:** the success of these blocks is increased substantially by the use of a nerve stimulator. A plexus or block needle is inserted at an angle of about 45° and directed rostrally just below the inguinal ligament and lateral to the pulsation of the femoral artery. Movement of the patella (quadriceps femoris) is the best indicator of correct placement (at around 0.5 mA). The mass of drug injected will depend on whether or not other nerves, such as the sciatic and obturator, are being blocked at the same time, but the general dose range is 15–20 ml of 0.5% levobupivacaine for a femoral nerve block, and 30 ml or more for a 3-in-1 block.

The sciatic nerve

Commentary

The sciatic nerve is the largest peripheral nerve in the body and it is accessible from a number of sites. Sciatic nerve block provides good analgesia for much lower limb surgery, and the variety of possible approaches provides an appropriate test of applied anatomy. As always with questions which include practical procedures, it will help the credibility of your answer if you can convince the examiner that you have done some of these blocks. You will not, however, be expected to be familiar with every single approach.

The viva

As an introduction to the topic you may be asked about the indications for sciatic nerve block.

- Sciatic nerve block alone will provide reliable analgesia for surgical procedures which involve the forefoot, the sole of the foot, and the lateral side of the foot and ankle. In conjunction with femoral and obturator nerve block, it provides good analgesia for major knee surgery (although some orthopaedic surgeons dislike it because the temporary loss of proprioception can delay early mobilization).

Alternatively, you might be asked in what situations the sciatic nerve is vulnerable.

- Sciatic nerve irritation can result from lumbar disc prolapse, leading to classic symptoms of sciatica in the distribution of the root that is affected. Impingement of the nerve can also occur in the pelvis where it crosses beneath or, in 15% of subjects, through the piriformis muscle. (The existence of the 'piriformis syndrome' remains controversial.) The nerve can be damaged by direct trauma, including surgical trauma, as well as by ill-directed intramuscular injections in the buttock. One of its peripheral branches, the common peroneal nerve, is particularly vulnerable as it winds round the fibular head.

You will then be asked to describe the anatomy.

- The sciatic nerve arises from the sacral plexus, which is formed by the union of the L_4, L_5, S_1, S_2 and S_3 nerve roots, and which lies separated from the anterior sacrum by the piriformis muscle.

- The nerve, which is the largest in the body, is about 2 cm in diameter as it exits the pelvis posteriorly via the greater sciatic notch.
- It continues its descent into the thigh between the ischial tuberosity and the greater trochanter, and then lies behind the femur before dividing in the popliteal fossa into the common peroneal and the posterior tibial nerves.
- The sciatic nerve provides a sensory supply to much of the lower leg via its main terminal branches (the tibial and common peroneal).
- It supplies the knee joint (via articular branches) and almost all of the structures below the knee.
- It does not supply a variable, but extensive, cutaneous area over the medial side of the knee, lower leg and ankle, and medial side of the foot around the medial malleolus. This area is supplied by the saphenous nerve (from the femoral).

Direction the viva may take

You may be asked to describe one method of blocking the sciatic nerve.

- **Posterior approach**
  — the patient lies in the supine position with the upper leg flexed to 90° at the hip and knee.
  — A line is drawn from the greater trochanter to the ischial tuberosity. The nerve can be located just medial to the mid-point of this line at a depth of around 6 cm. The depth clearly varies with the size of the patient.
  — The needle is inserted at right angles to the skin, attached to a nerve stimulator. A twitch in the lower limb (usually dorsiflexion of the foot) elicited at about 0.5 mA is a sign of accurate placement, and 20 ml levobupivacaine 0.5% is injected.
  — The stimulator technique and drug dose apply to the other proximal approaches to the sciatic nerve.
- **Posterior (classic approach of Labat)**
  — the patient lies in the decubitus position with the upper leg flexed to 90° at hip and knee.
  — A line is drawn from the greater trochanter to the posterior superior iliac spine. From the mid-point of this line a perpendicular is dropped 3–5 cm.
  — The needle is inserted vertically to the skin and the nerve is sought at around 6–8 cm. Alternatively, a line can be drawn from the greater trochanter to the sacral hiatus and the injection made at its mid-point.
- **Anterior approach**
  — The nerve emerges from the greater sciatic foramen and lies between the ischial tuberosity and the greater trochanter of the femur. Before it passes down behind the bone it is accessible medial to the femur and just below the lesser trochanter.
  — The patient lies supine and a line is drawn from the anterior superior iliac spine to the pubic tubercle. A line parallel to it is drawn from the greater trochanter. At the junction of the medial third and lateral two-thirds of the upper line, a perpendicular is dropped to meet the lower.
  — At this junction, a long (150-mm) needle is inserted vertical to the skin until it contacts the medial shaft of femur. It is then redirected medially to slide off the

femur before advancing another 5 cm or so to encounter the nerve in the region of the lesser trochanter.
— It is worth noting that in around 15% of patients the sciatic nerve lies immediately posterior to the femur at this point and so is inaccessible to the anterior approach.
● **Lateral approach**
— The patient lies supine.
— A long needle is inserted 3 cm distal to the most prominent part of the greater trochanter and seeks the nerve as it descends behind the femur. It is not as easy as it sounds and this approach is not commonly used in the UK.
● **Popliteal fossa block**
— The sciatic nerve can be blocked in the popliteal fossa before it divides into its tibial and common peroneal branches.
— The patient lies lateral or prone and the proximal flexor skin crease of the knee is identified.
— A line is drawn vertically for about 7 cm from the mid-point of the skin crease, and the injection is made about 1 cm lateral to this point.
— If dorsiflexion is elicited it may be the common peroneal nerve alone that is being stimulated, and the sciatic nerve may have already branched. Plantar flexion or inversion of the foot indicates successful location of the posterior tibial nerve.
— Drug dose: 10–20 ml levobupivacaine 0.5%.

Sensory innervation of the foot

Commentary

This is a predictable question about applied anatomy. There are several ways to provide analgesia for forefoot surgery and, although an ankle block does not necessarily provide the best analgesia, its applied anatomy has always made it a good topic for anatomical discussion. Five separate nerves need to be identified and your examiners may not have much practical experience of this block themselves unless they happen to work with a lower limb surgeon. Give yourself an advantage by observing or performing some ankle blocks so that you will have recent practical experience on which to draw.

The viva

You may be asked by way of introduction to the subject how you would provide analgesia for surgery on the foot (which can be disproportionately painful).

● **Possible local anaesthetic techniques:** these include subarachnoid (spinal) block, lumbar extradural (epidural) block, sacral extradural (caudal) block, sciatic nerve block at the hip, sciatic nerve block in the popliteal fossa, intraosseous nerve block (for procedures in the distal foot which cannot be performed under digital nerve (ring) block), intravenous regional anaesthesia (Bier's block, which needs high compression pressures and high volumes to obtain satisfactory analgesia), and local infiltration (this is unlikely to be satisfactory, but is included for completeness).

- **Indications:** these include forefoot surgery, typically Keller's procedure, metatarsal osteotomy, excision of neuromas, and foreign body removal.

You will then be asked about the anatomy and how you would block each nerve.

- **Ankle block:** this can provide effective and prolonged analgesia for the forefoot. Five nerves need to be blocked before local anaesthesia is complete. Concentrations may need to be reduced if the patient is frail or if the procedure is bilateral.
  — **Saphenous nerve:** this supplies a variable portion of the medial border of the foot and ankle. It is a terminal branch of the femoral nerve and is anaesthetized immediately anterior to the medial malleolus where it is superficial, close to the saphenous vein. It is blocked with subcutaneous local anaesthetic, for example, levobupivacaine 0.5% × 5 ml.
  — **Posterior tibial nerve:** this supplies the plantar surface of the foot. It is a branch of the sciatic nerve (which divides into tibial and common peroneal branches in the popliteal fossa) and is blocked behind the medial malleolus where it lies posterior to the posterior tibial artery. The needle is gently directed perpendicular to the skin until it encounters bone, and is then withdrawn 1–2 mm prior to injection of 3–5 ml levobupivacaine 0.5% on either side of the artery.
  — **Deep peroneal nerve:** this supplies only a small area of skin on the dorsum of the foot between the first and second toes. It passes beneath the extensor retinaculum at the front of the ankle joint and is most readily blocked between the tendons of extensor hallucis longus and extensor digitorum longus where it lies lateral to the dorsalis pedis artery. It is blocked with a total of 3–5 ml levobupivacaine 0.5% placed on either side of the artery and deep to the fascia.
  — **Sural nerve:** this supplies sensation to the fifth toe and the lateral border of the foot. It is a branch of the tibial nerve: at the level of the ankle it lies superficially behind the lateral malleolus. Subcutaneous infiltration of levobupivacaine 0.5% × 5 ml between the lateral malleolus and the tendo Achilles usually provides effective analgesia.
  — **Superficial peroneal nerve:** this supplies much of the dorsum of the foot (excepting the small area supplied by the deep peroneal nerve, and the lateral foot which is supplied by the sural nerve). It is a branch of the common peroneal nerve, which divides further into terminal branches at the level of the malleoli. It is blocked with a ring of superficial infiltration of levobupivacaine 0.5% × 10 ml between the anterior tibia and the lateral malleolus.

Direction the viva may take
You may be asked about complications.

- **Complications:** these are largely generic and include failure and partial failure, local anaesthetic toxicity (you may need to modify the concentrations quoted above to reduce the total dose), nerve and vessel damage, and intravascular and intraneural injection.

Cross-sectional areas of interest: eye, neck and lumbar region

Commentary

You may be asked to draw a cross-sectional diagram of anatomical interest which will then be followed by a discussion of an aspect of clinical relevance. Three such typical areas are the eye, the neck at the level of the sixth cervical vertebra, and the lumbar spine. (If you practise talking as you draw, and if you can include a little more anatomical detail than is strictly necessary, then you may be able to limit the examiner's opportunity for further questioning). The descriptions below are deliberately constructed in this way to try and reflect the way in which people might sketch the diagrams.

The viva

The eye (Figure 2.12)

- The anterior structures of the globe are more complex than the posterior and so the question is likely to include reference to the drainage of aqueous humour. The probable discussion about narrow angle glaucoma may extend to the pharmacological management of glaucoma and to determinants of intraocular pressure (page 151).
- **Outer layers:** the three layers of the eyeball consist of the outer fibrous *sclera*, the middle vascular *choroid* and the inner layer of the *retina*. The sclera is continuous posteriorly with the dural cuff that surrounds the optic nerve, and is continuous anteriorly with the cornea.

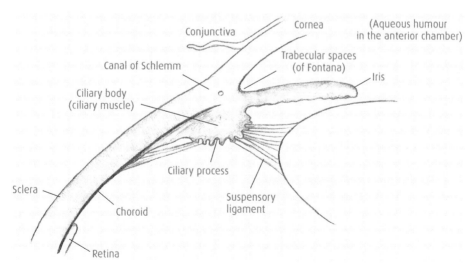

Fig. 2.12 The eye.

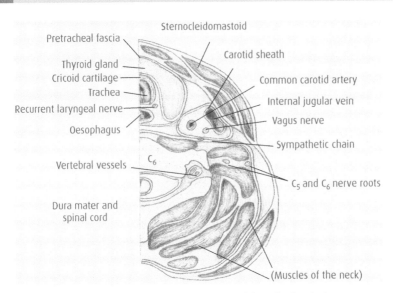

Fig. 2.13 Transverse section of the neck (right side) at the level of C₆.

- **Contents of the globe:** the posterior part contains *vitreous humour*, which is a colourless transparent gel and which constitutes about 80% of the total contents. Anteriorly, the vitreous body is bounded by the capsule of the *lens* and its suspensory ligaments. These ligaments extend to the *ciliary body*, which is a direct anterior continuation of the choroid and comprises the muscle involved in accommodation of the lens. The ciliary body also secretes *aqueous humour* into the anterior chamber, where it circulates before draining via spaces in the trabecular meshwork through the *canal of Schlemm*. The anterior chamber of the eye contains the *iris*, which itself is a forward continuation of the choroid via the ciliary body.

The neck at the level of C₆ (Figure 2.13)

- You may be asked to sketch a cross-sectional diagram of the neck at the level of C₆. This allows the examiner the choice of a number of follow-up questions which include central venous cannulation (page 17), the larynx (page 33), the phrenic nerve (page 54) and the vagus nerve (page 24).
- C₆ is the level of the *cricoid cartilage* whose lower border marks the beginning of the *trachea*. Immediately posterior is the *oesophagus*, which is separated from the body of the sixth cervical vertebra only by the *pretracheal fascia*. Immediately anterior is the isthmus of the *thyroid*. Posterolaterally is the *carotid sheath*, which encloses the common carotid artery, the internal jugular vein and the vagus nerve. Behind the sheath lies part of the *sympathetic chain*. Immediately lateral to the vertebral body are the *vertebral artery* and *vein*, beyond which are the *scalene* muscles. Between these lie the trunks of the *brachial plexus*.

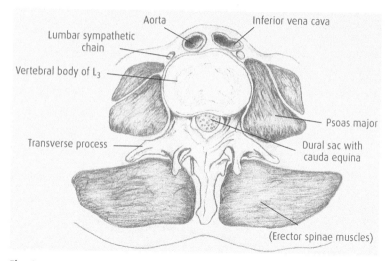

Fig. 2.14 Cross-sectional view at the level of the third lumbar vertebra.

The lumbar region at the level of L₃ (Figure 2.14)

- You may be asked to draw a cross-section of the lumbar area at the level of L₃. Questioning thereafter could include spinal anaesthesia (page 80), epidural anaesthesia (page 84), lumbar sympathectomy (page 64), or psoas compartment (lumbar plexus) block (page 65).
- Immediately anterior to the *vertebral body* are the *aorta* (on the left) and the *inferior vena cava* (on the right). On the lateral surface on each side lies the *sympathetic trunk*. Immediately lateral to the vertebral body at this level lies the *psoas major* muscle. Further lateral are the lower poles of the *kidney*. Posterior to the vertebral body is the *vertebral canal* which, at the level of L₃, contains the *theca* (comprising the dura and arachnoid maters), within which are *CSF* and the *cauda equina*. The theca is surrounded by the *epidural space*. This is minimal anteriorly because the dura is closely apposed to the vertebral body. The vertebral arch is completed by the *pedicles, transverse processes, laminae* and *spinous processes*.

Physiology

Pneumothorax

Commentary

Pneumothorax is an important complication in anaesthesia, trauma and medicine. This viva will concentrate both on the precise mechanisms by which pneumothoraces occur and on details of recognition and management. A pneumothorax can develop rapidly into a life-threatening emergency and so you must ensure that your management is competent.

The viva

You may be asked to list some of the common causes of pneumothorax, and explain how you would confirm the diagnosis.

Causes

- **Traumatic:** pneumothorax can follow penetrating injury, rib fracture or blast injury.
- **Iatrogenic (surgical):** it may occur during procedures such as nephrectomy, in spinal surgery, during tracheostomy (especially in children), laparoscopy, or as a consequence of oesophageal or mediastinal perforation.
- **Iatrogenic (anaesthetic):** pneumothorax may result from attempted central venous puncture and various nerve blocks, from barotrauma from mechanical ventilation at excessive pressures, and from high-pressure gas injector systems. Patients with emphysematous bullae are at risk.
- **Miscellaneous:** it may occur if the alveolar septa are weakened, as described above, and is associated with many pulmonary diseases, including asthma. There are some bizarre and unusual causes: recurring catamenial pneumothorax, for example, is a spontaneous pneumothorax, usually right-sided, which occurs in phase with the menstrual cycle. (By all means impress the examiners with this information, but do not cite it first.)

Diagnosis of pneumothorax in the awake patient

- Typical features (which are not invariable and which will depend on the size of the pneumothorax and whether or not it is expanding) include chest pain, referred shoulder tip pain, cough, dyspnoea, tachypnoea and tachycardia. There may be reduced movement of the affected hemithorax, hyperresonance on percussion, diminished breath sounds and decreased vocal fremitus. The coin test (bruit d'airain – 'noise of bronze') may be positive, as may Hamman's sign (auscultation reveals a 'crunching' sound of air in the mediastinum which occurs in time with the heartbeat). In the coin test the tapping of one coin against another placed flat on the chest wall can be heard on auscultation as a ringing sound. These signs are less definitive than chest X-ray which will confirm the clinical diagnosis.
- If the pneumothorax is expanding under tension, the clinical features are more dramatic because mediastinal compression by the expanding mass decreases venous return, impairs ventricular function and reduces cardiac output. Patients will complain of dyspnoea; signs include tachypnoea and eventual cyanosis. Cardiovascular compromise will manifest as tachycardia, hypotension and, ultimately, cardiac arrest. There may be tracheal deviation (which is not always easy to identify) and subcutaneous emphysema. Tension pneumothorax can be bilateral. The diagnosis of a tension pneumothorax should never await chest X-ray confirmation.

Diagnosis of pneumothorax in the anaesthetized patient

- Initial signs may be non-specific, with hypotension and tachycardia; others include diminished unilateral chest movement, wheeze, hyperresonance, decreased breath sounds and increased airway pressure. There may be tracheal deviation and elevated central venous pressure (if it is being monitored). Cyanosis, arrhythmias and circulatory collapse may supervene. If the diagnosis is suspected, treatment must not be delayed pending chest X-ray.

Direction the viva may take

The viva will then move to a discussion of the underlying mechanisms and so you will be asked how pneumothoraces may arise.

- By definition, a pneumothorax exists when there is air in the pleural space. This space is the area between the parietal and the visceral layers of the pleura which are usually in close apposition and separated only by a small amount of serous fluid.
- At the end of expiration there is no pressure differential between intra-alveolar and atmospheric pressure. However, the intrapleural, or transpulmonary, pressure is subatmospheric, and the slight negative pressure of around 4–6 cmH$_2$O (caused by the opposing elastic recoil of the lung and the chest wall) keeps the lungs expanded. This pressure differential also opposes the tendency of the thoracic wall to move outwards.
- When air gains access to the intrapleural space, the negative transpulmonary pressure is lost and the stretched lung collapses while the chest wall moves outwards.

- Air can enter the intrapleural space via a breach in the parietal or visceral pleura (or both), or via the mediastinal pleura as a consequence of intrapulmonary alveolar rupture. Gas insufflated into the abdomen under pressure may enter the interpleural space via the mediastinal pleura.

Damage to the parietal pleura

- This may occur as a result of open penetrating chest trauma, of oesophageal, tracheal or mediastinal perforation, or during operative procedures such as nephrectomy, tracheostomy and laparoscopy. It may also follow surgery to the thoracic spine.

Damage to the visceral pleura

- This is commonly iatrogenic and can be caused by needle punctures or vascular cannulation. It may follow attempted subclavian and internal jugular puncture, and is also a well recognized complication of some nerve blocks. These include supraclavicular, interscalene, intercostal and paravertebral blocks.

Intrapulmonary alveolar rupture

- Gas escapes from the alveolus, dissects towards the hilum and ruptures the mediastinal pleura. Causes include barotrauma from mechanical ventilation (caused by excessive pressures) or high-pressure gas delivery systems (injectors), and chronic obstructive pulmonary disease (COPD) with bullous emphysema. It is also caused by blast injury. It may occur in asthmatics and in patients in whom the alveolar septa are weakened or distorted by infection, collagen vascular disease or connective tissue disorders, such as Ehlers–Danlos and Marfan's syndromes. Severe hypovolaemia has been implicated as a risk factor for the same reason.

Further direction the viva could take

There may be time for the examiners to ask about management.

- **Management:** discontinue nitrous oxide (in the anaesthetized patient) and give 100% oxygen. Immediate management is decompression via needle thoracocentesis followed rapidly by insertion of a definitive chest drain (intravenous cannulae are too small to provide continued effective decompression). The traditional recommended site is the fifth intercostal space in the mid-axillary line. The British Thoracic Society (BTS) suggests that the drain should be inserted in the so-called 'safe' triangle, which is the area bordered by the lateral border of the pectoralis major muscle, by the anterior border of the latissimus dorsi, and by a line superior to the horizontal level of the nipple. Its apex is just below the axilla. The BTS recommend small size drains for simple pneumothorax (10–14 F), there being no evidence of benefit from larger diameter tubes; however, larger sizes (24–28 F) are recommended for drainage of blood or fluid.
- **Underwater seal drain:** air from the pneumothorax drains under water via a submerged tube in a sealed bottle and is then vented to the atmosphere. The depth of water is important: if it is too shallow, air may be entrained back into the

drainage tube; if it is too deep, the pressure may be too great to blow off the pneumothorax gas. The typical depth is 3–5 cm. Clamping a chest drain risks converting a simple pneumothorax to one that is under tension.

Central venous pressure and cannulation

Commentary

Central venous catheters are used widely in critical care and in major anaesthetic cases and so, although the underpinning principles are not complex, questions on the topic reappear. You will be expected to understand how to interpret measurements and the normal waveform, to know how to insert the devices, and to be familiar with most of the long list of potential complications. The topic may form part of an anatomy-based question on the internal jugular vein (page 15).

The viva

By way of introduction you may be asked to list the indications for central venous catheterization before going on to discuss central venous pressure (CVP) measurement.

- **Indications:** CVP catheters are used for the monitoring of CVP, for the insertion of pulmonary artery catheters, and to provide access for haemofiltration and transvenous cardiac pacing. Central venous lines also allow the administration of drugs that cannot be given peripherally, such as inotropes and cytotoxic agents, and the infusion of total parenteral nutrition. It is suggested that they can be used to aspirate air from the right side of the heart after massive air embolism, although very few anaesthetists have ever used them for this purpose.
- **Function of CVP monitoring – intravascular volume:** the CVP is the hydrostatic pressure generated by the blood within the right atrium (RA) or the great veins of the thorax. It provides an indication of volaemic status because the capacitance system, including all the large veins of the thorax, abdomen and proximal extremities, forms a large compliant reservoir for around two-thirds of the total blood volume. Hypovolaemia may be actual or effective, caused, for example, by subarachnoid block or sepsis, in which loss of venoconstrictor tone or venodilatation decreases venous return and reduces CVP. A single reading may be unhelpful, whereas trends are more useful, particularly when combined with fluid challenges.
- **Function of CVP monitoring – right ventricular function:** CVP measurements also provide an indication of right ventricular (RV) function. Any impairment of RV function will be reflected by the higher filling pressures that are needed to maintain the same stroke volume (SV).
- **Normal values:** the normal range is 0–8 mmHg, measured at the level of the tricuspid valve. The tip of the catheter should lie just above the RA in the superior vena cava.

- **CVP decreases:** if the blood volume is unchanged, then the CVP will alter with changes in cardiac output (CO). It will fall as the CO rises because the rate at which blood is removed from the venous reservoir also increases. This reflects the essentially passive volume–pressure characteristics of the venous vascular system. The major cause of a fall in CVP is depletion of effective intravascular volume. (Raising the transducer will lead to an apparent fall in CVP.)
- **CVP increases:** potential causes for an increase in CVP include a fall in CO (the converse of the effect described above). Ventilatory modes may also cause the increase which is seen with IPPV, PEEP and CPAP. The CVP also rises in response to volume overload, if there is RV failure, pulmonary embolus, cardiac tamponade or tension pneumothorax. Rarer causes include obstruction of the superior vena cava (assuming that the catheter tip lies proximally), and portal hypertension leading to inferior vena caval backpressure. (Moving the reference point and lowering the transducer will also lead to an apparent increase.)

The normal pressure waveform (Figure 3.1)

- This comprises three upstrokes (the 'a', 'c' and 'v' waves) and two descents (the 'x' and 'y') that relate to the cardiac cycle.
- **'a' wave:** this occurs at the end of diastole and is caused by increased **a**trial pressure as the atrium contracts (occurs at end-diastole).
- **'x' (or 'x'')** descent: this reflects the fall in atrial pressure as the atrium relaxes.
- **'c' wave:** this supervenes before full atrial relaxation, and is caused by the bulging of the closed tricuspid valve into the atrium at the start of isovolumetric right ventricular **c**ontraction.
- **'x' descent:** this is a continuation of the 'x'' descent (interrupted by the 'c' wave) and represents the pressure drop as the ventricle and valve 'screw' downwards at the end of systole.
- **'v' wave:** this is the increase in right atrial pressure as it is filled by the **v**enous return against a closed tricuspid valve.
- **'y' descent:** this reflects the drop in pressure as the right ventricle relaxes, the tricuspid valve opens, and the atrium empties into the ventricle.

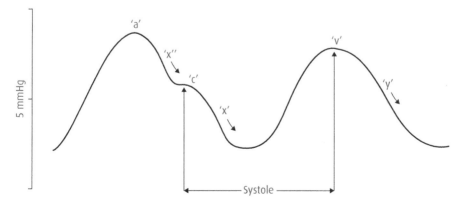

Fig. 3.1 Central venous pressure waveform.

- Any event that alters the normal relationship between the events above will alter the shape of the waveform. For example, in atrial fibrillation the 'a' wave is lost; in tricuspid incompetence, a giant 'v' wave replaces the 'c' wave, the 'x' descent and the 'v' wave. 'Cannon' waves are seen when there is atrial contraction against a closed tricuspid valve (as occurs at a regular interval if there is a junctional rhythm, or at an irregular interval if there is complete atrioventricular conduction block).
- **Complications of insertion:** these are numerous and include arterial puncture (carotid and subclavian), haemorrhage, air embolism, cardiac arrhythmias, pneumothorax, haemothorax, chylothorax, neurapraxia, cardiac tamponade and thoracic duct injury. Anatomically proximate structures such as the oesophagus and trachea can also be damaged. Parts of catheters or entire guidewires can embolize into the circulation. Ultrasound guidance can reduce complications associated with catheter insertion. Endocarditis and cardiac rupture have been reported. Venous thrombosis is common, but the risk may be reduced by the use of heparin-bonded catheters. Infection is a problem, and occurs in up to 12% of placements. Its risk is reduced by full aseptic precautions, by the use of antiseptic- and antibiotic-coated catheters (in high-risk patients), and by using the subclavian approach. There is no definite evidence of benefit for tunnelling, for prophylactic line changes or for the use of prophylactic antibiotics.

Direction the viva could take

CVP measurements are sometimes recorded as negative values. You may be asked to explain how this can happen.

- If the CVP is measured from the accurate reference point of the tricuspid valve, then a sustained negative intravascular pressure is impossible. Certainly, the negative intrathoracic pressure during inspiration will be transmitted to the central veins, and if there is respiratory obstruction this negative pressure will be high. It will, however, be transient. If a mean CVP reading is consistently negative it can only be because the transducer has been placed above the level of the right atrium.

Further direction the viva may take

You may be asked what information a CVP reading provides about LV function. (This is probably a sign that you are doing well.)

- The right atrial pressure reflects the right ventricular end-diastolic pressure (RVEDP) and it is frequently assumed that this also reflects the left ventricular end-diastolic pressure (LVEDP). This is not strictly true even in health, because the right ventricle ejects into a low pressure system and so the normal RV function curve (in which SV is plotted against filling pressure) is steeper than the LV curve (Figure 3.2). This means that, for a given fluid load, the increase in SV of each ventricle is identical, but the rise in filling pressure in the left ventricle exceeds that in the right. This discrepancy is accentuated by LV

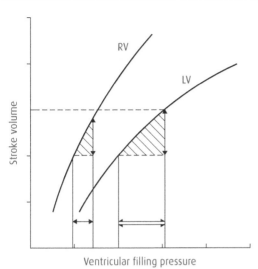

Fig. 3.2 Ventricular function curves. In response to a fluid challenge there is a differential rise in ventricular filling pressures although the increase in stroke volume is the same. RV, right ventricle; LV, left ventricle.

Stroke volume

Ventricular filling pressure

dysfunction, and under these circumstances accurate diagnostic information has to be obtained by other means.

Fluid therapy

Commentary

The optimum choice of fluids for many different clinical circumstances remains confusing and contentious, and you will not be expected to resolve the various controversies. Volume restoration, however, is such an important part of anaesthetic practice that you will be expected to demonstrate both an understanding of the fluid compartments of the body, as well as a logical appreciation of the characteristics of the different replacement fluids.

The viva

You may be asked first about the distribution of fluids within the body.

- **Normal body fluid compartments:** of the total body weight in men, 60% is water. In women, who have a higher proportion of body fat, it is 50–55%. These proportions change with age: total body water (TBW) as a percentage of body weight may be 80% in the neonate and 50% in the elderly. Two-thirds of TBW is intracellular water (ICW), the remaining third is extracellular fluid (ECF), which can be divided further into interstitial fluid (ISF) and the intravascular volume. There is a small volume of residual transcellular fluid, which has been secreted, but which remains separated from plasma, for example as cerebrospinal or intraocular fluid.

Direction the viva may take

You may then be asked how fluids can be lost from these compartments.

- **Blood loss:** this is straightforward. Intravascular volume may be depleted directly by trauma or during surgery. It may occur preoperatively, for example following the rupture of a varicose venous ulcer or an arterial aneurysm.
- **Pure dehydration:** this implies a loss of water alone, without electrolytes. This may be caused by prolonged lack of fluid intake, protracted preoperative fasting and as a result of any condition that may prevent swallowing. Dehydration depletes all the fluid compartments, and is corrected by a solution that equilibrates across all three, namely glucose 5%. Even in these situations there are always some electrolyte losses.
- **Dehydration:** in the context of clinical medicine, most water deficits are also accompanied by electrolyte losses. The causes are numerous and include inappropriate diuretic therapy, diarrhoea and vomiting, intestinal obstruction, preoperative bowel preparation, diabetes mellitus (and insipidus) and pyrexia. Insensible losses in a healthy individual in a temperate climate are of the order of $0.5\,\mathrm{ml\,kg^{-1}\,h^{-1}}$.
- **Perioperative fluid losses:** these include the fluid deficits accrued as a result of preoperative fasting, preoperative pathology, intraoperative haemorrhage and what are termed 'third space' losses. This refers to fluid that is sequestered at the site of injury. Losses are variable but, during the course of a long laparotomy through a large abdominal incision, fluid replacement may be needed by a balanced salt solution at a rate of up to $15\,\mathrm{ml\,kg^{-1}\,h^{-1}}$.

Further direction the viva could take

You will be asked which fluids you would use to restore volaemic status.

- **Crystalloids**
  — A crystalloid solution is defined chemically as one containing a water-soluble crystalline substance capable of diffusion through a semi-permeable membrane.
  — Crystalloids can be infused rapidly in large volumes, are readily available and are cheap. Disadvantages include their short duration in the circulation, with only about 50% of the infused volume remaining in the intravascular compartment at 20 minutes. This increases the potential for overinfusion, circulatory overload and pulmonary oedema. Crystalloids have no oxygen-carrying capacity.
  — *Normal saline (NaCl 0.9%):* this contains $154\,\mathrm{mmol\,l^{-1}}$ each of sodium and chloride ions and is isotonic. The excess of chloride ions means that if large volumes are infused a hyperchloraemic acidosis may supervene. This can be a particular problem in children.
  — *Hartmann's (compound sodium lactate):* this is a balanced salt solution whose composition approximates that of ECF. The lactate in Hartmann's is gluconeogenic and so it is recommended that the solution should not be used in diabetics. Some anaesthetists ignore this because they view NaCl 0.9% infusion as the greater problem.
  — *Glucose 5%:* this is effectively a means of giving free water. Isotonic glucose solutions are appropriate for resuscitation of the intracellular compartment, but will have minimal impact on intravascular volumes because they will equilibrate

throughout the 42 l of water in the body's fluid compartments. Fluids which contain glucose have no place in acute fluid resuscitation.

- **Colloids**
  - A colloid is defined chemically as a dispersion, or suspension, of finely divided particles in a continuous medium. It is not, therefore, a solution. A butterfly's wing is a colloid, as, more prosaically, are foam rubber and fog.
  - Colloids are theoretically more effective than crystalloids in resuscitation, but the evidence to support their superiority is equivocal. All contain NaCl 0.9%, and Haemaccel contains small amounts of potassium and calcium. Blood is also a colloid, but by convention is treated separately.
  - **Gelatins:** gelatins (Gelofusine and Haemaccel) contain modified gelatin of molecular weight between 30 000 and 35 000 Da, and have an effective half-life within the circulation of 3 hours. They carry a small risk of allergic reactions and have no oxygen-carrying capacity.
  - **Starches:** these consist of amylopectin that is etherified with hydroxyethyl groups. They comprise a wide range of molecular weights and remain within the circulation for much longer, with an effective intravascular half-life of 24 hours. Smaller molecular weight particles (less than 50 000) are excreted renally, but the average molecular weight of hetastarch is 450 000 Da and so much of it remains in the body after partial degradation by α-amylase. Some of the starch molecules are taken up by the reticuloendothelial system and may persist for over a year. Intractable pruritus has been reported as a complication of their use. Tetrastarches are newer preparations of lower molecular weight (130 000; degree of substitution 0.4). These appear to support the circulation well, do not accumulate in plasma, do not impair coagulation and cause minimal pruritus. Some anaesthetists remain cautious about advocating their widespread use but they are likely to supersede the higher molecular weight pentastarches and hexastarches. (Maximum volume is limited to $50\,ml\,kg^{-1}\,24\,h^{-1}$.)
  - **Dextrans:** these polysaccharides are classified according to their molecular weight: 40, 70 and 110×10^3. They also remain within the circulation for longer than crystalloids, with an effective half-life of 3 hours and upwards, but they have enjoyed only fitful popularity in the UK. They can also precipitate allergic reactions, may interfere with blood cross-matching (Dextran 70) and can cause renal problems (Dextran 40).
  - **Human albumin solution (HAS):** this was previously supplied as plasma protein fraction (PPF) and has an intravascular half-life of 24 hours. It is derived from pooled human plasma but is sterile. There remains uncertainty about prion diseases, vanishingly small though the risk may be, and there is controversy about its role in resuscitation. Some argue that if albumin crosses damaged cerebral and pulmonary capillary membranes; its use will only worsen outcome (by increasing interstitial fluid because of the osmotic pressure that it exerts). Albumin is not the 'killer fluid' identified by some meta-analyses, but is a useful volume expander that has been shown in other meta-analyses to improve survival.
- **Blood:** blood is also a colloid, but it is convenient to discuss it separately. In acute blood loss, fresh whole blood is arguably the ideal replacement: it has

oxygen-carrying capacity and expands the intravascular volume. Red cell concentrates, such as SAG-M, supply oxygen carriage but are not ideal intravascular expanders when given alone as each unit only has a volume of around 300 ml. Blood is the most physiological solution, but homologous transfusion has numerous potential disadvantages which must be set against the urgency of optimal intravascular resuscitation (page 371). Autologous transfusion is ideal but is impractical in unexpected major blood loss. Blood is also an expensive commodity.

Further direction the viva could take

You may finally be asked about alternative solutions that may potentially be of clinical value.

- **Perfluorocarbons:** these are inert, halogenated compounds which have the capacity to carry oxygen in solution according to Henry's Law (the amount of gas that is dissolved in a liquid at a given temperature is proportional to the partial pressure in the gas in equilibrium with the solution). Older preparations, such as Fluosol DA20, had limited usefulness because of the requirement for high inspired oxygen concentrations, their relative inefficiency of oxygen carriage and the potential for adverse reactions. Newer compounds, such as perfluoro-octobromide, allow the carriage of oxygen equivalent to a haemoglobin concentration of up to $7 \, g \, dl^{-1}$ and show more clinical promise.
- **Stroma-free haemoglobin solutions:** free haemoglobin is able to carry and deliver oxygen molecules, but to minimize the risk of toxicity it must be stroma-free (with no residual red cell debris). It has a higher affinity for oxygen than red cell haemoglobin (the P_{50} is 1.6 kPa compared to 3.6 kPa for red cell haemoglobin), and this marked leftward shift of the oxygen–haemoglobin dissociation curve reduces oxygen delivery to tissues. The molecules are also rapidly degraded in the body, may impair the immune response, and can cause renal failure.
- **Micro-encapsulated haemoglobin:** haemoglobin can be enclosed within artificial microspheres of diameter around 1 μm and which retain 2,3-DPG inside the membrane. Such solutions are experimental.

Compensatory responses to blood loss

Commentary

This is a standard but fundamental question about applied physiology. You need above all to be reassuringly confident about your handling of any of the clinical scenarios with which you may be presented. In addition, it must be clear that your management is rational, based both on an understanding of the homeostatic mechanisms involved and on familiarity with the characteristics of the fluids that you may give.

The viva

You will be asked about the normal compensatory responses to the loss of intravascular volume.

- The function of the circulation is to distribute the cardiac output to tissues sufficient to meet their metabolic demands. Any progressive loss of circulating volume is accompanied by a redistribution of flow aimed to ensure that the brain and myocardium continue to receive oxygenated blood.
- As blood loss continues, the decreases in venous return, right atrial pressure and cardiac output activate baroreceptor reflexes (mediated by stretch-sensitive receptors in the carotid sinus and aortic arch). This is an immediate response. The decreased afferent input to the medullary cardiovascular centres inhibits parasympathetic and enhances sympathetic activity.
- There follows an increase in cardiac output together with alterations in the resistance of vascular beds in an attempt to maintain tissue perfusion. These changes are mediated via direct sympathetic innervation, and by circulating humoral vasopressors such as adrenaline, angiotensin, noradrenaline and vasopressin, and by local tissue mediators, including hydrogen ions, potassium, adenosine and nitric oxide. (The renal vasculature is especially sensitive.) Hypovolaemia encourages movement of fluid into capillaries, the decreased capillary hydrostatic pressure favouring absorption of interstitial fluid with a resultant increase in plasma volume and restoration of arterial pressure towards normal (Starling forces). These mechanisms are particularly efficient in situations in which blood loss is slow and progressive.
- The hypothalamo–pituitary–adrenal response is also important, although it is slower. Reduced renal blood flow stimulates intrarenal baroreceptors which mediate renin release from the juxta-glomerular apparatus. Renin converts circulating angiotensinogen to angiotensin I, from which angiotensin II (AT II) is formed in the lung. AT II is a potent arteriolar vasoconstrictor that stimulates aldosterone release from the adrenal cortex and arginine vasopressin (ADH) release from the posterior pituitary. ADH release is also stimulated by atrial receptors, which respond to the decrease in extracellular volume. These changes enhance sodium and water reabsorption at the distal renal tubule as the body attempts to conserve fluid. Sympathetic stimulation also mediates secretion of catecholamines and cortisol.

Direction the viva may take

You may be asked why major blood loss is associated with a metabolic acidosis. A summary is likely to suffice but the detailed explanation is as follows.

- **Lactic acidosis:** decreased tissue perfusion causes a progressive decline in aerobic metabolism, which is accompanied by a compensatory increase in anaerobic metabolism. This shift to anaerobic metabolism results in a decrease in energy production and the development of a metabolic acidosis. In the aerobic tricarboxylic acid (TCA) cycle, the hydrogen ions which are produced are carried by NADH and $NADH_2$ to the electron transport chain in which the final acceptor is molecular oxygen, which is then converted to water. In the absence of molecular oxygen, the final acceptor is missing and so NADH accumulates. The lack of NAD^+ effectively blocks the TCA cycle and so pyruvate (CH_3-C=O-COOH) also accumulates (at the 'entrance' to the cycle). NADH and pyruvate react to form lactate (CH_3-HCOH-COOH) and NAD^+. The lactate then diffuses out of the cell to accumulate as lactic acid; NAD^+ meanwhile allows anaerobic glycolysis to proceed.

Further direction the viva may take

You are unlikely to be asked about the clinical features of hypovolaemia: unless your performance has been very shaky the examiners will take as read your ability to recognize a patient who is losing blood. Symptoms and signs of blood loss, however, may briefly be discussed in the context of responses to resuscitation, as you are asked about your fluid management.

- **Summary:** redistribution of blood flow is responsible for the typical pallor, cold peripheries, peripheral cyanosis and oliguria. Sympathetic stimulation explains the tachycardia and the increase in respiratory rate. Carotid chemoreceptors also stimulate ventilation in response to changes in PaO_2, $PaCO_2$, and pH. Systolic blood pressure is a relatively crude index which may show little change until substantial volumes have been lost. The pulse pressure may be more useful: as blood loss continues, it narrows and the mean arterial pressure may actually increase. This occurs because diastolic blood pressure is under the influence of catecholamines which rise in response to haemorrhage. Capillary refill time is a simple and effective measure. A delay of more than 2 seconds is abnormal, and trends can be used to gauge the effectiveness of fluid resuscitation. Confusion or other changes in mental state indicate cerebral hypoxaemia and hypoperfusion.
- **Fluid resuscitation:** see page 107.

Control of breathing

Commentary

This question has many potential complexities, but there will be insufficient time to cover these in any detail. The first part of the viva is likely to concentrate on disorders of respiration, most of which are straightforward.

The viva

You may be asked about disorders of respiration that you may see in the context of anaesthesia and critical care.

- **Apnoea and hypoventilation:** common primary causes include anaesthetic drugs such as opiates, neuromuscular blockers and inhalational agents. Hypocapnia will suppress respiratory drive, as will profound hypercapnia. It may follow hypoxic or traumatic brain injury and occurs in patients with type 2 respiratory failure who rely on hypoxaemic drive for respiration and who have been given supplemental oxygen ($>24\%$). Obstructive sleep apnoea is not strictly apnoea (defined as the 'suspension of respiration without movement of respiratory muscles'), but the terminology is too well established to quibble. Primary alveolar hypoventilation syndrome (Ondine's curse) is a rare disorder that is characterized by the loss of automatic respiration. Breathing becomes a voluntary activity and ceases when patients either stop concentrating or fall asleep.

- **Hyperventilation:** in the anaesthetized patient this may reflect inadequate anaesthesia or analgesia. It will occur in response to a rising CO_2 due to rebreathing. Rare causes include malignant hyperpyrexia, of which hyperventilation is a cardinal sign, and pontine haemorrhage. In the non-anaesthetized patient it may be due to pain or anxiety. Kussmaul respiration ('air hunger') is a form of hyperventilation characterized by increased tidal volume and reduced respiratory frequency. Typically it accompanies severe metabolic acidosis.
- **Abnormal respiratory patterns:** Cheyne–Stokes respiration (periodic breathing) is characterized by sequential increases and decreases in tidal volume interspersed with periods of apnoea. It is associated with conditions such as stroke, hypoxia, cardiac failure and altitude sickness, and appears to be caused by the failure of the respiratory centre to compensate rapidly enough for changes in PaO_2 and $PaCO_2$. Kussmaul respiration is described above. 'Fish-mouth' breathing occurs typically when a patient with chronic obstructive airways disease breathes out through pursed lips, thereby generating enough PEEP to keep alveoli open. 'Grunting' respiration in neonates is another example of the same phenomenon.

You will then be asked to describe how breathing is controlled.

- **Overview:** the control of breathing is coordinated by centres within the CNS, by receptors in respiratory muscles and the lung, and by specialized chemoreceptors such as the carotid bodies.
- **Respiratory centre:** a brain stem 'respiratory centre' mediates automatic rhythmic breathing, which is influenced by physical and chemical reflexes. Breathing is a complex activity, which can be interrupted by coughing, vomiting, sneezing, hiccoughing and swallowing. It is also subject to voluntary control from the cerebral cortex to allow activities such as singing, reading (during which the cortex computes the appropriate size of breath for the proposed segment), speech and vigorous exercise, during which expiration may be almost entirely an active process.
- **Inputs:** the 'centre' is in the medulla, where the respiratory pattern is generated and where the voluntary and involuntary impulses are coordinated. It contains receptors for excitatory neurotransmitters such as glutamate (whose activity is inhibited by opiates) and inhibitory neurotransmitters such as GABA and glycine. The centre receives a large number of afferents from the cortex, the vagus, the hypothalamus and the pons. An area in the upper pons, the pontine respiratory group (formerly known as the pneumotaxic centre), contributes to fine control of respiratory rhythm by influencing the medullary neurons, which comprise two main groups.
- **Dorsal respiratory neurons:** these are primarily inspiratory and are responsible for the basic ventilatory rhythm.
- **Ventral neurons:** these are predominantly expiratory.

- **Reciprocal innervation:** as activity increases in one or other of these groups of neurons, so inhibitory impulses are relayed from the other, resulting eventually in the reversal of the respiratory phase.
- **Central chemoreceptors:** these lie on the anterolateral surface of the medulla, and are acutely sensitive to alterations in H^+ ion concentration. A rise in $PaCO_2$ increases CSF PCO_2, cerebral tissue PCO_2 and jugular venous PCO_2 (which all exceed $PaCO_2$ by about 1.3 kPa or 10 mmHg). This rise in CSF PCO_2 decreases CSF pH. The acidosis stimulates chemosensitive areas by a mechanism not yet fully explained. Respiratory acidosis stimulates greater ventilatory change than metabolic acidosis despite the same blood–pH, because the blood/brain barrier is permeable to CO_2 but not to H^+ ions. Over a period of hours this CSF acidosis is corrected by the bicarbonate shift.
- **Peripheral chemoreceptors:** these are located in the carotid bodies, which are small structures, with a volume of only around 6 mm^3, which are found close to the bifurcation of the common carotid artery and in the aortic bodies along the aortic arch. Afferents from the carotid bodies travel via the glossopharyngeal nerve, while those from the aortic bodies travel via the vagus. These are sensitive primarily to hypoxia but, as sensors of arterial gas partial pressures, are less sensitive to a decline in oxygen content. This means that they mediate minimal respiratory stimulation in patients who are anaemic, or when there is carboxyhaemoglobinaemia. Their response time is of the order of 1–3 seconds. They are stimulated minimally by an increased CO_2. Acidaemia stimulates respiration, regardless of whether its cause is metabolic or respiratory. This rapid response is mediated via the peripheral chemoreceptors. Pyrexia is another stimulus mediated via the peripheral chemoreceptors, and which also enhances the responses to hypercapnia and hypoxia. Hypoperfusion is also a stimulant, presumably due to 'stagnant' hypoxia. Peripheral chemoreceptor stimulation may also mediate increases in bronchiolar tone, adrenal secretion, hypertension and bradycardia. Aortic body stimulation has a proportionately greater effect on the circulation. (The nerves to the carotid bodies may be lost during carotid endarterectomy. The subsequent loss of hypoxic ventilatory drive is not usually significant.)
- **Mechanoreceptors:** mechanical as well as chemical stimulation of pulmonary receptors leads to afferent input to the respiratory centre by the vagus nerve. Their importance remains contentious, since patients with denervated transplanted lungs or with (experimental) bilateral vagal block demonstrate normal ventilatory patterns. The inflation reflex comprises the inhibition of inspiration in response to an increased transmural pressure gradient with sustained inflation. In the deflation reflex, inspiration is augmented via a reflex excitatory effect in response to the decrease in lung volume.

Direction the viva may take

You may be asked about the ventilation response curves that can be drawn following changes in $PaCO_2$ and PaO_2.

- **$PaCO_2$/ventilation response curve** (Figure 3.3). In response to an increase in $PaCO_2$ there is an increase in respiratory rate and depth. This response is linear over the range of usual clinical values, although the slope varies. There is inter-individual

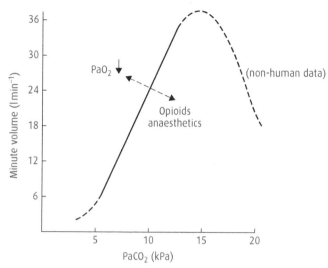

Fig. 3.3 PaCO$_2$/ventilation response curve.

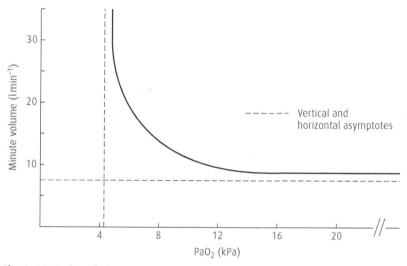

Fig. 3.4 PaO$_2$/ventilation response curve.

variation and the slope is also altered by disease, drugs and hormonal changes. The minute volume for a given increase in PaCO$_2$ is influenced by the PaO$_2$, so that a lower PaO$_2$ shifts the line up and to the left, leading to a greater increase in minute ventilation.

- **PaO$_2$/ventilation response curve** (Figure 3.4). This curve is a rectangular hyperbola, asymptotic to the ventilation at high PaO$_2$ (when there is zero hypoxic drive) and to the PaO$_2$ at which theoretically ventilation becomes infinite at around 4.3 kPa.

(The response is easier to gauge if it is linear, and a graph of ventilation plotted against oxygen saturation is linear down to about 70%.)

Further direction the viva could take

You may be asked about the influence of anaesthesia on these mechanisms.

- **Anaesthetics:** all anaesthetic agents have a depressant effect on the initial ventilatory response to hypoxia by the peripheral chemoreceptors. They also depress the response to increases in $PaCO_2$ (shifting the line of the CO_2 response curve down and to the right).
- **Hypoxia:** hypoxia has a direct depressant effect on the respiratory centre. Should the medulla be subjected to severe ischaemic or hypoxic hypoxia, then apnoea will result.
- **Opiates:** these exert a powerful central respiratory depressant action at the medulla.
- **Respiratory stimulants:** drugs such as doxapram and almitrine act at peripheral chemoreceptors. The mechanism of action remains unclear, but their effects may be mediated via products of their own metabolism.

Apnoea and hypoventilation

Commentary

Questions about breathing and gas exchange can come from different angles, and so you may be asked what happens during apnoea (either obstructed or non-obstructed) and about the consequences of hypoventilation. Neither of these patterns of respiration is uncommon in anaesthetic practice and so you will be expected to explain them with some clarity.

The viva

You may be asked about the clinical circumstances in which apnoeic oxygenation is used.

- **Apnoeic oxygenation:** this technique is used during the apnoea test for brain stem death testing, when $PaCO_2$ must rise to 6.6 kPa or above. Oxygenation can be achieved by simple insufflation. It can also be used during airway endoscopy and at critical points of complex upper airway surgery.

You will then be asked what happens to arterial blood gases during apnoea.

PaO_2

- **Obstructed apnoea:** the basal requirement for oxygen is around 250 ml min^{-1}. The functional residual capacity (FRC) in an adult is about 2000–2500 ml (21% of which is oxygen). Under normal circumstances, therefore, if a patient obstructs when breathing air, the oxygen reserves will be exhausted in about 2 minutes, and the partial pressure will fall from the normal 13 kPa down to about 5 kPa. The lung volume also falls, by the difference between the O_2 uptake and CO_2 output (which ceases).

- **Non-obstructed apnoea:** if the airway is patent the lung volume does not fall because ambient gas is drawn into the lungs by mass movement down the trachea. If the ambient gas is room air then hypoxia will occur almost as swiftly as it does in obstructed apnoea. If, however, the ambient gas is 100% oxygen then it will take about 100 minutes before hypoxia will supervene. (This assumes that the patient has effectively been pre-oxygenated by breathing 100% oxygen prior to becoming apnoeic.)
- **Rate of oxygen desaturation:** this depends on the alveolar oxygen (P_AO_2), the FRC and the oxygen consumption.
  - *Oxygen reserves:* these are mainly in the alveoli. The circulating oxygen is sufficient to maintain metabolism for only 2–3 minutes, and there is no real 'storage' capacity. Efficient pre-oxygenation (either for 3–5 minutes or with three vital capacity breaths) will replace alveolar air with 100% oxygen. If nitrogen washout has been completed, then 8–10 minutes may elapse before desaturation starts to take place.
  - *Lung volume:* the volume of the FRC decreases in pregnancy, in the obese and with some forms of pulmonary disease. FRC is decreased or is exceeded by closing capacity in children up to the age of 6 years and adults (in the supine position) over the age of 44 years.
  - *Oxygen consumption:* this is increased by any rise in metabolic rate such as is seen in children, in pregnancy, thyroid disease, sepsis and pyrexia. It is decreased by hypothermia, myxoedema and a range of drugs, including anaesthetic agents.

$PaCO_2$

- **$PaCO_2$:** during apnoea, CO_2 elimination stops and arterial CO_2 rises at a rate of between 0.4 and $0.8\,kPa\,min^{-1}$. (In patients in whom the metabolic rate may be low, as in a patient undergoing tests for brain stem death, this rate of rise may be slower.) The body stores of CO_2 total around 120 litres (compared with 1.5 litres of oxygen). In non-obstructed apnoea the CO_2 still rises, because elimination via convection or diffusion is opposed by the mass inward movement of ambient gas.
- This rise in $PaCO_2$ is inevitable and, should it reach too high a level, will lead to a respiratory acidosis and start to exert negative inotropic effects on the myocardium (at around 9–10 kPa). It also influences cerebral blood flow, which increases in a linear fashion by around $7.5\,ml\,100g^{-1}\,min^{-1}$ for each 1 kPa rise from baseline, to maximal at 10.5 kPa, above which no further vasodilatation is possible (see Figure 3.10). Carbon dioxide narcosis will occur at a $PaCO_2$ of around 12 kPa in non-habituated individuals.
- **Effect on oxygenation:** as the $PaCO_2$ and P_ACO_2 rise the P_AO_2 falls, by an amount that can be quantified by the alveolar gas equation, which states that the $P_AO_2 = P_IO_2 - P_ACO_2/RQ$ where RQ is the respiratory quotient. (The P_IO_2 is obtained by multiplying the inspired oxygen fraction (F_IO_2) by the atmospheric pressure (BPatm) and subtracting the saturated vapour pressure of water (SVP H_2O),

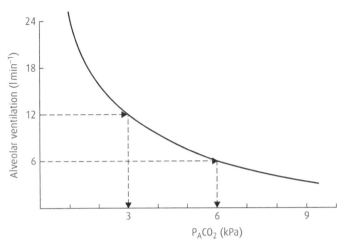

Fig. 3.5 Relationship of alveolar ventilation to P_ACO_2.

47 mmHg or 6.3 kPa. ($P_IO_2 = F_IO_2 \times$ BPatm – SVP H_2O.) This means that if a patient who is breathing room air has a P_ACO_2 of 12 kPa, their P_AO_2 will fall to only 5 kPa.

Further direction the viva could take
You may be asked about hypoventilation.

- The relations of alveolar gas tensions to alveolar ventilation are described by rectangular hyperbolas (concave upwards for eliminated gases such as CO_2 and concave downwards for gases that are taken up by the lung, such as O_2).
- In the case of the P_ACO_2 this relationship (which is given by the equation: $P_ACO_2 = CO_2$ output/alveolar ventilation) means that if the alveolar ventilation halves the P_ACO_2 will double (Figure 3.5). From the alveolar air equation above this makes it inevitable that a hypoventilating patient who is breathing air will become hypoxic. Oxygen enrichment to 30% will increase the P_AO_2 by almost 9 kPa, thereby restoring it almost to normal (while having no effect on the P_ACO_2). This can mask ventilatory failure because supplemental oxygen will ensure that oxygen saturations remain high even in the presence of a high P_ACO_2.

Compliance

Commentary
Compliance is an important concept with obvious implications for ventilatory management of patients, and this particular viva should divide quite evenly between the basic science and its clinical application. It is likely to be linked with a discussion of

management of a patient with deteriorating respiratory function (page 121). It will be useful if you are able to draw a typical pressure–volume curve.

The viva

You will be asked to define what is meant by 'compliance'.

- **Definition:** compliance is defined by the change in lung volume per unit change in pressure. It has two components: the compliance of the lung itself and the compliance of the chest wall. Lung compliance is determined both by the elastic properties of pulmonary connective tissue and by the surface tension at the fluid–air interface within alveoli. Both normal lung compliance and normal chest wall compliance are 1.5–2.0 $1\,kPa^{-1}$ (150–200 ml cmH_2O^{-1}). Total compliance is about 1.0 $1\,kPa^{-1}$ (100 ml cmH_2O^{-1}), and is determined from the sum of the reciprocals of the two values.
- **Static compliance:** a pressure–volume curve is obtained by applying distending pressures to the lung and measuring the increase in lung volume. The measurements are made when there is no gas flow. (The patient expires in measured increments and the intrapleural pressure at each step is estimated via oesophageal pressure.)
- **Dynamic compliance:** a pressure–volume curve is plotted continuously throughout the respiratory cycle.
- **(P–V curves:** pressure–volume curves are useful but they may oversimplify what is happening in the lung. In particular, accurate dynamic compliance curves can be difficult to generate in diseased lungs. The final curve also represents the total rather than the separate lung units, whose individual compliance may be very different. In acute respiratory distress syndrome (ARDS) about a third of the lung may remain normal. The curve can be used to set positive end expiratory pressure (PEEP) and to control ventilation (page 122).
- **Hysteresis:** the inspiratory and expiratory pressure–volume curves are not identical, which gives rise to a hysteresis loop. Hysteresis describes the process in which a measurement (or electrical signal) differs according to whether the value is rising or falling. It usually implies absorption of energy, for example due to friction, as in this case. The area of the hysteresis loop represents the energy lost as elastic tissues stretch and then recoil (viscous losses) and as airway resistance is overcome (frictional losses).
- **Specific compliance:** compliance is related to lung volume, and this potential distortion can be removed by using specific compliance, which is defined as compliance divided by the FRC. This correction for different lung volumes demonstrates, for instance, that the lungs of a healthy neonate have the same specific compliance as those of a healthy adult.
- **Factors which alter compliance:** ARDS and pulmonary oedema decrease respiratory compliance by reducing lung compliance. Restrictive conditions such as ankylosing spondylitis or circumferential thoracic burns reduce it by decreasing the compliance of the chest wall. Compliance is also decreased if the FRC is either higher or lower than normal. At high lung volumes, tissues are stretched to near their elastic limit, while at low volumes greater pressures are required to recruit alveoli. In acute asthma, therefore, patients are ventilating at a high FRC, at which the compliance is lower and the work of breathing correspondingly greater. Compliance is also affected by posture, being maximal in the standing position. Obesity may reduce compliance

both via a reduction in FRC and a decrease in chest wall compliance due to the cuirass of adipose tissue. Age has no influence.

Direction the viva may take

You may be asked about how different types of ventilator respond to a decrease in compliance.

- **Constant-pressure generators:** these ventilators generate an increase in airway pressure which produces inspiratory flow whose rate depends on the compliance and resistance of the whole system (patient and breathing circuit). The sudden initial mouth–alveoli pressure gradient produces high flow into the lungs, which then decreases exponentially as the lungs fill and the gradient narrows. In lungs with low compliance the alveolar pressure increases much more rapidly, the pressure differential reduces and inspiratory flow declines.
- **Constant-flow generators:** these ventilators produce an incremental increase in flow rate to generate a tidal volume that is a product of the flow rate and the inspiratory time. The pressure of the driving source is much greater than that in the airways, and so flow into the lungs is not affected by sudden decreases in pulmonary compliance or increases in airway resistance. The delivery of an unchanged tidal volume in the face of decreased compliance will be associated with a more rapid increase in alveolar pressure and a higher airways pressure.

Further direction the viva may take

Anaesthetic interest in compliance relates particularly to the ventilatory management of patients with acute lung disease. You may be asked about your approach to a patient with severely reduced compliance, such as that typically associated with ARDS (page 121).

The failing lung

Commentary

This is a question about the underlying theory of what has now become the routine management of patients whose respiratory function is deteriorating because of acute lung injury (ALI) and acute respiratory distress syndrome (ARDS). There has been considerable research effort aimed at providing an evidence base for lung-protective strategies, and what follows below is an abbreviated synthesis. It should, none the less, allow you to give a convincing overview of the main principles. The ARDS network has probably produced the most influential studies, but the structure of the viva will not really allow a detailed discussion of this research (some aspects of which have been criticized). Mention the trials if you are familiar with them, but you will not have to offer a rigorous critique.

The viva

You will be asked about the principles of ventilating critically ill patients.

Principles of ventilation

- **Conventional:** traditional methods of ventilating patients with ALI maximized oxygenation by using normal tidal volumes $(10-12 \, ml \, kg^{-1})$ which in non-compliant lungs were associated with very high peak and plateau airways pressures. The ventilatory mode was usually volume-controlled with synchronized intermittent mandatory ventilation (SIMV). A major concern was barotrauma. In the past decade it has become apparent that barotrauma is much less of a problem than *volutrauma* (caused by overdistension of the lung), *atelectrauma* (owing to cyclical shearing forces generated by alveoli closing and reopening), and *biotrauma* (so-called because of surfactant reduction and cytokine release in response to this repetitive injury).

- **'Lung-protective':** it has now become standard practice to try to minimize ventilator-associated lung injury (VALI) by using 'lung-protective' ventilation in which plateau airways pressures are limited to 30 cmH$_2$O by means of much reduced tidal volumes, typically of 6 ml kg^{-1}. There are two consequences of this technique: the minute ventilation may be insufficient for adequate removal of CO$_2$, and low tidal volumes will predispose to closure of alveoli and gas trapping. The first problem is dealt with by allowing the PaCO$_2$ to rise: this is 'permissive hypercapnia'. The second is addressed by adding PEEP to maximize the recruitment of alveoli.

- **Permissive hypercapnia:** this is a key part of current ventilatory strategies, and there are experimental data to suggest that it is safe (up to a PaCO$_2$ of ~9.0 kPa and pH of ~7.2) and that it might confer some protection in the context of lung injury and associated systemic organ damage. Hypercapnic acidosis (as opposed to metabolic acidosis) appears to attenuate VALI, particularly that associated with volutrauma rather than atelectrauma. It also has some myocardial protective effects, and although a PaCO$_2$ of >10 kPa does depress myocardial contractility, cardiac output can still increase as a result of a decrease in systemic vascular resistance. In other tissues, hypercapnic acidosis attenuates reperfusion brain injury and delays hepatocyte cell death. In addition, it appears to modifiy some key components of the inflammatory response (such as TNFa and IL-1). It reduces lung neutrophil recruitment as well as free radical production and oxidant tissue injury. In particular hypercapnic acidosis attenuates damage mediated by xanthine oxidase, a complex enzyme system whose production is increased during periods of tissue injury and which is a potent source of free radicals in the lung. However, its anti-inflammatory properties may also limit the host response to live bacterial pathogens, because free radical production is also central to the bactericidal activity of neutrophils and macrophages. This may be problematic with ongoing bacterial sepsis.

- **PEEP:** although PEEP increases airways pressures and may contribute to a fall in cardiac output, most clinicians consider it essential for alveolar recruitment and prevention of atelectrauma. It does not appear that outcomes are influenced by the use of 'high' (~13 cmH$_2$O) rather than 'low' PEEP (~8 cmH$_2$O). Typically PEEP is

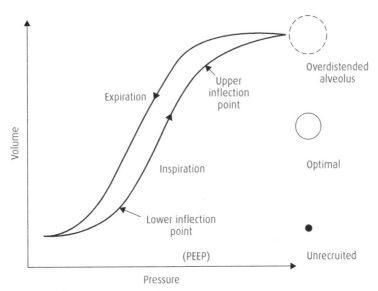

Fig. 3.6 Pulmonary pressure–volume curve.

set at 5–10 cmH$_2$O, but ideally this should be done with reference to the static pressure–volume curve (Figure 3.6). The upper inflection point represents probable encroachment on total lung capacity and so the distending pressure should be kept below this point to avoid overexpansion. The lower inflection point is where small airways and alveoli open (and is effectively the closing volume) and the inflation pressure should be just above this point to avoid de-recruitment of alveoli. Pressure-controlled ventilation on the steep linear part of the curve midway between the two points reduces the peak airway pressure for a given mean airway pressure and minimizes intrinsic PEEP. In practice, however, although modern ventilators will produce pressure–volume curves, the inflection points are often difficult to identify.

Direction the viva may take
You may be asked what else might improve gas exchange in a patient with severe ARDS.

- **High frequency ventilation:** ventilation at very high rates with low tidal volumes is theoretically 'lung-protective'. High frequency jet ventilation (HFJV) uses rates of between 60 and 300 min^{-1}, while high frequency oscillation (HFO) uses still higher rates of 300–1800 min^{-1}. HFJV is used for the management of ARDS in some units and can be useful in differential lung ventilation (via a double-lumen tube) and in patients with bronchopleural fistulae. HFO, in which there is considerable experience in children, is probably used more widely. HFO applies a constant mean airway pressure which prevents alveolar de-recruitment and minimizes peak pressures. Definitive evidence for benefit or otherwise is unlikely to appear before the end of the OSCAR trial (HF **O**scillation in **ARD**S) which is not due to complete until 2012.

- **Prone ventilation:** this reduces shunt and improves oxygenation by mechanisms which are thought to include better distribution of ventilation to previously dependent areas of lung, perfusion of less oedematous areas of lung, a rise in end-expiratory volume and an increase in diaphragmatic excursion. The optimal duration of prone ventilation has not been established and there is no evidence so far that it decreases mortality rates.
- **Inverse ratio ventilation:** changing the I:E ratio from 1:2 to 2:1 or even 3:1 will increase the inspiratory time sufficiently to allow ventilation of lung units with prolonged time constants. In effect, this may just be a way of increasing PEEP.
- **Nitric oxide:** inhaled NO is delivered to better recruited alveoli where it dilates the associated pulmonary vessels and reduces shunt fraction. It improves oxygenation but this is not mirrored by better outcomes.
- **Miscellaneous:** these include nebulized prostacyclin PGI_2 (less effective than NO in improving oxygenation), artificial recombinant protein C-based surfactant (evidence awaited of its benefit in adult patients), partial liquid ventilation with perfluorocarbons which preferentially fill and recruit dependent atelectatic areas of lung (no evidence as yet of improved outcomes), and interventional lung assist membrane ventilator devices (such as the Novalung®). Extracorporeal membrane oxygenation (ECMO) improves mortality in infants, but its effect on outcomes in adults awaits analysis of the MRC ('CAESAR') trial.

Bronchomotor tone (asthma)

Commentary
This is another topic that is central to anaesthesia but with a basic science component that is relatively well circumscribed. Much of the viva, therefore, should feel clinically relevant and you should be able to draw on your own experience of assessing and managing patients with acute severe asthma.

The viva
You will be asked about the factors which influence bronchomotor tone.
Changes in bronchial smooth muscle tone are mediated via the autonomic nervous system.

- **Parasympathetic:** this is dominant in the control of airway smooth muscle tone. Vagal stimulation of muscarinic cholinergic receptors causes bronchoconstriction, mucus secretion and vasodilatation of bronchial vessels. Increases in bronchial smooth muscle tone are mediated via the second messenger cyclic GMP under parasympathetic control.
- **Sympathetic:** sympathetic efferent nerves may control vasomotor tone but there is no direct sympathetic innervation of bronchial smooth muscle, despite the fact that β_2-adrenoceptors are abundantly expressed on human airway smooth muscle and

their stimulation leads to bronchodilatation. Smooth muscle fibre relaxation occurs via the production of cyclic AMP and the activation of myosin light chain kinase.

- **Non-adrenergic non-cholinergic (NANC) nerves:** the only neural bronchodilator pathways may be those of the inhibitory NANC nerves which contain nitric oxide and vasoactive intestinal polypeptide. In addition, there are excitatory NANC nerves which cause bronchoconstriction, vasodilatation, mucus secretion and vascular hyperpermeability.

- **Drugs:** β_2-agonists such as salbutamol, terbutaline and adrenaline cause bronchodilatation by increasing cAMP formation. Phosphodiesterase (PDE) inhibitors such as theophyllines do not inhibit intracellular PDE at therapeutic doses and their mechanisms of action remain speculative. Antimuscarinic drugs such as ipratropium antagonize cholinergic receptors. (This is non-specific antagonism of M_1–M_5 receptors.)

Direction the viva will take

You may then be asked what criteria you would use to decide whether an asthmatic patient needs respiratory support. Your own experience will tell you that essentially this is a clinical decision, so feel confident in emphasizing this rather than the various numerical criteria that are quoted. Measurements of peak expiratory flow rates (PEFR) and arterial blood gases are useful in quantifying the response to treatment but should not be the main criteria for ventilation.

- **Clinical features:** the patient with severe acute asthma is unable to talk in sentences and uses all the accessory muscles of ventilation. Their respiratory rate will be high ($>25\,min^{-1}$), as will the heart rate ($>100\,min^{-1}$). Oxygenation is usually maintained and the $PaCO_2$ is low. A normal $PaCO_2$ is ominous. The PEFR may be between 33% and 50% either of predicted or of the patient's recent best effort. Pulsus paradoxus (in which the arterial pressure changes in response to the large intrathoracic pressure swings) is no longer regarded as a useful sign. Life-threatening asthma is characterized by exhaustion, failing respiratory effort, a silent chest and sometimes confusion. Patients may be bradycardic, hypotensive and mentally obtunded. PEFR is below 33% of predicted; SpO_2 is less than 92% and the $PaCO_2$ is elevated.

You will then be asked to outline your management.

- **Treatment of bronchoconstriction:** this comprises humidified oxygen; nebulized salbutamol 5.0 mg and ipratropium 0.5 mg (both via an oxygen-driven device); and magnesium sulphate 1.2–2.0 g infused over 20 minutes. (Hydrocortisone 100 mg or other corticosteroids will also have been given.) These are British Thoracic Society (BTS) recommendations, but they do not include the use of drugs such as ketamine and volatile anaesthetics, which empirically some clinicians have found useful in refractory cases. The use of aminophylline is contentious; there is no firm evidence of additional benefit, although a $5\,mg\,kg^{-1}$ loading dose and infusion of around $0.5\,mg\,kg^{-1}\,h^{-1}$ may improve symptoms in a subgroup of patients whose response to other therapies has been poor.

- **Treatment of respiratory failure:** non-invasive ventilation has not yet established a place in management, and there is insufficient evidence to support the use of helium–oxygen mixtures. Patients will need general anaesthesia, administered cautiously because of the sudden loss of adrenergic stimulation. Traditional teaching has always held that these patients are dehydrated and need fluid resuscitation. The risk may have been exaggerated; there is some evidence in children at least that acute asthma attacks are accompanied by ADH release, and so hypovolaemia may be less of a danger. Ventilation can be problematic. Airways resistance is high and lung compliance is reduced by overdistension. High inflation pressures are almost inevitable and may lead to barotrauma. The distribution of ventilation in asthmatics is uneven, and high inflation pressures may be directed preferentially to relatively unobstructed bronchi. It is important to maximize expiration, if necessary by adjusting the ventilatory pattern, including the I:E ratio, so as to prevent further distension. It may be impossible to ensure minute ventilation that will clear CO_2, and so permissive hypercapnia may be necessary. It may even be desirable, because hyperventilation to reduce $PaCO_2$ can be associated with a substantial acute reduction in cardiac output.

Further direction the viva may take
If you have done well then you might be asked how the sound of wheeze originates. It is not a subject to which people give much thought and the usual answer is 'airway narrowing'. Asthma is associated with musical sounds, which a simple decrease in airways calibre would not produce. The noise is actually generated by the apposition of the bronchial walls, which vibrate together in response to airflow and act in effect like the reed of a wind instrument. It is the multiple different dimensions of the bronchi and bronchioles that make the sounds polyphonic.

Preoperative assessment of cardiac function

Commentary
Cardiac complications are a major cause of perioperative morbidity and mortality, and so there is much interest in methods of identifying, evaluating and protecting those patients who are at greatest risk. Such science as you will be asked in this viva will be largely descriptive and is of sufficient clinical relevance to keep most anaesthetists interested.

The viva
You may be asked first about clinical predictors of perioperative cardiac risk.

- **Cardiac risk:** this is usually defined as myocardial infarction, heart failure or death, and its incidence in adults undergoing non-cardiac surgery is in the order of 0.5–1%.
- **Clinical predictors:** minor predictors include advanced age, any abnormalities in the ECG, any rhythm other than sinus, reduced FRC, past history of cerebrovascular accident and uncontrolled systemic hypertension. Intermediate predictors include a

history of prior myocardial infarction, mild angina pectoris, diabetes mellitus, compensated cardiac failure and renal impairment. Major predictors of risk include unstable coronary syndrome, decompensated heart failure, any potentially malignant cardiac arrhythmia and severe valvular disease.

- **Risk classifications:** the Goldman index, which was first described in 1977, identified nine independent variables amongst which were recent myocardial infarction and heart failure. It was modified by Detsky but still remained cumbersome to apply. An index of risk that has since been validated in several studies is that described by Lee *et al.* in 1999. This is a further simplification of Goldman which identifies six independent predictors of adverse cardiac outcome. In outline summary, these are: 1) high-risk surgery, 2) ischaemic heart disease, 3) heart failure, 4) cerebrovascular disease, 5) type 1 diabetes mellitus, and 6) chronic renal impairment. (In patients with none of these factors the cardiac risk is 0.5%. In patients with three or more the risk is 9%.)
- **Surgery-specific risk:** high risk-surgery (>5% cardiac risk) includes all emergency major operations (especially in the elderly), prolonged procedures involving large fluid shifts or blood loss, major vascular and peripheral vascular surgery. Of intermediate risk (1–5%) are intraperitoneal and intrathoracic surgery, orthopaedic and prostatic surgery, carotid endarterectomy and other head and neck surgery. Low-risk procedures (<1%) include breast surgery, cataract surgery and endoscopic procedures.

You will then be asked how you would further evaluate and investigate a patient at risk.

- **Clinical assessment:** in addition to history and examination, the patient's functional capacity can be quantified by the metabolic equivalent level (MET). One MET represents the oxygen consumption of a resting adult ($3.5\,\mathrm{ml\,kg^{-1}\,min^{-1}}$), with four METs representing normal daily activities such as light housework or climbing a flight of stairs. Cardiac risks are increased in patients unable to meet a four-MET demand. Symptoms can be classified according to the New York Heart Association (NYHA) functional classification for patients with cardiac disease. In simplified outline:
  — Class I – ordinary physical activity causes no symptoms.
  — Class II – slight symptomatic limitation of physical activity.
  — Class III – marked limitation of physical activity.
  — Class IV – symptoms on minimal exertion; may have symptoms at rest.
- **Electrocardiography:** this is a routine investigation which may reveal ischaemic, hypertrophic and conduction abnormalities. A normal ECG, however, does not exclude cardiac pathology; hence the value of exercise ECG stress testing which may unmask ischaemic heart disease and establish thresholds at which symptoms appear.
- **Echocardiography:** this identifies impaired left ventricular function, determines the ejection fraction (EF), gives information about ventricular wall and septal motion abnormalities, and detects valvular heart disease. The EF as determined by echocardiography is not a good predictor of adverse perioperative cardiac events.

Lee TH *et al.* (1999). Derivation and prospective validation of a simple index for prediction of cardiac risk of major noncardiac surgery. *Circulation*, **100**, 1043–9.

- **Dobutamine stress echocardiography:** this is useful in patients in whom treadmill exercise testing is not possible and gives more information than the investigation performed at rest. Dobutamine increases cardiac output and myocardial oxygen demand, and a stress echocardiogram can identify regional wall motion abnormalities which may develop as the myocardium develops areas of focal ischaemia.
- **Dipyridamole–thallium scintigraphy scanning:** dipyridamole prevents the cellular uptake of adenosine and so potentiates its powerful vasodilatory effects on the small resistance vessels of the coronary circulation. In patients without coronary artery disease, bloodflow can increase fivefold, but if there is a significant coronary stenosis the distal vessels are already maximally dilated. Infusion of dipyridamole creates regional heterogeneity of bloodflow, with the diseased areas being underperfused. Thallium allows this heterogeneity of flow to be imaged using a gamma camera.
- **Coronary angiography:** although invasive, this investigation gives definitive information about the myocardial arterial supply in patients who are at such high potential risk that coronary revascularization should be considered.
- **Cardiopulmonary exercise (CPX) testing:** CPX testing identifies the anaerobic threshold (AT), which is the point at which the oxygen consumption of exercizing muscle outstrips aerobic supply and metabolism switches to anaerobic glycolysis with the production of lactic acid. An AT of less than $11\,\mathrm{ml\,kg^{-1}\,min^{-1}}$ is associated with significantly higher mortality rates, particularly if signs of myocardial ischaemia accompany the ergonomic test. A low AT indicates poor ventricular function and an inability to increase oxygen supply in response to the physiological stress of major surgery.

Direction the viva could take

You may be asked finally how you might reduce the risks of an adverse cardiac outcome.

- **Risk reduction:** the strategy may need to be tailored to the particular patient, but it could include pre-optimization, perioperative β-adrenoceptor blockade (page 239), and limiting the duration of surgery by staging procedures where appropriate. Important generic measures include maintaining normothermia, avoiding anaemia, delivering postoperative oxygen therapy and ensuring good postoperative analgesia.

Oxygen delivery

Commentary

An organism survives by means of effective oxygen delivery to mitochondria. There is continued interest in the concept of optimizing oxygen flux both in critically ill patients and in those undergoing major surgery. The examiners will not necessarily expect you to elucidate the finer points of the debate, but they will require an understanding of the basic principles which will allow you to deduce how the important variables can be influenced to increase oxygen delivery.

The viva

You may be asked what you understand by 'goal-directed therapy'(GDT).

- GDT is a term used to describe the use of specific indices to guide intravenous fluid, oxygen and inotrope therapy. Its origins lie in studies published in the 1980s (by, amongst others, Bland and Shoemaker), which suggested that survival in high-risk surgical patients was higher in those in whom supranormal levels of oxygen delivery (DO_2) were achieved. Subsequent trials and meta-analyses confirmed the benefit of this approach, which was also extended to the management of patients with sepsis and shock. Early goal-directed therapy (EGDT) has been shown to improve survival in the critically ill but, if delayed, it either makes no difference or worsens outcome.
- The strategy involves the manipulation of cardiac preload and myocardial contractility to optimize systemic oxygen delivery. Typical 'goals' include supra-normal DO_2 of $>600\,\mathrm{ml\,min^{-1}}$, central venous pressure (CVP) of 8–12 mmHg, mixed venous oxygen saturation (SvO_2) $>70\%$, mean arterial pressure >65 mmHg, urine output $>0.5\,\mathrm{ml\,kg^{-1}\,h^{-1}}$, oxygen saturation ($SpO_2$) $>93\%$ and haematocrit $>30\%$. The state of tissue perfusion is assessed best by measuring SvO_2, blood lactate concentration, base deficit and intramucosal gastric pH (pHi). (Normal oxygen utilization is around $110\,\mathrm{ml\,min^{-1}\,m^{-2}}$. This rises to over $170\,\mathrm{ml\,min^{-1}\,m^{-2}}$ following major surgery, which in patients of normal size is still well below the DO_2 that has been advocated.)
- The aim of sustaining a supranormal DO_2 may be an oversimplification. High global oxygen delivery does not exclude regional perfusion deficiencies. This is especially true of the splanchnic circulation, which is the first to falter and the last to recover. Any drop in cardiac output appears to be accompanied by a disproportionately large fall in splanchnic perfusion, which can lead to disruption of the enteric mucosal barrier, bacterial translocation and endotoxic triggering of the inflammatory cytokine pathways.

Direction the viva will take

You are then likely to be asked in more detail about the factors that determine oxygen delivery. You may also be asked in passing where oxygen is utilized (a simple question which has disconcerted some candidates).

- Oxygen is required for energy generation in mitochondria via the process of oxidative phosphorylation.
- Oxygen delivery (oxygen flux) to the tissues is governed by cardiac output (heart rate (HR) × stroke volume (SV)) and arterial oxygen content. Content is determined by:

$$[\text{Haemoglobin concentration}] \times [\%\ \text{saturation}] \times [1.31]$$

1.31 is the O_2-carrying capacity of haemoglobin. The theoretical figure of 1.39, which was based on a more exact determination of the molecular weight of haemoglobin, has been superseded by this figure of $1.306\,\mathrm{ml\,g^{-1}}$, derived from direct measurements of oxygen capacity and haemoglobin concentration. Dissolved oxygen ($0.003 \, \text{ml} \, \text{dl}^{-1} \, \text{mmHg}^{-1}$) is small and can be ignored unless hyperbaric therapy is contemplated.

- The formal equation relates delivery to cardiac index (cardiac output/body surface area (BSA)) and so is given by:

$$\text{O}_2 \, \text{flux} = [\text{HR} \times \text{SV} \, (l \, \text{min}^{-1}) / \text{BSA} \times \text{SaO}_2 \, (\text{SpO}_2)\%] / [100 \times [\text{Hb}](\text{g} \, l^{-1}) \times 1.31]$$

Direction the viva may take

The questioning is likely to concentrate on how oxygen flux might be manipulated.

- There are only four variables that can be manipulated: HR, SV, haemoglobin concentration ([Hb]) and oxygen saturation (SpO_2).
- **Cardiac output:** HR and SV are affected by various factors, including venous return and myocardial contractility. Ventricular preload can be improved by optimizing volaemic status, and contractility can be augmented by inotropes.
- **Measurement:** cardiac output determination is discussed on page 323.
- **Oxygen saturation:** this may be improved by enhancing cardiac performance as above. It will also be influenced by primary pulmonary factors affecting gas exchange, some of which may be amenable to treatment. Conditions that can be improved include chest infections, atelectasis and bronchoconstriction. Supplemental oxygen will increase PaO_2.
- **Haemoglobin concentration:** the oxygen delivery equation confirms the importance of haemoglobin: given a cardiac output of $5 \, l \, \text{min}^{-1}$ and an SpO_2 of 100%, O_2 delivery at a [Hb] of $10 \, \text{g} \, \text{dl}^{-1}$ is $670 \, \text{ml} \, \text{min}^{-1}$; at $15 \, \text{g} \, \text{dl}^{-1}$ it rises to $1005 \, \text{ml} \, \text{min}^{-1}$. It is clear, therefore, that oxygen flux can be improved significantly if a low haemoglobin is increased by transfusion. 'Low' in the context of anaesthesia and intensive therapy does not of course mean $10 \, \text{g} \, \text{dl}^{-1}$. An oxygen delivery of $670 \, \text{ml} \, \text{min}^{-1}$ is more than adequate, and few intensivists would wish to transfuse such a patient.
- **Dissolved oxygen:** at atmospheric pressure breathing air, the O_2 solubility coefficient ($0.003 \, \text{ml} \, \text{dl}^{-1} \, \text{mmHg}^{-1}$) means that dissolved O_2 content is around $0.26 \, \text{ml} \, \text{dl}^{-1}$. If a subject breathes 100% oxygen, this increases to $1.7 \, \text{ml} \, \text{dl}^{-1}$ and, at three atmospheres in a hyperbaric chamber, it reaches $5.6 \, \text{ml} \, \text{dl}^{-1}$. At this level, dissolved oxygen can make a significant contribution to delivery to the tissues.

Oxygen–haemoglobin dissociation curve

Commentary

This is a standard and predictable question relating to respiratory physiology, and will be viewed by most examiners as representing core knowledge that is basic to an

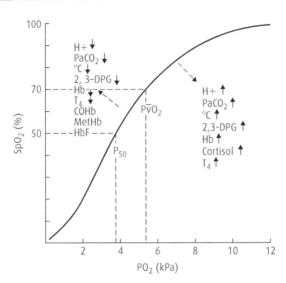

Fig. 3.7 Oxygen–haemoglobin dissociation curve. COHb, Carboxyhaemoglobin; MetHb, methaemoglobin; T_4, thyroxine.

understanding of respiratory physiology and monitoring. You will be expected, therefore, to answer it with some ease. You are almost certain to be invited to draw the curve, so make sure that you can do this with some facility, to reinforce the impression of complete familiarity with the subject.

The viva

This might start with a clinical or physiological scenario which demonstrates the relevance of the dissociation curve. You might, for instance, be asked about gas exchange in the fetus or about abnormal haemoglobins.

- **The oxygen–haemoglobin dissociation curve (OHDC)** (Figure 3.7). This defines the relationship between the partial pressure of oxygen and the percentage saturation of oxygen. In solutions of blood substitutes, such as perfluorocarbons, this curve is linear, with saturation being directly proportional to partial pressure. In solutions containing haemoglobin, however, the curve is sigmoid-shaped. This is because, as haemoglobin binds each of its four molecules of oxygen, its affinity for the next increases. Haemoglobin exists in two forms, an 'R' or 'relaxed' state in which the affinity for oxygen is high, and a 'T' or 'tense' state in which affinity for oxygen is low. As haemoglobin takes up oxygen this effects an allosteric change in the structure of the molecule, which increases affinity and enhances uptake with each of the combination steps.
- **Shifts in the OHDC:** the curve can be displaced in either direction along the x axis; movement that is usually quantified in terms of the P_{50}, which is the partial pressure of oxygen at which haemoglobin is 50% saturated. This is normally 3.5 kPa. The P_{50} is decreased (leftward shift) by alkalosis, by reduced $PaCO_2$, by hypothermia, and by reduced concentrations of 2,3-diphosphoglycerate (2,3-DPG). The curve for fetal haemoglobin (HbF) lies to the left of that for adult haemoglobin (HbA). A shift to the right is associated with acidosis, by increased $PaCO_2$, by pyrexia, by anaemia

and by increases in 2,3-DPG. In most instances, a shift to the right is accompanied by increased tissue oxygenation. A better reflection of this is the venous PO_2, which can be determined from the curve, assuming an arteriovenous saturation difference of 25%. At low PaO_2 levels, however (on the steep part of the curve), hypoxia may outweigh the benefits of decreased affinity and increased tissue off-loading. Under these circumstances, a rightward shift is actually deleterious for tissue oxygenation. At high altitude, with the critical reduction in arterial PO_2, the curve shifts to the left.

- **Haldane effect:** the deoxygenation of blood increases its ability to transport CO_2. In the pulmonary capillaries, oxygenation increases CO_2 release, while in peripheral blood deoxygenation increases uptake. The double Haldane effect applies in the uteroplacental circulation, in which maternal CO_2 uptake increases while fetal CO_2 affinity decreases, thereby enhancing the transfer of CO_2 from fetal to maternal blood.

- **Bohr effect:** this describes the change in the affinity of oxygen for haemoglobin which is associated with changes in pH. In perfused tissues, CO_2 enters the red cells to form carbonic acid and hydrogen ions ($CO_2 + H_2O \leftrightarrow H_2CO_3 \leftrightarrow H^+ + HCO_3^-$). The increase in H^+ shifts the curve to the right, decreases the affinity of oxygen and increases oxygen delivery to the tissues. In the pulmonary capillaries the process is reversed, with the leftward shift of the curve enhancing oxygen uptake. The double Bohr effect is a mechanism which increases fetal oxygenation. Maternal uptake of fetal CO_2 shifts the maternal curve to the right and the fetal curve to the left. The simultaneous and reverse changes in pH move the curves in opposite directions and enhance fetal oxygenation.

- **Carboxyhaemoglobin and methaemoglobin:** other ligands can combine with the iron in haemoglobin, the most important of which is carbon monoxide. Its affinity for haemoglobin is 300 times that of oxygen, and not only does it reduce the percentage saturation of oxygen proportionately, it also shifts the curve to the left. In methaemoglobinaemia the iron is oxidized from the ferrous (Fe^{2+}) to the ferric (Fe^{3+}) form, in which state it is unable to combine with oxygen. This happens when haemoglobin acts as a natural scavenger of nitric oxide (NO), when a subject inhales NO or when they receive certain drugs, including prilocaine and nitrates.

- **2,3-DPG:** this is an organic phosphate which exerts a conformational change on the beta chain of the haemoglobin molecule and decreases oxygen affinity. Deoxy-haemoglobin bonds specifically with 2,3-DPG to maintain the 'T' (low affinity) state. Changes in 2,3-DPG levels do alter the P_{50}, but the clinical significance of this seems to be small. It is true that concentrations of 2,3-DPG in stored blood are depleted (and are reduced to zero after 2 weeks) and that it can take up to 48 hours before pre-transfusion levels are restored. There is, however, little evidence that massive transfusion is associated with severe tissue hypoxia, and this is borne out by clinical experience with such patients.

- **Abnormal haemoglobins:** fetal haemoglobin is abnormal only if it persists into adult life, as in thalasssaemia. (It comprises two α-and two γ-chains, instead of the two α-and two β-chains in the normal adult.) Haemoglobin S, which is found in sickle cell disease, is formed by the simple substitution of valine for glutamic acid in position six on the β-chains. The P_{50} is lower than normal and the 'standard' OHDC for HbS is shifted leftwards. The anaemia that is associated with the condition then shifts the curve to the right. There are other haemoglobinopathies, including HbC and HbD (mild haemolytic anaemia without sickling), HbE, Hb Chesapeake and Hb Kansas. You will not be expected to know about these in any detail; they are rare conditions which most anaesthetists would wish to look up in a textbook of uncommon diseases should they encounter a case in clinical practice.

Hyperbaric oxygen

Commentary

This topic is clinically orientated, but in fact it also allows an exploration of some basic respiratory physiology. During the discussion you will have to make clear, for example, that you appreciate the difference between oxygen saturation, oxygen partial pressure and oxygen content. Be prepared to cite some figures to demonstrate that you understand the principles.

The viva

You will probably be asked first about the indications for hyperbaric oxygen therapy (HBOT). Many claims of benefit have been made; few have been supported by evidence. Cite them by all means, but not before you have discussed the mainstream indications, beginning with any that you may have encountered in clinical practice.

- **Decompression sickness:** recreational divers use compressed air mixtures which they breathe at hyperbaric pressures; each 10 metres of descent increases the pressure by one atmosphere. At depth the tissues become supersaturated with nitrogen. If the diver ascends too rapidly, the partial pressure of nitrogen in tissues exceeds the ambient pressure, and so the gas forms bubbles in the circulation and elsewhere. Most remains in the venous side of the circulation to be filtered out by the lung, but some may gain access to the arterial (and hence the cerebral) circulations via hitherto innocuous shunts. Hyperbaric treatment mimics controlled ascent from depth, and this allows the nitrogen to wash out exponentially without causing symptoms.
- **Infection:** the evidence supports the use of hyperbaric oxygen therapy as part of the management of patients with bacterial infections. The main indications are for anaerobic bacterial infections, particularly with clostridia, osteomyelitis and necrotizing soft tissue infections. Oxygen-derived free radicals are bactericidal.
- **Carbon monoxide (CO) poisoning:** the half-life of CO while breathing 100% oxygen is reduced to an hour. This is reduced further to about 20 minutes in a hyperbaric chamber but, unless the chamber is on site, the transfer time alone will make this benefit negligible. CO is, however, a cellular toxin, which appears to inhibit cellular respiration via cytochrome A_3, as well as impairing the function of neutrophils. The rationale for hyperbaric treatment rests on the presumption, as yet unproven, that it attenuates these toxic effects.
- **Delayed wound healing:** hyperbaric oxygen therapy may be of benefit to patients in whom wound healing is delayed by ischaemia. Its theoretical role in the treatment

of thermal injury has not been supported by recent studies. Angiogenesis is, however, stimulated at hyperbaric pressure by a mechanism that is unclear.

- **Anaemic hypoxia:** Jehovah's witnesses, and others in whom very low haemoglobin concentrations have compromised oxygen delivery to tissues, have been managed successfully using hyperbaric oxygen.
- **Soft tissue injuries:** early treatment has been used in elite sportsmen to treat soft tissue injuries and some fractures.
- **Multiple sclerosis:** hyperbaric therapy for this disease still has its enthusiasts, despite the many controlled trials that have shown no benefit.

Direction the viva may take

You will be asked about the principles underlying hyperbaric oxygen therapy. You might wish to start discussing it straight away, but the first two paragraphs below give some background which explains the rationale for its use.

- **Predicted PaO_2 from FiO_2:** there is a useful formula that predicts the partial pressure of oxygen in arterial blood (PaO_2) by multiplying the inspired oxygen percentage by 0.66. A young adult in good health and breathing room air, therefore, will have a PaO_2 of $20.93 \times 0.66 = 13.3$ kPa (100 mmHg). Vigorous hyperventilation can increase this to around 16 kPa (from the alveolar gas equation the fall in $PaCO_2$ allowing a rise in PaO_2), but further rises are possible only by enriching the inspired oxygen concentration. From the empirical formula above it can be seen that the maximum PaO_2 that can be achieved by breathing 100% oxygen is around 66 kPa. (In practice it may be slightly higher.)
- **Saturation, partial pressure and content:** at a partial pressure of oxygen of 13.3 kPa, haemoglobin is almost 100% saturated. Further increases in inspired oxygen (FiO_2) can therefore increase the oxygen saturation (SpO_2) only marginally, although the PaO_2 will rise substantially. The sigmoid shape of the OHDC, moreover, means that oxygen will start to be released to the tissues only when the PaO_2 is around 13.3 kPa. It is also important to note that, although the increase in PaO_2 is very high, the rise in oxygen content is relatively modest. If a subject changes from breathing room air to breathing 100% oxygen at barometric pressure, the arterial oxygen content rises from around 19 ml dl^{-1} to only 21 ml dl^{-1}. In practice, the venous oxygen content is probably more significant because this reflects more reliably the minimum tissue PO_2. In the situation described above, the venous arterial content rises from about 14 to 16 ml dl^{-1}. This is the same as the arterial rise, because the arteriovenous O_2 difference remains constant.
- **Hyperbaric oxygenation:** this is an example of an application of Henry's Law, which states that the number of molecules (in this case oxygen) which dissolve in the solvent (plasma) is directly proportional to the partial pressure of the gas at the surface of the liquid. It is the only means whereby very high arterial PaO_2 values (greater than 80 kPa) can be obtained. Thus, at 2 atmospheres the PaO_2 will be 175 kPa. However, even at these levels the venous content will only be of the order of 18 ml dl^{-1}, and it is not until the blood is exposed to oxygen at 3 atmospheres of pressure, at which the arterial content is 25.5 mldl^{-1} and the venous content 20.5 ml dl^{-1}, that all the tissue requirements can be met by dissolved oxygen. Content is determined by the product of the [Hb] × [% saturation] × [1.31]

(O_2-carrying capacity of Hb) plus dissolved oxygen. Dissolved oxygen (0.003 ml $dl^{-1} mmHg^{-1}$) is small and is usually ignored, except under these hyperbaric conditions when it assumes great importance.

Further direction the viva could take
You may be asked about the potential complications of hyperbaric therapy.
The main problem relates to oxygen toxicity.

Oxygen toxicity

Commentary
One of the most basic principles of anaesthesia and intensive care is the maintenance of oxygenation, and so it is paradoxical that a molecule which is essential to life can, under certain circumstances, be lethal. It is important that anaesthetists realize that oxygen is potentially toxic, and the viva is testing your recognition of that reality. It is a relatively sharply focused question and you will have to know some of the details to acquit yourself well.

The viva
You may be asked to describe the clinical features of oxygen toxicity.

Symptoms and signs
- These are most marked in conscious patients who are breathing oxygen under hyperbaric conditions.
- Initial symptoms include retrosternal discomfort, carinal irritation and coughing. This becomes more severe with time, with a burning pain that is accompanied by the urge to breathe deeply and to cough. As exposure continues, symptoms progress to severe dyspnoea with paroxysmal coughing.
- CNS symptoms may supervene, with nausea, facial twitching and numbness, disturbances of taste and smell. Convulsions may occur, preceded by a premonitory aura.
- In long-term ventilated patients in whom high inspired oxygen concentrations tend to be the norm, the non-specific clinical signs will be those of progressively impaired gas exchange with decreased pulmonary compliance.
- You may then be asked in more detail about the conditions under which oxygen may become toxic and the mechanisms whereby it does so.

Adverse effects at atmospheric pressure
- **Oxygen toxicity:** the major problem is dose-related direct toxicity. Dose–time curves have been constructed to allow the recommendation that 100% should be administered for no longer than 12 hours at atmospheric pressure; 80% for no longer than 24 hours, and 60% for no longer than 36 hours. An FiO_2 of 0.5 can be maintained indefinitely.

- **Pulmonary pathology:** oxygen causes pathological changes which begin with tracheobronchitis, neutrophil recruitment and the release of inflammatory mediators. Surfactant production is impaired, pulmonary interstitial oedema appears, followed, after around 1 week of exposure, by the development of pulmonary fibrosis. Toxicity also accelerates lung injury in the critically ill. In patients receiving certain cytotoxic drugs, particularly bleomycin and mitomycin C, ARDS and respiratory failure may supervene after 'normal' doses of oxygen.
- **Mechanism of toxicity:** this is complex and not fully elucidated, however, it is suggested that oxygen interferes with basic metabolic pathways and enzyme systems. It is known that hyperoxia increases production of highly oxidative, partially reduced metabolites of oxygen. These not only include hydrogen peroxide but also oxygen-derived free radicals (superoxide and hydroxyl radicals and singlet oxygen). The hydroxyl free radical is the most reactive and dangerous of these species. These substances appear particularly to affect enzyme systems which contain sulphydryl groups.
- **Defence mechanisms:** up to a partial pressure of oxygen of about 60 kPa, a number of endogenous antioxidant enzymes are effective. These include catalase, superoxide dismutase and glutathione peroxidase.

Adverse effects in obstetrics

- Conventional wisdom has always held that pregnant women undergoing operative delivery under regional anaesthesia benefit from supplemental oxygen, it being argued that this optimizes fetal oxygenation. This may not in reality be best practice. An FiO_2 as high as 0.6 is associated with only a small increase in umbilical venous oxygenation. However, what do rise are markers of oxygen free radical activity in both mother and baby. These radicals deplete intrinsic antioxidant systems. The placenta also increases its release of inflammatory mediators. Neonatal hyperoxia is known, moreover, to mediate tissue damage in conditions as diverse as retinopathy of prematurity, necrotizing enterocolitis, bronchopulmonary dysplasia and intracranial haemorrhage. Maternal cardiac function is also affected. In response to an FiO_2 of 0.4, the cardiac index falls and systemic vascular resistance rises, hyperoxia appearing to exert direct vasopressor effects.

Toxic effects under hyperbaric conditions

- This toxicity presents the major limitation of hyperbaric oxygen therapy. It is dose-dependent and affects not only the lung, but also the CNS, the visual system, and probably the myocardium, liver and renal tract.
- **Pulmonary toxicity:** oxygen at 2 atmospheres produces symptoms in healthy volunteers at 8–10 hours, together with a quantifiable decrease in vital capacity which starts as early as 4 hours. It persists after exposure ceases.
- **CNS:** oxygen at 2 atmospheres is associated with nausea, facial twitching and numbness, olfactory and gustatory disturbance. Tonic–clonic seizures may then supervene without any prodrome, although some subjects report a premonitory aura.
- **Eyes:** hyperoxia may be associated in adults with narrowing of the visual fields and myopia.

Direction the viva may take

You may then be asked under what other circumstances oxygen may have adverse effects.

- **Paediatrics:** neonates and infants of post-conceptual age less than 44 weeks may develop retrolental fibroplasia if they are allowed to maintain a PaO_2 greater than 10.6 kPa (80 mmHg) for longer than 3 hours. In practice, this means keeping the oxygen saturation (SpO_2) in these babies at around 90%. The condition is almost certainly multifactorial.
- **Absorption atelectasis:** this is an adverse effect of therapy.
- **Hypoventilation:** oxygen concentrations higher than 24% may suppress respiration in patients who are reliant on hypoxaemic ventilatory drive. This is another adverse effect of therapy. (It is a phenomenon that seems to worry physicians much more than anaesthetists, most of whom have seen it only rarely and who generally believe its importance to be overstated.)

One-lung anaesthesia

Commentary

Introduction to this topic may be via a question about desaturation during thoracic surgery or double-lumen tube placement, but the viva is likely to end up as a discussion about one-lung anaesthesia. This is a technique that is used mainly for complex and specialist procedures, but the physiological changes that ensue are of particular anaesthetic relevance, which make it an attractive science-based clinical topic. The examiners will not expect you necessarily to have had much direct experience but, as this is a standard and predictable question, you will have to show that you understand the basic principles.

The viva

You will be asked initially about the indications for, and the basic physiology of, one-lung anaesthesia.

- The indications for single lung anaesthesia (during which one lung is deliberately collapsed to facilitate surgical exposure) include pulmonary, oesophageal and spinal surgery. It may be necessary during surgery on the thoracic aorta, and is also used for relatively minor procedures such as transthoracic cervical sympathectomy and pleurodesis.

Physiological changes

- For the duration of anaesthesia the surgical side is uppermost, and the non-ventilated upper lung is usually described as the non-dependent lung.
- When ventilation is interrupted, the remaining blood flow takes no part in gas exchange, creating ventilation–perfusion mismatch and a shunt, which contributes to hypoxia.

- The shunt is partly reduced because gravity favours flow to the dependent lung, and because surgical compression and retraction may further decrease blood flow to the non-ventilated lung.
- The shunt will further reduce if non-dependent blood vessels are ligated surgically, and will largely disappear if the pulmonary artery is clamped prior to pneumonectomy.
- Hypoxic pulmonary vasoconstriction (HPV) decreases the flow to the non-dependent lung by around 50%, and may reduce the shunt from 50% down to 30% (which none the less is still significant).
- The dependent lung loses volume because of compression, but hypoxic vasoconstriction, should it occur, may compensate partially by diverting some blood to the non-dependent lung.
- Secretions may pool in the dependent lung, but suction removal via a double-lumen tube may be very difficult.

Direction the viva may take

You may be asked how you adjust ventilatory settings when the lung is collapsed.

- The ventilator settings are similar to those used for double lung ventilation with tidal volumes of around 10–12 ml kg^{-1}. Higher volumes increase both mean airways (P_{aw}) and vascular resistance, with the result that more blood may flow to the non-ventilated lung and increase shunt. Lower volumes are likely to lead to pulmonary atelectasis.
- Although shunt is not substantially improved by supplemental oxygen, many anaesthetists routinely increase the FiO_2 to 0.8–1.0.
- The respiratory rate is adjusted to keep the end-tidal carbon dioxide ($ETCO_2$) at around 5–6% or 40 mmHg.

Further direction the viva could take

You may then be asked how you would manage an episode of hypoxia.

- Pre-existing disease, either pulmonary or cardiac, may be an important contributory factor.
- You should check the FiO_2 and increase it if necessary. This may not help if significant shunt is the problem, but it is probably the swiftest intervention that you can make.
- You should check the tidal volume and other ventilator indices. Again, these are interventions that can be made rapidly. The $ETCO_2$ should be maintained at 5–6% because hypocapnia may decrease hypoxic pulmonary vasoconstriction, although small increases in tidal volume can help oxygenation.
- The double-lumen tube position should then be checked with a fibreoptic bronchoscope. Displacement to a suboptimal position is very common, particularly if the patient has been moved.
- If oxygenation still does not improve, then CPAP of around 5 cmH$_2$O can be added to the upper lung, but you will have to warn the surgeon that the lung may partially re-expand. Alternatively, oxygen can be insufflated in the upper lung, but many anaesthetists do this routinely from the start of surgery.

- You can also add around 5 cmH$_2$O of PEEP to the lower lung, which may increase volume in potentially atelectatic areas. This manoeuvre may, however, increase vascular resistance and divert blood to the non-ventilated upper lung.
- Both CPAP and PEEP can be increased in small increments.
- If none of these interventions is successful, intermittent inflation can be tried, or it may finally be necessary to revert to full double lung ventilation (with lung retraction which will allow surgery to continue).

Final direction the viva could take

At some stage during the viva you may be asked about the problems of using double-lumen tubes.

- Difficulties with double-lumen tubes are probably the most important cause of mortality and morbidity associated with one-lung anaesthesia. In the 1998 National Confidential Enquiry into Peri-operative Deaths (NCEPOD), which looked at oesophagogastrectomy, problems with double-lumen tubes were implicated in 30% of perioperative deaths. Studies have confirmed that critical malpositioning occurs in over 25% of cases, and general misplacements complicate over 80% of uses.
- This is not surprising: the anatomy may be distorted by tumour or effusion, and the tubes are bulky and more complex to insert than single-lumen tubes, requiring rotation within the airway of between 90° and 180°.
- Complications include failure to achieve adequate lung separation and one-lung ventilation, prolonged surgical retraction and associated pulmonary trauma, occlusion of a major bronchus with lobar collapse and secondary infection, contamination of the dependent lung by infected secretions from the upper lung, and trauma during insertion.
- A double-lumen tube is positioned correctly when the upper surface of the bronchial cuff lies immediately distal to the bifurcation of the carina. This tube position can be assessed clinically, but this may be unreliable. The average depth of insertion for a patient of height 170 cm is 29 cm, and the distance alters by 1 cm for every 10 cm change in height. This distance from the incisors can be used as an approximate guide. Auscultation of the lung fields during clamping and release can be performed, although findings may be equivocal if access to the chest wall is limited because surgery has begun. Oximetry and capnography will not give specific enough information about where the tube is sited. The tube position should therefore be checked using a fibreoptic bronchoscope.

Pulmonary oedema

Commentary

Pulmonary oedema is common in critical care, if less so in anaesthesia. This viva explores your understanding of the various forces that allow its development as well as your ability to apply that knowledge to its rational management.

The viva

You may be asked by way of introduction to outline some causes of pulmonary oedema.

- Pulmonary oedema, which is defined by the presence of fluid in the alveoli, may be caused by left ventricular failure, by direct lung injury (caused, for example, by smoke or toxin inhalation), by fluid overload, by endothelial damage associated with ARDS, by the high catecholamine output following neurological injury, and by obstruction to lymphatic drainage. It may also develop in response to acute airway obstruction.

You will then be asked what factors contribute to the formation of oedema by movement of fluid across capillary membranes.

- Fluid flux across the capillary into the interstitium and thence into the alveolus is governed by Starling's hypothesis for capillary fluid exchanges.
- **Starling equation:** fluid flux $= \kappa \, (p_{cap} - p_{is}) - \sum (\pi_{cap} - \pi_{is})$
  — κ: this is the capillary filtration coefficient, a proportionality constant which is a measure of the ease with which fluid traverses the endothelial boundary. It is the product of the area of capillary wall and its permeability to water. 'Leaky' capillaries have a high filtration coefficient.
  — p_{cap} **and** p_{is}**:** these are the capillary and interstitial hydrostatic pressures, respectively.
  — $\sum$ (also written sometimes as σ or δ): this is the reflection (or reflectance) coefficient, which is an indication of the permeability of the capillary barrier (acting as a semi-permeable membrane) to solute. A coefficient of 1 indicates total 'reflection', with no solute passing into the interstitium. A coefficient of zero indicates that the capillary wall allows free passage of solute.
  — π_{cap} **and** π_{is}**:** these are the capillary and interstitial oncotic pressures, respectively.
  — The net sum of the four forces is usually outwards, with the extravasated fluid being cleared by the lymphatics. This is despite the lower hydrostatic pressures in the pulmonary circulation. The normal clearance rate of 10–20 ml h^{-1} (in the lungs) can increase to 200 ml h^{-1} before the system is overwhelmed.
  — The oncotic pressure is the contribution made to total osmolality by colloids. (Hence the alternative term 'colloid osmotic pressure'.) The plasma oncotic pressure, at 25–28 mmHg, is only about 0.5% that of total plasma osmotic pressure, but is significant because, from the equation above, it can be seen that it is the only force whose effect is to retain fluid within the pulmonary capillary.

Direction the viva may take

You will be asked to explain how the different types of pulmonary oedema may arise.

- **Increased capillary hydrostatic pressure (p_{cap}):** this is common and explains the formation of pulmonary oedema as a consequence of left ventricular failure, fluid overload, mitral stenosis and any other condition that may cause pulmonary venous hypertension. Hydrostatic pressure is clearly greater in the dependent parts of the lung. Neurogenic pulmonary oedema (such as that associated with subarachnoid haemorrhage) may be caused by a sudden increase in hydrostatic pressure in response to a massive catecholamine surge.

- **Decreased interstitial pressure (p_{is}):** if interstitial pressure becomes acutely negative, pulmonary oedema may develop as the lymphatics are overwhelmed. This can occur with upper airway obstruction during which very high negative intrathoracic pressures may be generated, creating a gradient which favours transudation.

- **Decreased capillary oncotic pressure (π_{cap}):** this commonly worsens oedema that has another primary cause. Hypoproteinaemia, hypoalbuminaemia, haemodilution, liver failure and the nephrotic syndrome are all conditions which will decrease the gradient between the oncotic pressure and the pulmonary capillary occlusion (or 'wedge') pressure (PCWP). If this gradient does not exceed 4 mmHg, then oedema formation is inevitable. Albumin makes a substantial contribution to colloid oncotic pressure, and if the plasma albumin concentration × 0.57 does not exceed PCWP, then pulmonary oedema will supervene.

- **Decreased reflection coefficient ($\sum$):** capillary endothelial damage may reduce $\sum$ to zero, so that protein will diffuse freely across the wall such that no effective oncotic pressure can be exerted. This form of capillary leak characterizes ARDS. Capillary injury will also increase permeability to water, with a rise in the filtration coefficient, κ.

- **Decreased lymphatic clearance:** this is uncommon, but will accompany any disease process which obliterates lymphatic vessels. Examples include severe fibrosing lung disease, silicosis and lymphangitis carcinomatosis (lymphangitis obliterans).

- **Idiopathic:** other causes of pulmonary oedema include ascent to altitude and rapid lung re-expansion after collapse. The mechanisms are uncertain.

Further direction the viva could take

You may be asked to outline how you can apply these principles to the rational management of pulmonary oedema.

- Hydrostatic pulmonary oedema is treated by reducing left atrial pressure. This can be achieved by offloading the left ventricle using nitrates or ACE inhibitors to improve myocardial function. The emergency treatment of acute left ventricular failure commonly involves intravenous diamorphine and diuretic. These probably alleviate symptoms by the same mechanism. Myocardial contractility can be enhanced using positive inotropes.

- Decreased capillary oncotic pressure is usually contributory rather than primary. In theory, the restoration of the capillary oncotic pressure by giving albumin should be beneficial, but this is rarely done. Plasma albumin concentrations in the critically ill can be maintained only if the patient's condition begins to improve.

- Increased alveolar pressure: PEEP is now believed to increase the capacity of the interstitium to hold fluid. (The pulmonary interstitium can accommodate 500 ml with an increase in pressure of only 1.5 mmHg.) PEEP also increases alveolar recruitment.

Pulmonary hypertension (hypoxic pulmonary vasoconstriction)

Commentary

Pulmonary hypertension has myriad causes but for most anaesthetists it is a theoretical rather than a practical problem. The subject does, however, allow some discussion of pulmonary pathophysiology and its clinical implications. It may be linked to a question about hypoxic pulmonary vasoconstriction. This is one of several factors that influence ventilation–perfusion relationships in the lung, and anaesthetists rarely intervene directly to exploit the mechanism. So this is theoretical, yet because the mechanism is influenced by anaesthetic drugs and because it has relevance for special situations such as one-lung anaesthesia, it remains of interest to examiners.

The viva

You may be asked first about pulmonary hypertension; some causes and its implications for anaesthesia.

- **Diagnosis:** definitive diagnosis requires determination of pulmonary arterial pressures (PAP). The normal mean PAP is 12–16 mmHg: pulmonary hypertension is defined by mean pressures at rest of >25 mmHg or >30 mmHg with exercise.
- It can be caused by excessive pulmonary blood flow. This '*arterial*' hypertension is associated with conditions such as congenital cardiac anomalies involving left to right shunts, and with collagen vascular disease.
- It can also result from increased resistance to pulmonary venous drainage. This '*venous*' hypertension occurs typically as a result of chronic left ventricular failure and mitral valve disease. The rise in left atrial pressure is transmitted backwards through the pulmonary circulation.
- Pulmonary hypertension occurs commonly in response to alveolar hypoxia with obliteration of part of the capillary bed. Causes of this '*hypoxic*' hypertension include chronic obstructive pulmonary disease (COPD), obstructive sleep apnoea syndrome (OSAS) and interstitial lung disease.
- It is associated with thrombotic disease. '*Thrombotic*' hypertension may develop as a consequence of chronic proximal embolic disease or as a result of obstruction of distal vessels by thrombus. (These vessels can also become occluded by parasites, such as schistosomes, or by foreign material, as can happen in intravenous drug abusers.) Acute proximal obstruction owing to pulmonary emboli leads to only moderate rises in pulmonary artery pressure, because without chronic adaptation the right ventricle can generate a systolic pressure no greater than about 50 mmHg. The right ventricle may therefore fail acutely in the presence of massive pulmonary thromboembolism.
- '*Drug-induced*' hypertension may follow the use of appetite suppressants such as fenfluramine (definite link), amphetamines and L-tryptophan (probable link) and cocaine (possible link).

- Pulmonary hypertension can be idiopathic. It is also associated with HIV infection and inflammatory conditions such as sarcoidosis and schistosomiasis.
- **Anaesthetic implications:** cardiac output from the right ventricle is crucially dependent on right ventricle filling pressure and on PAP. Thus it is compromised by any decrease in venous return or any increase in pulmonary vascular resistance. The aims of any anaesthetic technique, therefore, should be to avoid tachycardia which may reduce ventricular filling, to maintain sinus rhythm and to optimize preload. A reduction in afterload is acceptable as long as the pulmonary hypertension is not secondary to a left-to-right shunt which has the potential to reverse (Eisenmenger syndrome).
- **Increase in pulmonary vascular resistance (PVR):** PVR rises with hypoxia, hypercapnia, acidosis, nitrous oxide (in the presence of pre-existing pulmonary hypertension), catecholamines and exogenous pressors which increase systemic vascular resistance.
- **Falls in PVR:** agents that can reduce PVR include oxygen, calcium-channel blockers, prostacyclin, nitric oxide, and phosphodiesterase-5 inhibitors such as sildenafil. Specific endothelin receptor antagonists such as bosentan both reduce PVR and improve exercise capacity. (Endothelin is a potent vasoconstricting peptide.)

Direction the viva may take

You may then be asked to describe the phenomenon of hypoxic pulmonary vasoconstriction (HPV).

- **Definition:** HPV is a mechanism that diverts bloodflow away from areas of the lung where the alveolar oxygen tension is low, shunting it to better ventilated zones and improving the ventilation–perfusion ratio. (Elsewhere in the circulatory system, hypoxia always results in the vasodilatation of vascular beds.)
- **Significance:** HPV is of little importance in health, but it is more significant in disease. It explains, for example, the upper lobe diversion characteristic of left ventricular failure, as blood in the congested and hypoxaemic lower parts of the lung is diverted away. It is significant during one-lung anaesthesia.
- **Response:** the response occurs via the constriction of small arterioles. This is not neurally mediated. It is seen, for example, in denervated lungs (following transplantation). Nor is it mediated by humoral vasoconstrictors but by pulmonary mixed venous oxygenation and, more importantly, by alveolar oxygenation. Larger blood vessels may be affected globally, as in the fetal pulmonary circulation in which the low PaO_2 reduces pulmonary blood flow to about 15% of the cardiac output.
- **Onset:** this is within seconds of the decrease in PaO_2, and lobar blood flow may halve within minutes from its value during normoxia. The phenomenon is biphasic, with the vascular resistance returning almost to baseline before the onset of a second phase of slower and sustained vasoconstriction that reaches a plateau at 40 minutes.
- **Mediators:** the mechanisms have not been fully identified. The pulmonary vasculature is maintained in a state of active vasodilatation to which nitric oxide may contribute, and so suppression of endothelial nitric oxide production will lead to vasoconstriction. In addition, hypoxia stimulates production of endothelin. It is

also known that pulmonary blood vessels have oxygen-sensitive potassium channels such that the membrane potential alters in response to hypoxia, with opening of calcium channels and smooth muscle contraction. This phenomenon is not seen in the systemic vasculature.

- **Influences:** acidosis and hypercarbia potentiate HPV, while alkalosis either attenuates or abolishes it and causes pulmonary vasodilatation.

Direction the viva may take
You may be asked about the influence of anaesthesia on HPV.

- **Anaesthesia:** all inhalational anaesthetics inhibit HPV. The effect is dose-dependent and is similar for all the agents apart from nitrous oxide, whose action is less potent. The dose–response curve is of typical sigmoid shape; the ED_{50} is just under 2 MAC, and the ED_{90} is around 3 MAC. At 1.3 MAC, HPV is diminished by around 30%. Intravenous induction agents have little effect.
- **Oxygen:** a high FiO_2 may inhibit HPV by maintaining higher PaO_2 even in underventilated alveoli.
- **Cardiac output:** any factor which depresses cardiac output will reduce mixed venous PO_2 and so may enhance HPV.
- **Drug effects:** drugs such as calcium-channel blockers, sodium nitroprusside, glyceryl trinitrate, bronchodilators, nitric oxide and dobutamine all attenuate HPV. It is potentiated by cyclo-oxygenase inhibitors, propranolol and by the respiratory stimulant almitrine. (This is not used in the UK, but acts by stimulating carotid body chemoreceptors. It also enhances the effect of HPV in situations in which it is deficient.)

Intracranial pressure

Commentary
There are several variations on this question about intracranial pressure (ICP). The viva may concentrate on ICP itself or divert to include the concept of cerebral perfusion pressure (CPP), or the protection of the brain against hypoxic or ischaemic brain injury. The diagnosis and rational management of raised ICP are important and so you will need to know about basic underlying mechanisms.

The viva
You may be asked about the clinical features of raised ICP.

- **Symptoms:** these depend on whether the ICP rise is acute or chronic. Typically, patients complain of headache, nausea and vomiting. These symptoms are worse in the morning both because of increased hydrostatic pressure effects and because the $PaCO_2$ may be raised. Patients may have changes in level of consciousness and visual disturbances (see below).

- **Signs:** patients may exhibit neurological signs caused by brain distortion or by one of the brain herniation syndromes (see below), including pupillary changes and failure of upward gaze. There may be papilloedema, hypertension, bradycardia and abnormal respiration. These last three constitute Cushing's triad.
- **Cerebral herniation:** several syndromes have been described, including central, cingulate and uncal herniation.
  — **Central herniation:** in this situation (which is the most important), the raised ICP forces the brain downwards through the foramen magnum as the cerebellar tonsils herniate and compress the medulla. This is known colloquially as 'coning'.
  — **Cingulate herniation:** the cingulate gyrus and part of the hemisphere are displaced beneath the falx cerebri. This primarily affects the anterior cerebral vessels.
  — **Uncal herniation:** the uncus (which is part of the hippocampal gyrus) herniates through, and is then compressed against, the tentorium.

Specific clinical signs (ICP can rise without these)

- **Cushing's reflex:** the triad comprises hypertension, bradycardia and abnormal respiration. This is a late and ominous sign that coning is imminent, as the carotid body receptors attempt to mediate an increase in perfusion pressure that is doomed to fail.
- **Pupillary signs:** these may follow uncal compression or kinking of the oculomotor nerve by distorted vessels. There is ipsilateral pupillary dilatation followed by motor paralysis of the extraocular muscles (excluding the superior oblique and lateral rectus muscles which are supplied by the fourth and sixth cranial nerves, respectively).
- **Eye signs:** the lateral rectus is also affected because of the displacement of the sixth cranial nerve (abducens), which has a long intracranial course. As it leaves the posterior margin of the pons, it is crossed by the anterior inferior cerebellar artery. Displacement of the cerebellum may distort these vessels such that they compress the abducens nerve. The clinical effect of such compression is failure of lateral gaze.

Direction the viva may take

You will be asked about the factors that may influence ICP.

- The skull of an adult is in effect a rigid box which contains brain tissue, blood and CSF. The brain itself has minimal compressibility and so there is very limited scope for compensation. An increase in the volume of one component invariably results in an increase in ICP unless the volume of another component decreases. (This is the Monroe–Kellie hypothesis.) These intracranial contents comprise brain tissue (1400–1500 g), blood (100–150 ml), CSF (110–120 ml) and extracellular fluid (<100 ml). The intracranial compliance curve is shown in Figure 3.8.
- Normal ICP is 10–12 mmHg. Any increase may be significant because of the potential impact upon cerebral perfusion. The CPP is determined by mean arterial pressure (MAP) minus the sum of the central venous pressure (CVP) and the ICP. $CPP = MAP - (CVP + ICP)$.
- **Mass lesions:** ICP is raised by mass lesions which increase the volume of brain, bone or meninges. These include tumours of all three structures, as well as infection (with abscess formation).

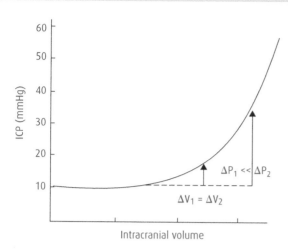

Fig. 3.8 Intracranial pressure–volume curve.

- **Volume increases:** ICP is raised by conditions which increase non-CSF fluid volume. Intracranial aneurysm, arteriovenous malformation and trauma are all relatively common causes of subarachnoid or subdural haemorrhage. ICP is raised by cerebral oedema, which itself has many causes, including trauma, infection, metabolic dysfunction (such as hepatic encephalopathy or Reye's syndrome), hypoxia, venous obstruction and increased hydrostatic pressure (such as is caused by a steep or prolonged Trendelenberg position on the operating table). It may also be idiopathic, as in benign intracranial hypertension. This is a clinical entity defined by an ICP greater than 15 mmHg (but which can reach three times that figure) in the presence of normal CSF composition, normal conscious level and with no evident pathological process. It may be caused by a rise in intracranial venous pressure which is offset by intracranial and CSF pressure increases that restore the required gradient for CSF absorption into the venous system. Some cases can be managed with corticosteroids, diuretics and acetazolamide, but severe cases may require the insertion of a lumbo(thecal)–peritoneal shunt.
- **Impaired drainage:** ICP is also raised by conditions which impede drainage of CSF (which is produced at $0.4\,\mathrm{ml\,min^{-1}}$) and thus increase its intracranial volume. These include congenital and acquired hydrocephalus, which may also be associated with trauma, tumour or infection. A blocked ventricular shunt is another important cause.
- **Pathophysiology:** in the presence of raised ICP, CPP is given by MAP − ICP. Perfusion will be maintained until CPP starts to fall below 50 mmHg, with the onset of critical ischaemia at 30–40 mmHg. There may also be focal ischaemia in the region of a mass lesion. Raised ICP attenuates cerebral autoregulation to the point at which it is lost completely, after which cerebral blood flow follows MAP passively.

Further direction the viva may take

You may be asked about the management of raised ICP.

Management

- Moderate head-up position will reduce venous pressure without unduly affecting the MAP (provided there is no physical constriction to drainage by artefacts such as tracheal tube tapes). Moderate hypocapnia will reduce ICP, but the benefit is short-lived, and there is a risk of rebound hyperaemia. Mannitol 20% in a dose of $0.5 \, \text{g} \, \text{kg}^{-1}$ has a marked but transient effect. It may shift the patient back down the intracranial compliance curve and gain sufficient time for definitive treatment before a catastrophic rise in ICP (Figure 3.8), but it too is associated with rebound hypertension. If the blood–brain barrier is affected, mannitol may also cross into brain parenchyma and exert a reverse osmotic effect. High-dose dexamethasone reduces oedema secondary to intracranial tumours, but has no effect on raised ICP following trauma. It is important to avoid hyperthermia, which will increase the cerebral metabolic rate for oxygen ($CMRO_2$) and cerebral blood flow. Hypothermia has the opposite effect and may confer some benefit.
- ICP can be measured by subdural or extradural transducers or via an intraventricular catheter. All these methods are invasive, requiring a burr hole, but they allow quantification of CPP.

Further direction the viva could take

You may be asked finally about CSF. This could form a question on its own, and would be linked to the topic of postdural puncture headache and its management (page 85).

- **Formation:** its total volume is around 150 ml, about 80% of which is intracranial. Most of the extracranial (spinal) CSF is found distal to the conus medullaris. The choroid arterial plexuses form CSF either by secretion or by the quantitatively much less significant process of ultrafiltration. It is produced in the lateral, third and fourth ventricles, at a rate of around $0.4 \, \text{ml} \, \text{min}^{-1}$ ($575 \, \text{ml} \, 24 \, \text{h}^{-1}$). The rate of production is constant and is not related to ICP unless it is sufficiently high to compromise CPP and reduce blood flow to the choroid plexus.
- **Circulation:** CSF passes through the cerebral aqueduct to the fourth ventricle and thence through the midline foramen of Magendie and the two lateral foramina of Luschka to communicate with the subarachnoid space of the brain and spinal cord. It is either absorbed directly into cerebral venules (10%) or absorbed by the arachnoid villi (90%).
- **Functions:** it has a cushioning effect which protects the brain from injury. Supported by CSF, the effective cerebral weight is only 50g. CSF can partly buffer increases in ICP by translocation from the intracranial to the extracranial subarachnoid space.
- **Composition:** it has a higher PCO_2 than plasma and a lower pH (7.33). The mean specific gravity is 1.006, with a range of 1.003 to 1.009. Its protein content is low (0.2 $g \, l^{-1}$), so buffering capacity is negligible. Glucose concentration is lower than in plasma. Sodium and chloride are higher, while potassium is lower (40%). This is because the formation of CSF requires the active transport of Na^+, Cl^- and K^+ into the ventricles. Further Na^+ is then added in exchange for K^+ (mediated by Na^+/K^+ ATPase). The influx is maintained by the further exchange of H^+ and HCO_3^- for Na^+ and Cl^-. H^+ and HCO_3^- are generated from H_2CO_3 in a reaction catalysed by carbonic anhydrase.
- **Factors affecting rate of production:** acetazolamide, which is a carbonic anhydrase inhibitor, may reduce CSF production by as much as 50%. High-dose diuretics also

reduce it by affecting the sodium transport process. Corticosteroids may increase production, but not consistently enough to make them a reliable treatment for postdural puncture headache.

Cerebral blood flow

Commentary

This is a standard question which has obvious relevance for general anaesthesia, for head injury, for techniques such as induced hypotension and for anaesthesia in patients with hypertensive disorders, including pre-eclampsia.

The viva

You will be asked about the factors which influence cerebral blood flow.

- The brain weighs 2% of the human organism yet receives 15% of the cardiac output. The intracranial contents consist of brain tissue (approximately 1400–1500 g), blood (100–150 ml), CSF (110–120 ml) and extracellular fluid (<100 ml).
- **Normal cerebral bloodflow (CBF):** normal CBF is 50 ml 100 g^{-1} of brain tissue per minute, and is determined by the CPP. The CPP = MAP – (CVP + ICP) (page 371). The normal CPP is 70–80 mmHg. Blood flow to grey matter is more than twice that to white matter.
- **Autoregulation:** over a wide range of MAP, typically between 50 and 150 mmHg, autoregulation maintains normal flow. The process is not instantaneous, and may take some seconds to complete. The classic cerebral autoregulation curve is an oversimplification: there is not a neat linear relationship between MAP and CBF at each end of the curve, and changes in perfusion pressure may be regional. Chronic hypertension shifts the autoregulatory curve to the right; drug-induced hypotension shifts it to the left (Figure 3.9). The mechanisms which underlie

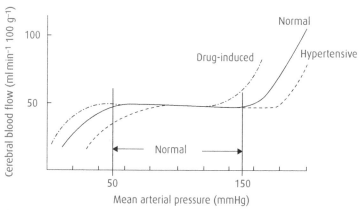

Fig. 3.9 Cerebral autoregulation.

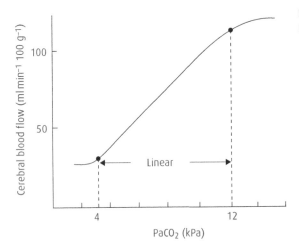

Fig. 3.10 Cerebral blood flow and $PaCO_2$.

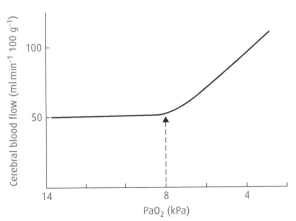

Fig. 3.11 Cerebral blood flow and PaO_2.

autoregulation are primarily myogenic, modulated by stretch receptors in vascular smooth muscle, and metabolic, in which hydrogen ions and substances such as nitric oxide and adenosine accumulate in the tissues at low flow and mediate vasodilatation.

- **$PaCO_2$:** there is a linear relationship between $PaCO_2$ and CBF in the range of partial pressures from 3.5 to 10.0 kPa. Below 3.5 kPa, cerebral vasoconstriction leads to tissue hypoxia (with subsequent reflex vasodilatation); at around 10.0–12.0 kPa there is a ceiling at which blood flow is maximal (at around 120 ml 100 g^{-1} min^{-1}) (Figure 3.10).
- **PaO_2:** decreases in the partial pressure of oxygen below 8 kPa are associated with sharp increases in CBF up to around 110 ml 100 g^{-1} min^{-1}. At 4.0 kPa, CBF is doubled. Hyperoxia is associated with decreases in CBF (Figure 3.11).

- **Temperature:** changes in temperature are associated with altered requirements for cerebral oxygen (the cerebral metabolic rate for oxygen, $CMRO_2$), although the relationship is not linear but exponential. Thus, while at 37°C a 1°C drop in temperature is accompanied by a fall in $CMRO_2$ of 6–7%, at a brain temperature of 15°C (during deep hypothermic circulatory arrest, for example), a further 1°C drop results in a decrease in $CMRO_2$ of only 1%.
- **$CMRO_2$:** CBF is linked to $CMRO_2$ by a mechanism that has not yet been fully elucidated. There is a short lag time of 1–2 minutes.
- **Rheology:** lower plasma viscosity is associated with enhanced capillary flow, although there is a balance between optimal rheology and oxygen delivery. A haematocrit above 50% risks intravascular sludging and a reduction in CBF, while a haematocrit below 30% is associated with decreased oxygen flux.
- **ICP:** The formula for CPP confirms that CBF is compromised by increases in ICP from its normal 10–12 mmHg (page 143).

Direction the viva may take

You may be asked how you would measure cerebral flow.

- **Kety–Schmidt method:** this is an application of the Fick principle, which states that flow is equal to the amount of a substance taken up or excreted by an organ, divided by the arteriovenous (AV) concentration difference. (Hence CBF = Quantity of substance taken up by the brain/AV difference.) Nitrous oxide is used as the diffusible tracer. The subject breathes 10% N_2O for 10 minutes, during which time paired peripheral arterial and jugular venous bulb samples are taken. At the end of 10 minutes the concentrations are equal, at which point the venous concentration is the same as brain. The speed at which the arterial and venous curves equilibrate is a measure of N_2O delivery to the brain. The technique is invasive and gives only a global measure of flow. It is not a technique for clinical use.
- **Transcranial Doppler ultrasonography:** this gives a measure of the velocity of red cells flowing through large cerebral arteries, most commonly the middle cerebral, and can be used in clinical practice. The velocity can give an index of flow provided that the diameter of the artery is determined independently, and provided that this diameter changes little (as is the case with the major cerebral arteries).
- **Positron emission tomography (PET):** this (research) technique monitors the uptake by different areas of the brain of 2-deoxyglucose, which is labelled with a positron emitter.
- **Scintillography and SPECT scanning:** these techniques use radioactive xenon to trace regional blood flow, with or without enhancement by CT or MR imaging.

Further direction the viva could take

You may be asked what effect anaesthesia has on CBF.

- **Intravenous induction agents:** all except for ketamine reduce $CMRO_2$ and as a result CBF falls in tandem. Autoregulation is not affected. Ketamine increases MAP which leads to a rise in blood flow.

- **Volatile anaesthetic agents:** these uncouple CBF and $CMRO_2$. They reduce $CMRO_2$ but are associated with a rise in CBF secondary to their capacity to vasodilate the cerebral circulation and abolish autoregulation. The response to changes in $PaCO_2$ is unchanged. This action is dose-dependent but can partly be offset by the vasoconstrictor effect of hyperventilation. Autoregulation is abolished by 1.5 MAC of all the agents bar sevoflurane. This has only 30% of the vasodilatory potential of isoflurane and does not impair autoregulation. Nitrous oxide increases CBF by increasing the $CMRO_2$, while also affecting autoregulatory mechanisms.
- **Opiates:** opiates have little direct effect, but CBF will rise in response to CO_2 retention should respiratory drive be depressed.
- **Arterial pressure:** chronic hypertension shifts the autoregulatory curve to the right, while drug-induced hypotension shifts it to the left (Figure 3.9). If autoregulation is attenuated by the use of volatile anaesthetics, then CBF and ICP will rise in parallel with an increase in MAP.
- **Venous pressure:** Any of the many factors which increase venous pressure, such as position, coughing, straining against a ventilator, impeded drainage from the head and neck, volume overload, or the use of IPPV and PEEP, will decrease CPP and reduce CBF.
- **Steal and inverse steal:** there will be focal areas of injured brain in which autoregulation is lost, while elsewhere it is retained. Cerebral vasodilatation may further compromise these areas by diverting blood away ('cerebral steal'); conversely, the vasoconstriction associated with hyperventilation may divert blood from normal to damaged brain, where vasoconstrictor responses have been lost ('inverse steal').

Intraocular pressure

Commentary

Successful intraocular surgery requires a still, soft and quiet eye. Attention to the principles outlined below should allow you to satisfy the examiners that you can provide this safely. However, remember that theory is not always mirrored by practice. Cataract surgeons will operate uncomplainingly on a patient breathing spontaneously through a laryngeal mask airway whose high end-tidal CO_2 should in theory raise intraocular pressure (IOP) to the point at which surgery is impossible. Your considered clinical answers can reflect this reality, and if you do suggest that general anaesthesia for cataract surgery in the elderly should involve high-dose opiates and IPPV to hypocarbia you may not prosper.

The viva

You may be asked first about the principles of emergency anaesthesia in a patient with a penetrating eye injury. This is a standard question which seems to have been around since exams began, but it is a means of establishing whether you understand the basic concepts of IOP.

- Anaesthesia for a patient with a penetrating eye injury involves balancing the risks of pulmonary aspiration of gastric contents against the risks of causing a rise in IOP that may further threaten sight. (The possibility of failed intubation is another consideration.) Assuming that the procedure is a surgical emergency and that the patient is not fasted there are two main problems: the first is the use of suxamethonium and the second is the rise in IOP that may accompany laryngoscopy and tracheal intubation.
  — **Suxamethonium:** this causes a transient increase in IOP (see below) and in theory therefore should be avoided. In practice, there are no published reports of further eye damage associated with its use under these circumstances. However, most anaesthetists would prefer an alternative for rapid sequence induction, and high-dose rocuronium ($0.9\,mg\,kg^{-1}$) will provide satisfactory conditions for intubation within 60 seconds.
  — **Laryngoscopy:** the sympathetic response to laryngoscopy also increases IOP (see below). Many different methods have been described for attenuating this pressor response and if you try to embark on a detailed account of these then the examiner will almost certainly move you on. However, you may be asked to give one or two examples. The long list of possible techniques includes pre-treatment with a β-adrenoceptor blocker, high-dose intravenous induction agent, nebulized lignocaine or intravenous lignocaine ($2\,mg\,kg^{-1}$), topical local anaesthetic to the hypopharynx, intravenous opiate (such as alfentanil $20–40\,\mu g\,kg^{-1}$ or remifentanil $1\,\mu g\,kg^{-1}$), and clonidine ($5\,\mu g\,kg^{-1}$).

Direction the viva will take

You will already have discussed some anaesthetic aspects of IOP during the clinical discussion but you will be asked in more detail about its prime determinants.

- **Definition:** IOP is the pressure exerted by the contents of the globe on the scleral envelope that encloses them. Normal pressure is quoted as $16\pm5\,mmHg$.
- **Choroidal blood volume:** the choroid is a thin, but dense, capillary plexus which covers most of the posterior chamber of the globe. It also contains small arteries and veins. Autoregulation maintains blood flow over a wide range of pressures and only acute large rises in systolic blood pressure affect choroidal blood volume (CBV). It rises in response to elevations of venous pressure and is also very sensitive to increases in $PaCO_2$ and to hypoxia. Hypocarbia reduces CBV and also inhibits carbonic anhydrase.
- **Aqueous humour:** the production and drainage of aqueous humour are in dynamic equilibrium. Aqueous is produced under the influence of carbonic anhydrase, and is secreted via the ciliary processes in the posterior chamber. It circulates freely through into the anterior chamber before draining through spaces in the trabecular meshwork (the spaces of Fontana) to the canal of Schlemm. This drainage can be affected by increases in venous pressure or by any decrease in the area of the trabecular spaces. This is one of the mechanisms underlying chronic open-angle

glaucoma. Relaxation of the iris can narrow the iridocorneal angle and impair drainage. In subjects in whom this angle is already narrow the use of mydriatics can precipitate acute ('narrow-angle') glaucoma (see Figure 2.12). Drainage can be restored by constricting the pupil with miotic drugs such as pilocarpine and carbachol.

- **Central venous pressure:** this rises acutely (to as much as 40 mmHg) with coughing, straining, retching and the Valsalva manoeuvre. Other precipitants include head-down posture, obstruction to venous drainage from the head and neck, hypervolaemia, breathing against a ventilator and the use of IPPV and PEEP. This increase in pressure both reduces aqueous drainage and also increases CBV.
- **Extrinsic compression:** IOP rises as a result of direct extrinsic pressure on the globe, caused, for example, by retrobulbar haemorrhage or by undue pressure on the eye when a patient is anaesthetized in the prone position.
- **Extraocular muscle tone:** any increase (such as is caused by a depolarizing muscle relaxant) is reflected in a rise in IOP; otherwise this is not a significant component.

Further direction the viva may take

The viva may then move on to the anaesthetic implications of IOP.

- **Laryngoscopy and tracheal intubation:** if measures are not taken to obtund the sympathetic responses to laryngoscopy, the IOP can rise by 20 mmHg or more.
- **Drugs used in anaesthesia:** all intravenous anaesthetic agents except ketamine will reduce IOP, as will inhalational agents, assuming that the $PaCO_2$ is not allowed to rise. Etomidate can cause myoclonus and so should probably be avoided. Involuntary extraocular muscle contraction associated with suxamethonium transiently increases IOP by around 10 mmHg. In addition, the fine muscle intraocular muscle fibres demonstrate tonic contraction which lasts as long as the neuromuscular block. (The rise in IOP is not purely mechanistic; an increase is seen even if the four recti muscles have been sectioned.)
- **Nitrous oxide:** N_2O will diffuse into gas-filled spaces, and this will include the eye if the vitreous has been replaced by a gas such as sulphur hexafluoride (SF_6). N_2O is over 100 times more diffusible than SF_6 and enters the vitreal cavity, thus increasing gas volume and IOP.
- **The open eye:** when the eye is open (either surgically or due to trauma) the IOP is lower than normal and so the transluminal pressure on the choroidal vessels is greater. This means that any sudden increase in pressure in the choroidal circulation may be associated by prolapse of intraocular structures such as the iris and the lens, or by expulsive haemorrhage with almost certain loss of vision. Anaesthetic techniques should be such as to minimize this risk.
- **Drugs used to lower IOP:** these work mainly by reducing aqueous humour formation and include topical β-adrenoceptor blockers such as timolol, and systemic carbonic anhydrase inhibitors such as acetazolamide. Dorzolamide and brinzolamide are also sulphonamide derivative carbonic anhydrase inhibitors, but both can be used topically.

The neuromuscular junction

Commentary

If you are asked about the neuromuscular junction it is almost inevitable that the viva will include questions about neuromuscular blockers and the assessment of neuro-muscular blockade. If, on the other hand, you are asked about either of the two latter topics you may not be required to discuss the neuromuscular junction in any detail. It is for this reason that the account below is somewhat simplified. The subject may be introduced by a discussion about disorders affecting neuromuscular transmission.

The viva

You may be asked about myasthenia gravis and related disorders. None is common, except perhaps in medical exams.

- **Myasthenia gravis:** this is an autoimmune disease in which antibodies are formed to the postjunctional acetylcholine (ACh) receptor. (This is a simplification but will suffice for this exam.) The resulting decrease in the population of effective receptors means that muscles fatigue rapidly on repetitive exertion. Clinically, this can be demonstrated by asking a patient to chew gum; the muscles of mastication do not fatigue in normal individuals. Electromyographic stimulation of myasthenic patients will reveal fade.

- **Anaesthetic considerations:** patients may clinically be weak and postoperative ventilatory support may be required in as many as 30% of subjects. Myasthenic patients demonstrate some resistance to depolarizing neuromuscular blockers, but a dose of suxamethonium $2\,mg\,kg^{-1}$ will allow good conditions for intubation. Acute sensitivity to the effects of non-depolarizing blockers means that initial doses should be around one-tenth of normal. In practice, combinations of drugs such as propofol and remifentanil mean that muscle relaxants can usually be avoided.

- **Crises:** a myasthenic crisis, which can be precipitated by various physical and emotional stresses or which can be spontaneous, is manifest by an exacerbation of symptoms severe enough to cause respiratory failure. A cholinergic crisis is pre-cipitated by an overdose of anticholinesterase. In addition to stimulating muscarinic receptors, the excess ACh acts as a neuromuscular blocker at the diminished number of receptors, thereby leading to muscle weakness and respiratory compromise. Edrophonium, which is a short-acting anticholinesterase with effects which last for about 5 minutes, will transiently improve a myasthenic, and transiently worsen a cholinergic, crisis.

- **Eaton–Lambert syndrome:** in around two-thirds of cases this condition is associated with malignancy, classically with bronchogenic carcinoma. It appears to reduce the number of pre-synaptic quanta of ACh that are released (possibly by antibodies to voltage-gated calcium channels and to the associated protein synaptotagmin), but the post-synaptic membrane sensitivity is normal. Unlike myasthenia gravis, the muscle weakness improves with activity; however, these patients are acutely sensitive to the effects both of depolarizing and non-depolarizing muscle relaxants.

Direction the viva will take

You will then be asked about the generation of a muscle action potential.

- ACh is formed in the motor nerve terminal (by the acetylation of choline, catalysed by choline-O-acetyltransferase). Much of the synthesized ACh is stored in vesicles containing around 10 000 molecules and which lie just within the axonal prejunctional membrane.
- ACh release is triggered by the motor nerve action potential. In response to depolarization, voltage-gated channels permit an inward flux of calcium which stimulates release into the junctional gap. (This itself is complex, involving the activation of a number of improbably named proteins which facilitate the process: synaptotagmin, syntaxins, synaptophysin and synaptobrevin. Synaptobrevin is of passing interest because it is inhibited by botulinum toxin which thereby prevents ACh release and muscle contraction.)
- Prejunctional nicotinic cholinergic receptors modulate further ACh mobilization and release via a positive feedback mechanism.
- ACh acts at the postjunctional nicotinic receptor, whose structure has been fully identified. It consists of five glycoprotein subunits characterized as α (2), β, δ and ε which form a central ionophore (ion channel). Binding of one molecule of ACh to one of the two α units facilitates the binding of a second, during which the receptor undergoes an evanescent conformational change and the ionophore opens. A net influx of sodium ions then depolarizes the muscle cell membrane.
- The ACh in the cleft will interact with an α unit only once before being broken down within 100 μsec by the acetylcholinesterase in the junctional folds of the muscle membrane.

Direction the viva may take

You may be asked about the action of neuromuscular blocking agents (pages 209 and 211).

- **Structures:** all are quaternary amines, whose potency is increased if the molecule contains two quaternary ammonium radicals. (Pancuronium is bisquaternary whereas vecuronium is monoquaternary.)
- **Depolarizing block:** suxamethonium is the only therapeutic depolarizing neuromuscular blocker, but agonists at nicotinic cholinergic receptors can have a similar effect. Anticholinesterases given in the absence of non-depolarizing block, for example, may themselves cause blockade. Following depolarization of the muscle membrane, suxamethonium remains bound to the receptor for some minutes, during which time muscle action potentials are prevented.
- **Phase II block:** this is a postjunctional non-depolarizing ion channel block which accompanies the prolonged action or accumulation of suxamethonium. The block is also characterized by impairment of prejunctional PCh release. This probably explains why anticholinesterases may reverse the block, although the advice to do so is not universal.
- **Non-depolarizing block:** non-depolarizing blockers are competitive inhibitors of ACh at the postjunctional nicotinic receptors. They bind to one or both of the α units to prevent ACh access, but they induce no conformational change in the

receptor. Receptor occupancy needs to be at least 80%, depending on the surgery that is planned, and it is important to recognize that the sensitivity of muscle groups is very different. The pattern appears to be the same across all mammalian species such that the muscles of facial expression, including the ocular muscles, and the muscles of the distal limb (including the tail) are much more sensitive than the diaphragm. Thus only 20% receptor blockade is sufficient to paralyse the tibialis anterior muscle, whereas the diaphragm requires 90%.

Further direction the viva could take

You are likely to be asked to describe how neuromuscular block may be assessed.

- **Clinical signs:** grip strength, the generation of a tidal volume of between 15 and 20 $ml\,kg^{-1}$, the ability to keep the head lifted from the pillow for 5 seconds, and the capacity to retain a tongue depressor gripped between the teeth are cited as useful indicators of recovery from neuromuscular block.
- **Nerve stimulators:** the degree of block can be assessed using a battery-operated nerve stimulator that is capable of delivering different patterns of square wave pulses of uniform amplitude. The stimulus that is delivered should be supramaximal to ensure recruitment of all the muscle fibres. The stimulus is usually transcutaneous.
- **Single twitch:** a decrease in twitch height will be apparent only after 75% or more receptors are blocked, so this is of limited use in monitoring non-depolarizing block. It can be used for assessing block caused by depolarizing relaxants (which do not exhibit fade or post-tetanic facilitation).
- **Train-of-four (TOF):** four identical stimuli are delivered at 2 Hz and repeated every 10 seconds. The number of twitches observed corresponds approximately to the percentage receptor blockade. (0 twitches = 100% blockade; 1 twitch = 90%; 2 twitches = 80%; 3 twitches = 75%; 4 twitches = <75%). The ratio of twitch heights can be quantified to give an objective measure of block. The $T_4:T_1$ ratio must be 90% before it can be assumed that protective airway reflexes are intact.
- **Double burst stimulation (DBS):** two tetanic bursts at 50 Hz and separated by 750 ms are applied every 20 ms. The muscle response is detectable as two twitches which show a more exaggerated fade than that of the TOF. DBS is more sensitive at detecting residual block, which makes it of particular value at the end of surgery.
- **Tetanic stimulation:** stimuli of 50 or 100 Hz for 5 seconds may produce fade in situations when the twitch response after TOF or DBS has returned to normal. It is therefore a more sensitive means of detecting low levels of receptor blockade. It cannot be used in the conscious patient who may be aware of marked residual discomfort even if the stimulus has been applied during anaesthesia.
- **Post-tetanic count (PTC):** a tetanic stimulus as above is followed by single stimuli at 1-second intervals. Tetany triggers supranormal Ach release (post-tetanic facilitation) which transiently overcomes the neuromuscular blockade. The twitches which result comprise the PTC. The technique is used to monitor significant degrees of block (for example, in neurosurgery during which any patient movement could be disastrous), and a PTC of less than 5 indicates profound block. A PTC of greater than 15 approximates to two twitches following TOF stimulation, at which point pharmacological reversal should be possible.

- **Mechanomyography, electromyography and acceleromyography:** these methods allow much more accurate measurement of neuromuscular blockade during onset and offset of effect. Whether or not such (expensive) accuracy is necessary during routine clinical practice remains contentious, but at present these instruments are used mainly in research, and details of their function will not be expected of you.

Physiological changes of late pregnancy relevant to general anaesthesia

Commentary

This is not designed to be a question about general anaesthesia for caesarean section, but as few other surgical procedures are performed at or around term, it will be a difficult subject to avoid. However, the examiners will initially try to do so, which will free you to take a standard systems approach to the subject. As all anaesthetists in training are exposed regularly to obstetric anaesthesia you will be expected to have a good understanding of its principles and practice.

The viva

You will be asked about the changes in late pregnancy pertinent to general anaesthesia. A discussion of the various systems is an appropriate start. Most of the information is little more than a list and you will be unlikely to cover any single aspect in great detail.

- **Cardiovascular system:** during pregnancy there is a total weight gain that averages 12 kg. Half of this is accounted for by an increase in plasma volume and interstitial fluid. Plasma volume increases by up to 40% and total body water by around 7–8 Litres. This volume loading is associated with mild cardiac dilatation, and so heart murmurs (for example, that of mitral regurgitation) are common. Cardiac output increases by 40–45% to near maximal at 32 weeks' gestation. The resting heart rate increases by 15% and tachyarrhythmias are more common. The ECG shows left axis deviation caused by mechanical displacement by the gravid uterus, and minor T wave and ST segment changes may be seen. Blood pressure falls, with the diastolic drop of 10–15 mmHg making a bigger contribution than the systolic, and there is a decrease in systemic vascular resistance. There is reduced sensitivity to circulating vasopressors, although it appears that the uterine circulation may be more sensitive to these than the systemic.
  - *Aortocaval compression (supine hypotension syndrome):* this is important. Compression by the gravid uterus of the great vessels affects mainly venous return, but it can also compromise aortic flow. Symptoms of decreased venous return occur in at least 10–15% of mothers. The problem is attenuated by the use of a wedge or by lateral tilt, but there are some women in whom only the full lateral position will prevent hypotension. The uteroplacental unit does not autoregulate and so blood flow is crucially dependent on the pressure gradient.

— *Anaesthetic implications*: there must be careful positioning to avoid aortocaval compression. Cardiac output and systemic blood pressure must be maintained to ensure continued perfusion of the uteroplacental unit, but equally the anaesthetist must be aware of the consequences of fluid-loading a mother who is effectively waterlogged already.

- **Respiratory system:** some of the data are contentious and much is based on older studies of small numbers of subjects, which are unlikely ever to be repeated. There is an increase in minute volume by 40% at term, but this is initiated early in pregnancy when progesterone-induced hyperventilation reduces $PaCO_2$ by around 1 kPa. This is associated with a mild respiratory alkalosis. This would shift the oxygen–haemoglobin dissociation curve downwards and to the left were it not for an increase in maternal 2,3-DPG which offsets this effect. Increased metabolic demand for oxygen increases by around 50%, along with an increase in the work of breathing and a decrease in both chest wall and lung compliance. The increased demand for oxygen is more than compensated by the increase in cardiac output and so there is a small rise in PaO_2 of about 1 kPa. There are anatomical changes which influence the upper airway: general fluid retention and oedema of pregnancy may complicate laryngoscopy and intubation. With regard to pulmonary volumes, the most important change is the 20% decrease in FRC, which, by the third trimester, may fall in the supine position to half its predicted value.

  — *Anaesthetic implications:* the FRC must be filled with oxygen prior to induction to minimize risk of desaturation. This can be achieved either by pre-oxygenating the mother for 3 minutes with 100% O_2, or by asking her to take three vital capacity breaths. Slight head-up position will reduce encroachment of the closing volume on the FRC. The reduced FRC means that the onset of the effect of volatile anaesthetic agents will be more rapid.

  — Relative hyperventilation and low normal $PaCO_2$ should be maintained, although it is not until the $PaCO_2$ falls below about 2.7–3.3 kPa (20–25 mmHg) that uterine blood flow is compromised.

  — The congested and more oedematous upper airway may be traumatized during instrumentation. A smaller tracheal tube (7.0) may be required.

- **Gastrointestinal system:** by the third trimester some 70% of mothers have symptoms of gastro-oesophageal reflux and heartburn. Oesophageal barrier pressure decreases with the loss of lower oesophageal sphincter tone, and there is also a fall in intestinal transit time and some duodenal gastric reflux. Gastric emptying itself, however, is not delayed in late pregnancy. Gastric residual volumes are increased, as is placental gastrin secretion. Whether this translates into maternal gastric hyperacidity remains disputed.

  — *Anaesthetic implications:* the airway must be protected against the risk of pulmonary aspiration of gastric contents by antacid prophylaxis (H_2 antagonists, proton pump inhibitors and sodium citrate). Effective cricoid pressure applied during a rapid sequence induction is also essential.

- **CNS:** under the influence of progesterone and endogenous β-endorphins, the MAC of anaesthetic agents decreases by about one-third, and there is an increased sensitivity to all drugs which act centrally. (Requirements for local anaesthetics also decrease, which may be related to an increased availability of free drug and to hormonally enhanced neural sensitivity.)

— *Anaesthetic implications*: reduction in the doses of anaesthetic agents, sedatives and analgesics may be possible. Interpatient variability, however, is so great that it would be unwise to assume that anaesthetic awareness or severe postoperative pain are less likely.

- **Musculoskeletal system:** pregnancy increases ligamentous laxity owing to the rises in the hormones progesterone and relaxin. There is also an increased lumbar lordosis which helps to accommodate the enlarging uterus.
  — *Anaesthetic implications*: scrupulous positioning of the patient with appropriate supports and protection may minimize the risk of postoperative backache or other joint problems.

- **Haematological:** pregnancy is a hypercoagulable state. There is an increase in all clotting factors, except for Factor XI, and fibrinolysis is impaired by a plasminogen inhibitor that is derived from the placenta.
  — *Anaesthetic implications*: the risk of venous thromboembolism is increased fivefold and routine preventative measures should be used (page 262). Should a mother have additional risk factors, then pharmacological intervention may be necessary.

- **Metabolic:** there is a 30% fall in the levels of plasma cholinesterase.
  — *Anaesthetic implications*: this fall has the greatest implications for those patients with atypical cholinesterases. It is often claimed that this decrease does not produce a clinically important increase in the duration of suxamethonium. Clinical experience would suggest, however, that the actions of suxamethonium are prolonged in many pregnant patients and that rapid offset with the resumption of spontaneous respiration is by no means guaranteed.

- **Drug handling:** increased renal blood flow and glomerular filtration enhances the clearance of drugs excreted renally. The reduction in maternal albumin may increase the amount of free drug present in plasma, which may enhance its effects.

Direction the viva may take

Discussion of the factors above is likely to take up much of the time available. If you have covered many of the points above then the viva may move on to related topics. Be prepared, for example, to discuss traditional rapid sequence induction and the role of cricoid pressure. Rocuronium has its advocates, particularly with the likely arrival of its reversal agent Sugammadex (possibly in 2008), but there are others who cite the rapidity of suxamethonium's action (up to 35 s quicker) as the prime reason for its continued use in obstetrics. You would be brave to argue against the routine use of cricoid pressure in obstetric anaesthesia. It has often been argued that it is not used commonly in France, but this is something of an urban myth: by 1998 some 88% of French anaesthetists were employing the technique in obstetric general anaesthesia. Certainly, cricoid deformation can make intubation more difficult, but equally the backwards, upwards and rightwards pressure manoeuvre may well improve the view. Take a balanced approach in the discussion, enough to show that you are at least aware of the opposing arguments.

Non-obstetric surgery in the pregnant patient

Commentary

It is not uncommon for pregnant women to require surgery for non-obstetric reasons such as acute appendicitis, torsion of ovarian cysts and trauma. There are implications both for mother and fetus of which anaesthetists should be aware, but the questions in the viva will be predictable. For a mother whose pregnancy is well advanced the anaesthetic considerations are those which apply to caesarean section under general anaesthesia. For a mother in the first trimester the main concerns relate to teratogenesis.

The viva

You will be asked about the implications of anaesthetizing a pregnant woman for non-obstetric surgery.

- Non-obstetric surgery is required in 0.5–2.0% of women (the incidence varies with the survey). Acute appendicitis occurs in 1 in 2000 confinements, and other surgical procedures include ovarian cystectomy and cervical cerclage. Maternal trauma may also necessitate surgery. The anaesthetic considerations vary according to gestational age.

General principles

Maternal safety considerations are as for any general anaesthetic. In respect of the fetus, the timing of surgery should be such as to maximize fetal viability. The techniques used should minimize the risks of teratogenesis or the onset of premature labour, and prevent uterine hypoxia or hypoperfusion. The same principles apply to postoperative analgesia and to fluid and oxygen therapy.

First trimester

- The major concerns are of teratogenesis and of spontaneous abortion. There is very little evidence that any of the long established anaesthetic agents are teratogenic in humans. The teratogenic effects of nitrous oxide have been demonstrated only in rats. The developing fetus is most vulnerable up to 8 weeks' gestational age.
- **Drug effects:** single doses of established agents as used during a general anaesthetic are unlikely to cause problems. Regular NSAIDs should be avoided because of the risk of premature closure of the ductus arteriosus. (Aspirin, however, appears to be safe.)

Later pregnancy

- From about the third trimester of pregnancy the anaesthetic considerations are little different from those which apply to caesarean section. As fetal delivery is not imminent, however, there is less concern about giving drugs such as opiates which might otherwise cause neonatal respiratory depression.
- The general physiological changes are described above (page 156).

- **Summary of anaesthetic considerations:** avoidance of aortocaval compression (significant from around 20 weeks, depending on individual size); maintenance of uteroplacental perfusion; pre-oxygenation prior to induction; airway congestion so consider smaller endotracheal tube; antacid prophylaxis and rapid sequence induction; quicker onset of volatile effect owing to reduced FRC; reduced MAC; ligamentous laxity so care with moving and positioning; and hypercoagulability and increased risk of venous thromboembolism so thromboprophylaxis is indicated. The physiological changes associated with laparoscopic surgery are more marked when superimposed upon the maternal alterations imposed by pregnancy.

Direction the viva may take

You may be asked what you would tell a mother about the risks of damage to the baby.

- **Teratogenesis:** major organogenesis is completed by the eighth week of pregnancy and, although the risk of other malformations persists briefly beyond that period, you could reassure a mother who was 10 weeks into pregnancy that the risks were negligible. Were she to require an anaesthetic in very early pregnancy, you could explain that you would use agents whose risks of causing fetal defects were extremely small. In practice, this would mean using the older agents which have been in long established use.
- **Spontaneous abortion:** the increased risk of miscarriage is also very small, and probably bears no relation to anaesthesia. It is more likely that direct surgical stimulation might provoke premature uterine activity, but in practice this is unusual, even after pelvic surgery. The exception is following cervical cerclage, but in this case it should be the obstetric team rather than the anaesthetist who explains the risks and benefits.

Further direction the viva could take

You may be asked about factors which affect the transfer of drugs across the placenta to the fetus.

- The placenta is in effect a lipid bilayer. Some nutrients cross this membrane by active transport processes, but drugs cross only by passive diffusion.
- Small hydrophilic molecules (up to a molecular weight of around 100) will diffuse across the placenta, but transfer of larger compounds that are poorly lipid-soluble depends largely on the concentration gradient (according to Fick's law of diffusion), on the permeability and on the area available for transfer. Permeability is inversely proportional to molecular weight.
- Lipophilic substances will cross the placenta according to flow-dependent transfer, according to the rate at which they are delivered to the placental circulation.
- Transfer depends on the diffusion gradient, and this in turn is affected by the degree of protein binding and ionization on either side of the membrane. Local

anaesthetics, for example, may concentrate on the fetal side of the circulation, due to ion-trapping. The relative fetal acidaemia increases the proportion of drug in the ionized form, thereby reducing its transfer back across the placental membrane. The same is true of pethidine.

Circulatory changes at birth (congenital heart disease)

Commentary

This is not an area of clinical practice that involves anaesthetists very directly. Although congenital heart disease (CHD) is common, occurring in as many as 1 in 125 live births (the figure is from North American data), most abnormalities are identified early and the problems are referred on to specialist paediatric cardiac teams. Occasionally, patients do present later in life, but it is the applied patho-physiology itself which seems to be of particular interest to examiners, who will want to discover whether or not you understand the principles of rational management.

The viva

You may be asked first about CHD. This is a highly specialized area of practice and so you will not be expected to do more than give one or two examples of acyanotic and cyanotic conditions.

- **Acyanotic:** the commonest conditions are atrial septal defect (ASD), accounting for 5–10% of all congenital lesions, and ventricular septal defect (VSD), occurring in up to 25%. Others include patent ductus arteriosus, coarctation of the aorta, aortic and pulmonary stenosis, and atrioventricular septal defect (AVSD).
- **Cyanotic:** The tetralogy (tetrad) of Fallot is the most frequently occurring cyanotic lesion (10%). Others, such as transposition of the great vessels (5%), hypoplastic left heart syndrome (1–2%), total anomalous pulmonary venous drainage (1%), truncus arteriosus (<1%), tricuspid atresia, hypoplastic right ventricle and Ebstein's anomaly, are much less common. The details of these complex lesions do not matter; what is of importance is the principle that deoxygenated blood bypasses the lungs and shunts directly into the systemic arterial circulation.
- (Some of these terms have been superseded in the specialist literature by a nomenclature that is based on following the blood flow through the heart and on *concordant* (normal) or *discordant* (abnormal) anatomical relations. According to this system, transposition of the great vessels, for example, is described as 'ventriculo-great arterial discordance'. By all means describe CHD in this way if you have this expert knowledge, but be aware that most examiners will still be much more familiar with the traditional terminology.)

Direction the viva will take

You will then be asked in more detail about the transition from the fetal to the neonatal circulation that occurs at birth.

Circulatory changes at birth (Figure 3.12)

- **Fetal circulation:** umbilical venous blood (SpO_2 80%) passes into the IVC (SpO_2 ~67%) via the ductus venosus (which traverses the liver). Most of this blood crosses into the left atrium via the foramen ovale. By the time that this blood reaches the ascending aorta its saturation has fallen but some of this flow is destined for the cerebral circulation and its saturation of around 62% is still higher than that in the ductus arteriosus (50%) and descending aorta (58%). These figures emphasize the fact that the fetus exists in a relatively hypoxic environment. Only about 10% of the cardiac output traverses the pulmonary vascular bed.
- In utero the right and left hearts pump in parallel. There are connections between the systemic and pulmonary circulations via the ductus arteriosus (which links the pulmonary artery to the aorta) and the foramen ovale (which is a communication between the left and right atria). The pulmonary circulation has high resistance and the right and left ventricular pressures are equal, although the right ventricle ejects 66% of the combined ventricular output.

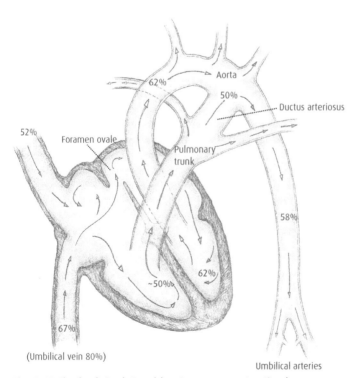

Fig. 3.12 The fetal circulation (showing oxygen saturations).

- With clamping of the umbilical cord there is a sudden rise in systemic vascular resistance (SVR) and aortic pressure.
- Respiration expands the lungs, and pulmonary vascular resistance (PVR) decreases in response to expansion, respiratory movements, increased pH and increased oxygenation. (PVR continues to decrease with recruitment of small arteries, and the reduction over weeks of pulmonary vascular smooth muscle.) Pulmonary blood flow increases. Enhanced pulmonary venous return into the left atrium raises the left atrial pressure above the right, and the foramen ovale closes by a flap valve effect. It is a functional closure which can be reversed if there is a sudden increase in right atrial pressure.
- The increase in left-sided pressure and the fall in right-sided pressures decrease, or even reverse, the shunting through the ductus arteriosus.
- The ductus closes in response to oxygen, to decreasing prostaglandin levels, to bradykinin and acetylcholine. The process takes up to 14 days to complete. It can be accelerated should the duct remain patent by giving a prostaglandin antagonist such as indomethacin. In duct-dependent congenital cardiac disease it is important that the duct should be prevented from closing. Alprostadil (prostaglandin E_1) is the agent of choice. The dose in neonates, should the examiner pursue it this far, is 50–100 nanograms kg^{-1} min^{-1} titrated against effect.

Further direction the viva may take

The practical application of this information may lie in the rational management of children, and later adults, with uncorrected lesions. It is unusual to encounter adults with cyanotic CHD.

Acyanotic CHD

- The main problem in acyanotic heart disease is pulmonary hypertension, which develops as the circulation attempts to 'protect' itself from high pulmonary bloodflows caused by intracardiac left-to-right shunting (for example, through a septal defect) by developing hypertrophy of the media of vascular smooth muscle.
- With progressive disease the resistances in the left and right circulations become finely balanced so that an increase in PVR or a decrease in SVR may reverse the shunt (from left to right, to right to left). This is Eisenmenger's syndrome.
- **Principles of anaesthesia:** rises in PVR or falls in SVR must be avoided.
  — *PVR:* the resistance in the hyperreactive pulmonary vascular tree is increased by hypoxia, hypercapnia, acidosis, nitrous oxide and catecholamine release.
  — *SVR:* this is decreased by various factors, among them sympathetic block, most forms of general anaesthesia, some anti-hypertensive drugs and vasodilators, high ambient temperatures and pyrexia.
- Left ventricular function is also impaired by chronic hypoxia and by increased pulmonary venous return. Mechanical efficiency may be impaired by the loss of some of the stroke volume through a VSD.
- There is substantial risk of paradoxical embolus and so filters should be attached to intravenous lines to ensure that even the smallest amount of air does not gain access to the circulation. The risk of bacterial endocarditis has probably been

overstated, and guidelines for antibiotic prophylaxis are currently under review. Meanwhile their use is still recommended (as with any cardiac structural abnormality).

Cyanotic CHD

This will be identified more commonly in children, and exists when there is:

- Right-to-left shunt with pulmonary oligaemia, as in the tetrad of Fallot (VSD, overriding aorta, pulmonary stenosis and right ventricular hypertrophy).
- Parallel left and right circulations (transposition of the great arteries).
- Mixing of oxygenated and deoxygenated blood without decreased pulmonary blood flow (double outlet RV, single ventricle, total anomalous pulmonary venous drainage (TAPVD), truncus arteriosus).

Problems

- The chronic hypoxia stimulates polycythaemia. This leads to suboptimal rheology which worsens with dehydration (sludging and thrombosis is possible), and a significant risk of cerebrovascular accident (CVA) at a haematocrit of greater than 65%.
- There is a risk of paradoxical emboli, as described above.
- There is a risk of bacterial endocarditis, as described above.
- If there is pulmonary oligaemia, inhalation induction will be slower.

Final direction the viva could take

You may be able to entice an examiner who will be unable to resist asking why you have described the condition as the 'tetrad' rather than the 'tetralogy' of Fallot. This will be your opportunity to widen their education.

- A 'tetralogy' is any series of four related literary or dramatic compositions, just as a 'trilogy' is a set of three. A 'tetrad' is a group of four, as a 'triad' is a group of three. The condition associated with Fallot may be dramatic, but it is not a composition, and whoever named it, you can state loftily, was disappointingly imprecise in their use of language. (Unfortunately prolonged usage has legitimized this illiteracy, but you still might as well look like an intellectual.)

Physiology and clinical anatomy of the infant and neonate

Commentary

The scope for asking basic science questions that are directly related to paediatric clinical practice is quite restricted, and so topics tend to be limited to aspects of infant anatomy and physiology. With the exception of questions about the paediatric airway, physiology is probably asked more commonly than anatomy because it is inherently more complex. The discussion may include overall physiological aspects but is more likely to concentrate only on one or two. Examiners will expect theoretical rather than practical knowledge because they will assume that you have not anaesthetized children as young as this.

The viva

A common physiology question relates to normal fluid requirements in children (who, it will be assumed, are in hospital).

- **Fluid balance – children:** maintenance fluid requirements in children can be calculated according to a simple formula: $4\,ml\,kg^{-1}\,h^{-1}$ ($100\,ml\,kg^{-1}\,day^{-1}$) for the first 10 kg body weight; $2\,ml\,kg^{-1}\,h^{-1}$ ($50\,ml\,kg^{-1}\,day^{-1}$) for the next 10 kg body weight; and $1\,ml\,kg^{-1}\,h^{-1}$ ($20\,ml\,kg^{-1}\,day^{-1}$) for each additional kg body weight. This is only a guide; illness, pyrexia and prematurity are among many factors that influence fluid replacement (which should be oral wherever possible).
- **Fluid balance – neonates/infants:** the calculation above does not apply to neonates and young infants. By the fifth day of life, term neonates of weight >2.5 kg require $150\,ml\,kg^{-1}\,day^{-1}$. However, newborns have a relative excess of total body water and extracellular fluid, and in the first few days their requirements are much less. A typical regimen would be $60\,ml\,kg^{-1}\,day^{-1}$ on day 1; $75\,ml\,kg^{-1}\,day^{-1}$ on day 2, $90\,ml\,kg^{-1}\,day^{-1}$ on day 3, $120\,ml\,kg^{-1}\,day^{-1}$ on day 4 and $150\,ml\,kg^{-1}\,day^{-1}$ thereafter.
- **Fluid resuscitation:** the immediate management of a child with moderate or severe volume loss is a bolus of $20\,ml\,kg^{-1}$ of colloid or NaCl 0.9% repeated as necessary. Infants not only have high total body water of 70–80% compared with around 60% in the adult, but also have a higher proportion of extracellular fluid ($>50\%$ in the neonate compared to 33% in the adult). This increases their vulnerability to dehydration.

Other common topics are the paediatric airway and paediatric respiration.

- **Airway:** a number of characteristics have implications for airway management. The head is disproportionately large in comparison with adults; the angle of the jaw is 140° (120° in adults); and the dimensions of the upper airway are reduced by a larger tongue, by lymphoid tissue, and by narrower nasal and pharyngeal passages. The epiglottis is U-shaped and, although it is stiffer than in the adult, lies more horizontally (at an angle of 45°). The larynx is higher (the cricoid cartilage lies at the level of C_4) and not only lies more anteriorly but is also tilted anteriorly. The ring of the cricoid cartilage forms the narrowest part of the airway up to at least the age of 8 years. The trachea is short (around 4 cm in the infant) and narrow (about 5–6 mm). The angles of the left and right main bronchi are approximately equal, so that left endobronchial intubation is as likely as right.
- **Respiration:** the high basal metabolic rate (BMR) of infants is associated with a high respiratory rate. Respiratory compensation occurs via an increase in respiratory frequency more than increases in tidal volume. Infant ribs are more horizontal and so are mechanically less efficient. The compliant chest wall is unable

effectively to oppose the action of the diaphragm to maintain the FRC, and the soft sternum retracts rather than providing support for respiration. Respiration is predominantly diaphragmatic and the intercostal and accessory muscles are relatively weak, being deficient in type 1 muscle fibres until around the age of 2 years. (Tidal ventilation is $7\,ml\,kg^{-1}$, the same as in older children and adults.) Infants respond to hypoxia with bradypnoea rather than tachypnoea.

- Alveoli at birth number 20–50 million, and they are structurally underdeveloped. By 18 months they total 300 million, and thereafter grow in size rather than number. The FRC is small and desaturation occurs quickly.
- Decreased compliance (because of poorly developed elastic tissue) means that ventilatory units have short time constants, so alveolar ventilation is maintained at the expense of a high respiratory rate, high work of breathing and high oxygen consumption (15% of the total).
- Closing capacity exceeds FRC (up to the age of 6 years) and infants generate physiological CPAP (of around 4 cmH$_2$O) by partial adduction of the cords during expiration. The 'grunting' of a premature neonate in respiratory difficulty is an exaggeration of this mechanism.
- Pre-term infants are at risk of sudden apnoeic episodes (defined as cessation of breathing for 15 seconds or more). This applies up to around 60 weeks of post-conceptual age, and is a manifestation of poor maturation of ventilatory control.
- More than 50% of total airways resistance in infants (and children up to the age of around 6 years) is provided by peripheral airways less than 2 mm in diameter. This is why conditions such as bronchiolitis are so problematic in this age group.

Direction the viva may take

You could be asked to describe the general physiological characteristics of the infant (defined as a child aged between 1 month and 1 year). Make reference to the neonate, by all means, because the youngest children exemplify the differences between paediatric and adult practice.

Surface area to mass ratio

- The smaller the child the larger is the ratio of surface area to mass, so that in the neonate it is 2.5 times that of the adult. This difference explains many of the physiological characteristics.

Cardiovascular system

- **Anatomical features:** at birth there is right ventricular hypertrophy (owing to the fetal circulation). The limbs are smaller in relation to the body, so there is less reserve blood volume to mobilize from the periphery. The foramen ovale closes functionally at birth although it remains anatomically patent.
- The need to maintain body temperature via heat production results in a higher BMR and higher tissue oxygen consumption which, at $7\,ml\,kg^{-1}\,min^{-1}$, is twice that of an adult.
- Cardiac output, which at birth is $200\,ml\,kg^{-1}\,min^{-1}$ ($100\,ml\,kg^{-1}\,min^{-1}$ in the adult), increases predominantly by an increase in heart rate rather than stroke volume.

- Blood volume is $80 \, \text{ml kg}^{-1}$ at term and $75 \, \text{ml kg}^{-1}$ at age 2 years. The haemoglobin concentration at birth is $16–18 \, \text{g dl}^{-1}$ (80% HbF), dropping to $10 \, \text{g dl}^{-1}$ at 3 months and rising again to $12–14 \, \text{g dl}^{-1}$ at 1 year.
- Infants demonstrate increased sensitivity to vagal stimulation.

Respiratory system (as above)
Temperature control

- Thermoregulation is immature in the infant. A large surface area is associated with increased heat loss, and neonates are especially vulnerable to rapid hypothermia. Infants aged less than 3 months do not shiver, but generate heat via non-shivering thermogenesis from brown fat, which comprises up to 6% of the body weight of the term fetus. Heat is generated by the catecholamine-mediated metabolism of fatty acids.

Energy metabolism

- Fetal, pre-term and neonatal glucose homeostasis is complex. It should be sufficient to know that the infant does not have the same capacity to mobilize glucose as the adult. Illness, trauma or the stress of preoperative fasting can all combine with the high BMR to deplete glycogen stores and produce hypoglycaemia (defined as a blood glucose concentration below $2.2 \, \text{mmol l}^{-1}$). Restricted fat reserves also reduce the mobilization of free fatty acids and the production of ketones (which are an important energy substrate).

Renal system

- Infant kidneys have a reduced glomerular filtration rate (which, at $65 \, \text{ml min}^{-1}$, is half that of the adult), diminished tubular function and sodium excretion, and a decreased concentrating ability. Sodium loss is inevitable and there is limited ability either to conserve or excrete water, so infants tolerate hypovolaemia or overtransfusion badly. The excretory load is mitigated partially by 50% of the nitrogen that is incorporated into growing tissue. Renal function is mature at about 2 years of age.

CNS

- Neurological development continues in the early years of life with the completion of myelination of the brain and spinal cord. The sympathetic nervous system is also incompletely developed, which explains the tolerance of central neuraxial blockade. The blood–brain barrier is immature, which increases the neonate's, and to a lesser extent the infant's, sensitivity to opiates and other CNS depressants. By 6 months of age the response to morphine is probably the same as in adults.

Gastrointestinal system

- The incidence of neonatal gastro-oesophageal reflux is high (coordination of swallowing with respiration does not mature until around 4–5 months), but this rarely proves to be a problem in clinical practice.

Drug effects

- A combination of factors influences the response of the neonate and infant to drugs. CNS depressants may have enhanced effects both because the blood–brain barrier is less effective and because cerebral blood flow accounts for a greater proportion of the cardiac output. Total body water is higher and so water-soluble drugs have a larger volume of distribution and may require higher initial doses. (Suxamethonium is an example.) Fat-soluble drugs may have a longer clinical effect because lower stores of body fat decrease redistribution. Plasma proteins are lower and so free diffusible drug levels may be higher. Enzymatic function, particularly that associated with hepatic phase II conjugation reactions, is also immature. This may delay metabolism and excretion of drugs.

Postoperative nausea and vomiting

Commentary

Postoperative nausea and vomiting (PONV) is a common problem and this is a standard question which can follow a predictable course. It combines physiology and pharmacology, and you will be expected to demonstrate that you understand the underlying physiological principles and that you can recognize patients who are at risk. You may also be asked about treatment, although this in itself is a large subject. If the examiner wants to cover all three areas, then time constraints mean that the questioning will be relatively superficial. Do not be surprised, however, if instead you are examined in more depth on one or other aspects of the topic.

The viva

You may be asked which groups of patients are particularly at risk of PONV. The answer lends itself readily to some form of classification, an example of which is found below.

- **Factors related to patients**: a positive history of PONV is the most reliable predictive factor and increases its likelihood threefold. The incidence of PONV in women exceeds by two to four times that seen in men. It is also more marked during the second half of the menstrual cycle (when progesterone levels are high). It is greater in obese subjects, in the young, and if ambulation after surgery is premature. It is increased by preoperative anxiety. Smoking appears to exert a protective effect (acting as a potent inducer of the cytochrome P450 system); so, to a lesser extent, does regular alcohol consumption.
- **Factors related to surgery:** intra-abdominal, intracranial, middle ear and squint surgery are all associated with a higher incidence of PONV, as are laparoscopic and gynaecological procedures. Moderate to severe postoperative pain can also be a potent precipitant.
- **Factors related to anaesthesia:** opiates and all inhalational agents, including nitrous oxide, predispose patients to PONV. The same applies to agents with sympathomimetic actions such as ketamine. Hypoxaemia is a stimulus to vomiting.
- **Factors related to disease:** the list of potential causes is long and includes intestinal obstruction, hypoglycaemia, hypoxia, uraemia and hypotension.

Direction the viva may take

You may then be asked about the neural pathways which mediate nausea and vomiting.

Neural pathways

- Nausea and vomiting are reflexes. The afferent and efferent pathways by which they are mediated are linked to a central integrator, the vomiting centre, which is an anatomically ill-defined area located in the medulla oblongata.
- **Vomiting centre:** this receives afferents from a large number of sources, including the cerebral cortex, the viscera and the chemoreceptor trigger zone (CTZ). Its receptors are primarily cholinergic (muscarinic M_3) but it also contains some histaminic (H_1) receptors.
  - *Cortical afferents:* nausea and vomiting may be provoked by pain, fear and anxiety, as well as by association and by other psychological factors. It may also be precipitated by visual and olfactory stimuli. Cortical stimulation of the vomiting centre may also result from organic disturbance such as raised or lowered ICP, hypoxia (of which nausea is a sensitive early sign), and the vascular derangement that accompanies migraine.
  - *Visceral afferents:* the vomiting centre responds to stimuli such as peritoneal irritation, as well as a variety of visceral disorders, including inflammation, distension and ischaemia. Obvious causes include intestinal obstruction or perforation, gastric stasis and gastric irritation. Cardiac pain is also a potent stimulus to vomiting.
  - *CTZ afferents:* see below.
- **CTZ:** this is also located in the medulla, in the area postrema on the floor of the fourth ventricle. It lies outside the blood–brain barrier and receives afferents from various sources. Its receptors are primarily dopaminergic (D_2) and serotoninergic (5-HT_3).
  - *Vestibular afferents:* inputs are received from the vestibular apparatus via the cerebellum. Its receptors are cholinergic (muscarinic M_3) and histaminic (H_1).
  - *Drug effects:* numerous drugs exert a direct action on the CTZ. These include opiates (which also sensitize the vestibular apparatus to motion), cytotoxic drugs, cardiac glycosides, volatile anaesthetic agents and numerous others, including drugs with sympathomimetic effects.

Further direction the viva could take

It is likely that you will also be asked about the management of PONV. The main emphasis will be on pharmacology and the sites of actions of the agents that you suggest.

- **Overall management:** this includes prevention by avoidance of emetic drugs (including nitrous oxide), by the use of total intravenous anaesthesia (TIVA), by vigorous hydration, and (contentiously) by high inspired oxygen concentrations. There are also complementary techniques such as acupressure on the P_6 acupuncture point at the wrist. Mention these only at the end for completeness; the examiner may otherwise think that you are stalling for time.
- **Drug treatment:** the pharmacology is considered in detail on pages 249–250. The multimodal approach uses combinations of H_1-antagonists (phenothiazines such as

prochlorperazine), anticholinergic M_3-antagonists (atropine, glycopyrrolate), anti-dopaminergic D_2-antagonists (domperidone, metoclopramide, haloperidol), 5-HT$_3$ antagonists (ondansetron, granisetron), and, experimentally, NK_1-antagonists (aprepitant). Other drugs with a useful anti-emetic effect include corticosteroids, cannabinoids and propofol.

Obesity

Commentary

This topic is a perennial favourite, possibly because the nation is getter fatter, with some 20% of adults being classified as obese, and with 10% satisfying the criterion for morbid obesity. There is potentially much to cover in the time available but, equally, this is a topic on which it is quite difficult to fail. There is a lot of information to convey, but most of it is relatively soft, and in reality there is little in the subject for the examiner to use as a discriminator. You will none the less be expected to address those areas where safety is crucial: the risk of regurgitation and aspiration, perioperative respiratory problems and prophylaxis against venous thromboembolism.

The viva

You may first be asked about anaesthesia for bariatric surgery.

- **Bariatric surgery:** ('baro-' comes from the Greek for 'weight'). The financial costs of obesity are such that bariatric surgery may become more common in the NHS. There is evidence that it can reverse some of the complications such as hypertension and diabetes. Procedures include laparoscopic gastric banding, in which an adjustable band encircles the upper part of the stomach to create a small pouch; surgical gastroplasty, which reduces the effective size of the stomach; gastric bypass surgery, which causes weight loss by malabsorption; and intragastric balloon insertion.
- **Anaesthetic considerations:** these follow from the long list of potential complications associated with the various systems of the body.

It may first be helpful to define obesity.

- **Classification:** the most widely used method of classifying obesity is the body mass index (BMI), which is determined by the weight (kg) divided by the square of the height (m^2). A BMI of 18–25 is normal, 26–30 is overweight, 31–35 is obese, and over 35 is morbidly obese. There are further categories of 'super obesity' (patients with a BMI of 50–60) and 'super-super obesity'. At this point the terminology risks becoming faintly ridiculous but this latter category defines any patient with a BMI of more than 60.
- **Ideal weight:** there are simple empirical formulae to approximate a patient's 'ideal' weight. One such estimates the optimum weight by subtracting from the height in centimetres 105 (for women) and 100 (for men).

- **Abdominal obesity:** there has been more interest recently in abdominal obesity as a predictor of cardiovascular disease, hypertension and diabetes. In patients with a BMI of 25 or less the waist circumference should not exceed 102 cm (40 in) in men and 88 cm (34.5 in) in women. Waist to hip ratios are also used and ideally should not exceed 0.9 in men and 0.85 in women.
- **Mortality:** the morbidly obese individual has only a 1 in 7 chance of reaching a normal life expectancy, and their mortality for all forms of surgery averages twice that of the non-obese population. Problems affect most systems.

Physiological and anaesthetic implications.

- **Cardiovascular:** hypertension is found in 50–60% of subjects, and is severe in 5–10%. There is increased blood volume, with increased cardiac work. Although adipose tissue is relatively avascular, it has been calculated that each additional 1 kg of fat contains 0.6 km of blood vessels. (This piece of peculiar information may at least momentarily entertain your examiner.) There is an increased incidence of coronary artery disease and cardiomyopathy. The risk of deep venous thrombosis and pulmonary embolus doubles. Obese patients have less water per unit of body weight; they tolerate hypovolaemia badly and they may also compensate poorly for changes of position during anaesthesia.
- **Respiratory problems:** the increased adipose tissue of the neck and upper chest may increase problems with tracheal intubation as well as making it much more difficult to maintain the airway with a facemask. The work of breathing is increased because of the mass effect of chest weight, which reduces chest wall compliance. Spontaneous respiration is restricted, and the large abdominal mass can cause diaphragmatic splinting. There is a reduction in the FRC together with an increase in closing volume. Other lung volumes decrease (total lung capacity, inspiratory capacity and expiratory reserve volume), and there is also an increase in pulmonary 'shunting' with mild hypercapnia and perioperative hypoxia. Equilibration with inhaled volatile anaesthetic agents may be slow. Some 5% of obese subjects have obstructive sleep apnoea. Seriously obese patients may hypoventilate and manifest the 'Pickwickian syndrome', which consists of obesity, somnolence, polycythaemia, pulmonary hypertension and right heart failure. (This is not named after Mr Pickwick in *The Pickwick Papers* by Dickens, but after the fat boy Joe.)
- **Gastrointestinal system:** obesity predisposes to hiatus hernia, gastro-oesophageal reflux with potential pulmonary aspiration of gastric contents, and cholelithiasis.
- **Endocrine:** there is a fivefold increase in the likelihood of developing diabetes mellitus. There is an increase in plasma insulin levels which is linked to high calorie intake, but binding to cell receptors decreases (this is insulin resistance).
- **Miscellaneous physical and technical problems:** these patients are difficult to move, lift and nurse. Venepuncture is challenging, and all practical procedures, including local and regional anaesthetic blocks, can be technically demanding. The accurate estimation of drug dosage is problematic, and non-invasive arterial pressure monitoring may be inaccurate. Surgeons as well as anaesthetists face technical problems, and the duration of surgery is frequently prolonged.

- **Summary of anaesthetic problems:** potentially difficult airway; high risk of regurgitation of gastric contents; problematic determination of drug dosage (should titrate against lean body mass rather than total body weight); difficulty in maintaining perioperative oxygenation; increase in difficulty of all practical procedures; problems with manual handling; wide range of potential co-morbidities; risk of venous thromboembolism.

Physiology of ageing

Commentary

This subject, like obesity, is another question which is quite difficult to fail. In this topic also there is a lot of information that can be conveyed, but much of it is predictable and again there may be little in the subject for the examiner to use as a discriminator. It will help if you can quote some numerical data; it may appear otherwise that you are simply recounting the obvious fact that every physiological variable deteriorates. An alternative strategy is to make clear that you are focusing your answer on the areas of higher anaesthetic priority.

The viva

You will be asked about changes in physiology with increasing age.

This lends itself to a systems-based approach.

- **General points:** progressive and global decline in physiological function is measurable after about the fourth decade of life, and more rapid deterioration occurs when patients reach their seventies.
- **CNS:** there is progressive structural change with cerebral atrophy (the weight of the brain decreases by over 10%), a decrease in neurotransmitter concentrations, diminished cerebral blood flow and a fall in oxygen consumption. MAC decreases with age both for general and for local anaesthesia. It declines by about 5% per decade after the age of 40 years, and if this curve is extrapolated it reaches zero at the age of 137. BMR is said to decline by 1% per year after the age of 30 years. There may be some increase in receptor sensitivity, for example to benzodiazepines, while the effect of opiates may be enhanced because of decreased protein binding.
- **Autonomic nervous system:** there is a gradual functional decline as evinced by orthostatic hypotension owing to impairment of baroreceptor function. This occurs in 25% of subjects older than 65 years. Temperature control is impaired, and heat generation is reduced by the decline in BMR. The frail and elderly may also have less subcutaneous fat for insulation. The autonomic changes have been described as 'physiological beta blockade'.
- **Cardiovascular system:** there is gradual functional decline: cardiac output decreases (by 20% at age 60), with decreases in heart rate, stroke volume and myocardial

contractility. A decline in receptor numbers means that there is decreased sensitivity to inotropes. The risk of pulmonary thromboembolism is increased, both because of age itself, and because of the nature of the surgery for which elderly patients may present, particularly orthopaedic fractures and intra-abdominal procedures. Anaemia is common.

- **Respiratory system:** there is a progressive decline with age. The closing volume matches FRC in the upright position at around the age of 65 years but encroaches on FRC by age 44 if supine. Increased V/Q mismatch leads to a widening of the alveolar–arterial oxygen gradient (A–aDO$_2$), there is decreased sensitivity to hypoxia and hypercapnia, and there is a decrease in lung compliance.
- **The airway:** elderly patients are likely to be edentulous, with mandibles that are osteoporotic. Oropharyngeal muscle tone is lax, and cervical spondylosis and osteoarthritis are common problems.
- **Gastrointestinal system:** elderly subjects have slower gastric emptying, parietal cell function is impaired, and hiatus hernia and gastro-oesophageal reflux are more common.
- **Renal system:** renal blood flow diminishes and glomerular filtration rate is decreased by 30–45% in the elderly. Renal concentrating function is diminished, fluid handling is impaired, and preoperative dehydration is more likely.
- **Drugs:** hepatic and renal function decline with a decrease in the clearance of drugs, protein binding is reduced and receptor sensitivity alters. It is increased for CNS depressants, but decreased for inotropes and for β-adrenoceptor blockers.

Direction the viva will take

You may be asked to outline factors of particular relevance to anaesthesia.

- **Coexisting disease is common:** the list is potentially very long and includes ischaemic heart disease, hypertension, chronic airways disease, cerebrovascular disease, osteoarthritis, diabetes mellitus, dementia (which has an incidence of 20% in those aged over 80 years), Parkinson's disease, physical frailty, malnutrition, polypharmacy, and sensory impairment.
- **Surgical mortality is high:** about 15% of the population of the UK is aged over 65, and the population is continuing to age. This is a group in whom surgery is more common, and in whom mortality rates are higher. In the 1999 CEPOD report, which looked at the extremes of age, 75% of reported deaths were over 70 years and the overall mortality rate was 10%.
- **Summary of anaesthetic considerations:** high probability of coexisting disease; increased regurgitation risk (but not enough to mandate rapid sequence induction); increased sensitivity to effects of hypnotic and opiate drugs; greater difficulty in maintaining perioperative oxygenation; skin fragility and high susceptibility to pressure effects of prolonged immobility; reduced temperature control; increased likelihood of POCD (see below) and thromboembolic events.
- **Postoperative cognitive dysfunction (POCD):** this describes a spectrum of deficits which include short-term memory lapses, acute disorientation and confusion,

longer-term personality changes, and difficulties with tasks requiring organization of thought. Some form of POCD occurs in about 25% of the elderly surgical population. Intuitively, it would be easy to attribute this to alterations in cerebral perfusion and oxygenation associated with anaesthesia and surgery, but there is no evidence to support this contention. POCD is almost certainly multifactorial.

The 'stress response' to surgery

Commentary

The stress response to injury is a subject of continued, although perhaps diminishing, interest to anaesthetists, if not to examiners. There is no consensus about the desirability of abolishing it, but considerable research effort has been expended into studying the attenuating effects of general and regional anaesthesia. Much remains speculative and so the subject eludes focus. You will be able to give the impression of knowing sufficient about the topic if you have grasped the overall picture and can reproduce some of the key words, and it should not be difficult to provide a broad overview.

The viva

You will be asked for a definition of the stress response followed by an outline of its important features.

- The 'stress response' is the term used to describe the widespread metabolic and hormonal changes which occur in response to trauma, including surgical trauma. It is a complex neuroendocrine response whose net effect is to increase catabolism and release endogenous fuel stores while conserving body fluids. In evolutionary terms, it is a natural mechanism which increases an injured animal's chances of survival.
- The degree of catabolism is related to the severity of the surgical insult or traumatic tissue injury. In practice, the plasma concentrations of most substances increase, and it is unlikely that the examiner will ask you specifically about a single hormone. If this does happen, and you do not immediately know the answer, or you suspect that it is a trick question, then try to answer it from first principles. Do not be concerned if your reply does not seem that logical; it is not clear, for example, why prolactin concentrations should increase while thyroid hormone should rise little, if at all.

Endocrine response

- **Autonomic nervous system – sympathoadrenal response:** this is mediated via the hypothalamus with the stimulation of adrenal medullary catecholamines. There is also increased presynaptic noradrenaline release. This leads to cardiovascular stimulation with tachycardia and peripheral vasoconstriction. The renin–angiotensin system stimulates aldosterone release, leading to sodium and water retention.

- **Hypothalamic–pituitary–adrenal (HPA) axis:** hypothalamic releasing factors respond to major surgical trauma by stimulating the anterior pituitary. This in turn leads to increases in adrenocorticotrophic hormone (ACTH) which stimulates adrenal glucocorticoid release, and somatotrophin (growth hormone). This enhances protein synthesis and inhibits breakdown, stimulates lipolysis and antagonizes insulin. Prolactin release is also evident, although its purpose is not obvious. The other anterior pituitary hormones, including thyroid hormone, change little. The posterior pituitary produces increased amounts of arginine vasopressin (antidiuretic hormone, ADH).
- **Cortisol:** release from the adrenal cortex after stimulation by ACTH may increase fourfold, and this leads to intense catabolism in which there is protein breakdown, increased gluconeogenesis and lipolysis, with inhibition of glucose utilization. Cortisol is anti-inflammatory: it inhibits leucocyte migration into damaged areas and inhibits synthesis of various inflammatory mediators, including prostaglandins.
- **Insulin:** this is the major anabolic hormone of which there is a relative perioperative deficiency. Its effects are unable to match the catabolic response.
- **Inflammatory response:** after major tissue trauma, a number of cytokines are released (including IL-1, IL-6, TNF and interferons). IL-6 is the cytokine mainly responsible for the development of the systemic 'acute phase response'.

Direction the viva may take

You may be asked about the significance of the stress response for anaesthesia, whether or not anaesthetists should modify it, and the techniques that can be used.

Modification of the response by anaesthesia

- Catabolism provides endogenous fuel from carbohydrate, fatty acids and amino acids, with the loss of body nitrogen. The process is accompanied by sodium and water retention. As an evolutionary process this may have conferred a survival benefit, but this must apply less in the context of modern surgery and anaesthesia. In the elderly surgical population with patients with significant co-morbidity, the stress response may have obvious adverse effects. Whether or not anaesthetists should be trying to ablate the response, however, remains contentious.
- **Opiates:** these suppress hypothalamic and pituitary secretion, and high-dose opiates (for example, morphine in a dose of $4\,\mathrm{mg\,kg^{-1}}$ or fentanyl in a dose of $100\,\mu\mathrm{g\,kg^{-1}}$) may attenuate the response substantially, but this is at the cost of profound sedation and respiratory depression. The effect does not endure.
- **Etomidate:** this drug is an effective inhibitor of cortisol and aldosterone synthesis via its inhibition of the $11\text{-}\beta$ and $17\text{-}\alpha$ hydroxylase steps of steroid synthesis. This inhibition persists for 6–12 hours after a single dose. It might be logical to use etomidate deliberately to attenuate the response, although this has never been done, presumably because of anxieties about an agent whose use as an infusion in intensive care patients is associated with increased mortality.
- **Benzodiazepines:** these also inhibit cortisol production, probably via a central effect.
- **α-2 agonists:** these attenuate the sympathoadrenal responses, and lead indirectly to a decrease in cortisol production.

- **Regional anaesthesia:** this is of continued interest because it has been demonstrated that extensive extradural block ablates the adrenocortical and glycaemic responses to surgery. It may be more difficult to achieve in upper gastrointestinal tract and thoracic surgery, but there is increasing acceptance of the claim that targeted and sustained regional anaesthesia has beneficial effect on surgical outcome. This, however, may be related as much to earlier ambulation and improvements in respiratory function as to the abolition of the stress response itself.

The glucocorticoid response to surgery

Commentary

The stress response to injury may be important in patients who are receiving corticosteroids. The traditional concern relates to the danger of precipitating an Addisonian crisis in patients whose HPA axis is suppressed. Many clinicians believe that these anxieties are overstated. Certainly there is now little justification for the use of potentially dangerous supraphysiological replacement regimens.

The viva

The viva may be introduced by a question about the problems of anaesthetizing patients who are being treated with steroids (glucocorticoids). It will go on to the normal steroid response to surgery.

- Patients who are receiving corticosteroids are often assumed to have suppression of the HPA axis. This occurs via a feedback inhibition of hypothalamic and pituitary function.
- This adrenal suppression means that patients cannot mount a normal steroid response to surgery, and may develop an Addisonian crisis in the postoperative period. This is characterized by cardiovascular instability and electrolyte derangement. Patients have hypotension, which may be refractory to routine treatment, and can be hypokalaemic, hyponatraemic and hypoglycaemic.

Steroid response to surgery

- **Sympathoadrenal response:** this is an autonomic response which is mediated via the hypothalamus, and which results in an increase in medullary catecholamines. There is also an increase in the presynaptic release of noradrenaline. Aldosterone release is stimulated by the renin–angiotensin system, leading to sodium and water retention.
- **HPA axis response:** hypothalamic releasing factors stimulate the anterior pituitary, with resultant increases in ACTH via corticotrophin-releasing hormone (CRH).
- **Cortisol production:** ACTH stimulates adrenal glucocorticoid release. This is mediated by a specific cell-surface receptor, with G protein activation, adenyl

cyclase stimulation and increased intracellular cAMP. The effects of cortisol are catabolic, with protein breakdown, gluconeogenesis, inhibition of glucose utilization and lipolysis. The hormone is also anti-inflammatory; it inhibits leucocyte migration into damaged areas and decreases the synthesis of inflammatory mediators such as prostaglandins.

- **Cortisol output:** This varies according to the degree of surgical stress. There is normally a maximal rise at 4–6 hours with peak cortisol usually subsiding within 24 hours. After major surgery it may be sustained for up to 72 hours. Normal blood levels are around 200 nmol l^{-1}, but the increase following surgery may range from 800 to more than 1500 nmol l^{-1}. Normal 24 hour cortisol output is around 150 mg; minor surgery such as hernia repair will stimulate extra production of less than 50 mg in 24 hours, whereas following thoracotomy or laparotomy, between 75 and 100 mg will be released.

Direction the viva may take

You will be asked to describe your approach to perioperative steroid replacement.

- Ideally a replacement regimen should be based on laboratory evaluation of the HPA axis (by conducting short synacthen or insulin tolerance tests if possible) and an assessment of the likely degree of surgical stress. Corticosteroid supplementation minimizes the risk of perioperative cardiovascular instability.
- Patients who are taking less than prednisolone 10 mg daily (or the equivalent) have a normal response to HPA testing and require no supplementation. Patients who have previously been taking an HPA suppressant dose, but have discontinued this within 3 months from surgery, should be assumed to have residual suppression. They should be tested wherever possible because exogenous steroid supplementation is not innocuous. Patients on high immunosuppressant doses must continue these perioperatively.
- If taking more than 10 mg prednisolone daily and undergoing minor to moderate surgery:
  — Continue the usual dose preoperatively.
  — Give hydrocortisone 25 mg iv at induction.
  — Prescribe hydrocortisone 100 mg in the first 24 hours (by continuous infusion).
- If taking more than 10 mg daily and undergoing major surgery:
  — Continue the usual dose preoperatively.
  — Give hydrocortisone 25 mg iv at induction.
  — Prescribe hydrocortisone 100 mg per day for 48–72 hours (by continuous infusion).

Further direction the viva could take

You may be asked finally about the dangers of supraphysiological doses of exogenous corticosteroids. Complications of steroid therapy make for a long list, although this question pertains to problems related to acute administration.

- **Complications of acute therapy:** increased catabolism, hyperglycaemia, immuno-suppression, peptic ulceration, delayed wound healing, myopathy (which can occur acutely), steroid psychosis (which is related to sudden large increases in blood levels), fluid retention and electrolyte disturbance, including hypokalaemia.

If there remains time you may be asked to fill it with a list of the numerous complications related to long-term treatment.

- **Complications of chronic therapy:** in addition to the above, these include immunosuppression, hypertension, increased skin fragility, posterior subcapsular cataract formation, osteoporosis, hypocalcaemia caused by reduced gastrointestinal absorption; negative nitrogen balance and Cushing's syndrome.

Adrenaline (epinephrine)

Commentary

Adrenaline is a key drug in anaesthesia, intensive care and resuscitation. The questioning will include some clinical aspects of its use, but these are rooted firmly in the basic physiology of the compound and so it is this with which you must be familiar.

The viva

You might be asked a straightforward introductory question about indications for its use.

- **Cardiac resuscitation:** adrenaline is the main drug in the cardiac arrest algorithms. Its main action is to constrict the peripheral circulation into which the much reduced cardiac output produced by external cardiac compression is being delivered. (CPR delivers at best around 10–15% of normal output.) This central redistribution of the available cardiac output increases coronary perfusion pressure and coronary arterial flow. The standard dose in adults is 1 mg (10 ml of 1 in 10 000).
- **Circulatory support:** its use to support the failing circulation is popular in some intensive therapy units. Some cardiologists also favour it as the drug of choice for cardiogenic shock. It is given by continuous infusion via a central vein at a rate of 0.05–2.0 μg kg^{-1} min^{-1}.
- **Bronchodilatation:** adrenaline can be used in acute severe and refractory asthma in a dose range similar to that used for circulatory support.
- **Anaphylaxis:** adrenaline is the drug of first choice. It is given either by deep intramuscular injection in a dose of 500 μg (0.5 ml of 1 in 1000), or by intravenous injection at a rate of 100 μg min^{-1} until the patient responds.
- **Upper airway obstruction:** nebulized adrenaline can reduce upper airways oedema, due, for example, to croup in children or allergic reactions in adults. A dose of 1–2 mg diluted with saline can be used in adults, while children may receive 400 μg kg^{-1} up to a maximum dose of 5 mg.
- **Vasoconstriction:** adrenaline can be added to solutions of local anaesthetic to reduce local bleeding, to prolong the duration of action and to reduce the rapidity with which the drug is absorbed. Surgeons may use pre-prepared solutions containing adrenaline 1 in 80 000 up to 1 in 200 000, but they may also prepare their own

mixtures for use, for example, in plastic surgical procedures in which large areas of subcutaneous tissue are infiltrated. It is important to be aware of how much adrenaline is being given in these circumstances. The total dose should not exceed 500 μg. (Solutions of 1 in 1000 contain 1000 μg ml^{-1}; 1 in 10 000 contain 100 μg ml^{-1}; 1 in 80 000 contain 12.5 μg ml^{-1}; 1 in 100 000 contain 10 μg ml^{-1}; and 1 in 200 000 contain 5 μg ml^{-1}.) Some surgeons may also use vasoconstrictors such as cocaine (in nasal surgery) and phenylephrine. The pressor effect of these drug combinations can be very hazardous.

Direction the viva will take

You will then be asked about the basic pharmacology of adrenaline.

- Adrenaline is one of the body's principal catecholamines (a catechol is a benzene ring with two adjacent hydroxyl groups) and is produced via a short biosynthetic pathway in the adrenal medulla, from where it is secreted. Phenylalanine undergoes two hydroxylation steps to form first tyrosine, and then dihydroxyphenylalanine (dopa). Dopa is decarboxylated to form dopamine, which is hydroxylated to produce noradrenaline. Methylation of noradrenaline produces adrenaline. In summary: phenylalanine $\rightarrow$ tyrosine $\rightarrow$ dopa $\rightarrow$ dopamine $\rightarrow$ noradrenaline $\rightarrow$ adrenaline (dihydroxyphenylmethyl aminoethanol).
- Adrenaline is inactivated by oxidative deamination (monoamine oxidase) and methylation (catechol-O-methyltransferase, COMT). COMT is much the more significant pathway. Metabolism is very rapid and adrenaline's elimination half-life is <60 s.
- Unlike noradrenaline, which is responsible for maintaining normal sympathetic tone, it is not a 'routine' neurotransmitter, but is released instead in response to physiological crisis.
- Adrenaline has effects at both α- and β-adrenoceptors, of which there are several subclasses: α_1, α_2 (each with a further three subtypes) and β_1, β_2 and β_3.
- These adrenoceptors are G protein-coupled, and are associated with different second messenger systems. α_1 effects are mediated via phospholipase C, and α_2 effects via a decrease in cyclic AMP. β effects are all mediated via an increase in cAMP.
- **Cardiovascular effects:** in lower doses, the β_1 effects predominate, but there is still a rise in systolic blood pressure caused by the increase in cardiac output. Even at low blood concentrations (the normal level is around 25 pg ml^{-1}) there is still a β-receptor-mediated fall in diastolic pressure, and so the pulse pressure widens with only a small rise in mean arterial pressure. α_2 vasodilatation in skeletal muscle and in the liver also counteracts any rise in peripheral vascular resistance. There is an α_1-mediated increase in the force and rate of myocardial contraction, coupled with an increase in stroke volume secondary to enhanced venous return. Cardiac output increases. Direct myocardial stimulation is partially opposed by inhibitory baroreceptor reflexes which act to modify the rises in blood pressure. The transplanted heart, which is denervated, shows a more exaggerated response to circulating adrenaline than would otherwise be the case. The same is true if the actions of the vagus nerve have been blocked by high doses of atropine, or if ganglion-blocking drugs have been given. (In both normal and denervated hearts, adrenaline enhances the excitability of myocardial cell membranes.)

As the dose of adrenaline increases so both a and β effects are seen, while at high doses a_1 vasoconstriction predominates. It may also cause a_1-mediated vasoconstriction in the main coronary arteries, which is offset by β_2-mediated vasodilatation in the smaller vessels. From an evolutionary point of view it would seem curious were the net effects of adrenaline to compromise the coronary circulation, although the evidence for that proposition remains elusive.

- **Respiratory effects:** adrenaline is a potent bronchodilator, acting via β_2 receptors to inhibit smooth muscle contraction in the airways.
- **Metabolic effects:** adrenaline increases oxygen consumption by up to 30%. Blood glucose rises both because of increased glycogenolysis in muscle and liver, and also because of decreased insulin secretion. This is an a_2 effect.
- **CNS effects:** in higher doses adrenaline is a cerebral stimulant which causes arousal. If administered intrathecally, adrenaline acts on a_2 receptors to produce analgesia.
- **Gastrointestinal effects:** smooth muscle of the gastrointestinal tract relaxes, although the sphincters contract (a_1 effect).

Further direction the viva could take

You may be asked about potential problems.

- **Ischaemic necrosis:** injection of adrenaline-containing solutions into digits or appendages may jeopardize the blood supply.
- **Cardiac arrhythmias:** adrenaline appears to increase the automaticity of the ventricular conducting system. The ECG may show runs of ventricular premature beats, leading in the worst case to ventricular fibrillation. This effect is enhanced by hypercapnia, by hypoxia and by acidosis. In conjunction with the use of some volatile agents, particularly halothane, this could be a fatal combination, although newer agents are much safer.
- **Cardiac disease:** adrenaline should be infiltrated with caution in those patients who have pre-existing hypertension or ischaemic heart disease. The combination of adrenaline and monoamine oxidase inhibitors (MAOIs) may also be hazardous.
- **Alternative vasopressors:** these include agents such as felypressin (Octapressin), which is a vasopressin (ADH) analogue. This is a potent local vasoconstrictor which is less likely to provoke cardiac arrhythmia.

5-Hydroxytryptamine (serotonin)

Commentary

This is a basic science topic that you might expect to encounter in the Primary FRCA rather than the Final. Although serotonin does mediate a large number of physiological functions via a family of receptors and subtypes, the direct anaesthetic applications nonetheless are quite limited. Much remains to be elucidated about the receptor types, which, as always, will relieve the pressure on you to deliver precise factual answers. You cannot, for example, be expected to know details of 5-HT$_6$ and 5-HT$_7$ receptors when their functions remain unclear. You might even succeed in bluffing your way through part of this question. At one sitting of the exam just after this topic first appeared, a candidate approached it with as much confidence as if serotonin had been the subject of his MD thesis. So when he announced resolutely that there were at least 27 5-HT receptors (rather than the 14 that have so far been characterized) the uneasy examiner (me) felt that he had little choice but to let him proceed. If you adopt this strategy only to find, alas, that serotonin actually was the subject of the examiner's MD thesis, then it is easy enough to retreat with the excuse that you must have confused it with some other receptor subset. The examiner will not pursue you, because to do so would mean that they were using their highly specialist knowledge to unfair advantage.

The viva

There are a number of clinical directions which the viva may follow although none concern conditions that are common. So, the questioning may begin with a discussion of the carcinoid syndrome.

- **Carcinoid syndrome:** this occurs as a result of enterochromaffin tumours which secrete not only 5-HT but other neuropeptides such as substance P, vasoactive intestinal polypeptide (VIP), prostaglandins, histamine and bradykinin. More than 80% of these tumours originate in the gut and so symptoms do not appear until they metastasize to the liver. Prior to metastasis these substances are degraded to inactive metabolites. Once they gain direct access to the circulation, either from primary sites in the lung or from metastases, then the problems of flushing, hypotension, tachycardia, wheeze, abdominal cramps and diarrhoea may supervene. Endocardial and valvular fibrosis (which affects the right side of the heart more frequently than the left) may also complicate the condition, as may pellagra. This is due to nicotinamide (vitamin B2) deficiency, which is caused by the excessive consumption of dietary tryptophan by the tumour. The symptoms of carcinoid are due not solely to serotonin secretion, but those which are mediated via 5-HT can be treated with the 5-HT$_2$ antagonist cyproheptadine. Octreotide, which is a long-acting somatostatin analogue which suppresses 5-HT and other hormone secretion, can also be used.

You will then be asked in more detail about serotonin.

- 5-HT, or serotonin, is one of four aminergic neurotransmitters (the others being dopamine, noradrenaline and histamine) which has its highest CNS concentrations in the midbrain. At 1% this is a tiny proportion of total body 5-HT, the remainder of which is found peripherally. It is most abundant in the enterochromaffin cells in the walls of the stomach and the small bowel, and it is also found in platelets. In the gastrointestinal myenteric plexus it functions as an excitatory neurotransmitter.
- 5-HT is synthesized by hydroxylation and decarboxylation of tryptophan (an essential amino acid, the dietary intake of which can influence 5-HT levels), and is metabolized by monoamine oxidase. It is stored in cytoplasmic vesicles. Reuptake is the primary mechanism whereby the compound is recovered following release.
- There are numerous receptor subtypes, further examples of which continue to be characterized. Currently there are 5-HT$_1$ (with five subtypes 1_A, 1_B, 1_D, 1_E, 1_F),

5-HT$_2$ (with subtypes 2$_A$–2$_C$), 5-HT$_3$, 5-HT$_4$, 5-HT$_5$ (with subtypes 5$_A$–5$_B$), and 5-HT$_6$ and 5-HT$_7$ receptors, totalling 14. All of these, apart from 5-HT$_3$ receptors, are coupled to G proteins. The effects of the 5-HT$_3$ receptor are mediated via a rapid sodium/potassium ligand-gated ion channel. The receptors are variously presynaptic and postsynaptic depending on subtype. They appear to mediate a large number of different and sometimes contradictory effects.

- **CNS:** these include mood and affect, arousal, circadian rhythms and CSF. Serotoninergic pathways are similar to noradrenergic systems which inhibit some dorsal horn pain tracts. Discharge in the dorsal raphe nucleus precipitates migraine. 5-HT influences autonomic function, including temperature and blood pressure.
- **Cardiovascular system:** 5-HT causes platelet aggregation and can mediate both vasoconstriction and vasodilatation. Intravenous serotonin causes a fall in blood pressure owing to arteriolar vasodilatation, which is preceded by an initial rise. In blood vessels, 5-HT$_{2A}$ receptors mediate vasoconstriction. (5-HT$_1$ agonism leads to constriction of larger intracranial vessels.) Other 5-HT receptors, however, cause vasodilatation which is mediated via the release of nitric oxide (NO) and by the inhibition of noradrenaline release from sympathetic nerve terminals.
- **Respiratory system:** 5-HT causes bronchial smooth muscle contraction.
- **Gastrointestinal system:** 5-HT increases gastrointestinal secretion and peristalsis. It is also involved with nausea and vomiting.
- **Genitourinary system:** 5-HT increases uterine muscle tone.

Direction the viva may take

The above gives an overview of the diverse functions of serotonin. You may be asked about some of the receptor subtypes, mainly because there is some evidence relating to the site of action of various drugs.

- Many, but not all, 5-HT$_1$ receptors are inhibitory in effect. 5-HT$_{1A}$ receptors are the main target of drugs used to treat depression, thus drugs such as fluoxetine (Prozac) are selective serotonin re-uptake inhibitors (SSRIs) at these sites. Buspirone, which is a 5-HT$_{1A}$ agonist, is used as an anxiolytic. Sumatriptan and related drugs are 5-HT$_{1D}$ agonists which are effective treatments for migraine, 5-HT$_1$ receptors mediating intracranial vasoconstriction.
- 5-HT$_2$ receptors appear to exert excitatory postsynaptic effects and are abundant in the cortex and the limbic system (the hallucinogen LSD is a potent agonist). Platelet aggregation and smooth muscle contraction is mediated by 5-HT$_{2A}$ receptors, and CSF production by 5-HT$_{2C}$. Gastrointestinal secretion and peristalsis is enhanced by a 5-HT$_2$ stimulatory effect on smooth muscle. 5-HT$_{2A}$ receptors mediate vascular smooth muscle contraction and vasoconstriction. Methysergide, which is an ergot alkaloid used to treat refractory migraine as well as diarrhoea associated with carcinoid syndrome, is a 5-HT$_{2A}$ and $_{2C}$ antagonist. (The use of this drug is limited by its well recognized potential to cause devastating endocardial, valvular and retroperitoneal fibrosis.)
- 5-HT$_3$ excitatory ionotropic receptors in the area postrema mediate nausea and vomiting. They are also excitatory to enteric neurons. Ondansetron, ranisetron and tropisetron are effective 5-HT$_3$ antagonists.

- 5-HT$_4$ receptors are found in the gut, and centrally in the striatum of the brain. They may have a presynaptic facilitatory effect on acetylcholine release, and so may be involved in cognitive function. They are also excitatory to enteric neurons. Metoclopramide is a 5-HT$_4$ agonist.

- The remaining receptor types have functions which remain incompletely understood. 5-HT$_5$ and 5-HT$_6$ receptors in the limbic system appear to be involved with the control of mood, and 5-HT$_6$ receptors in particular have a high affinity for antidepressants. 5-HT$_7$ receptors may have some role in sleep and arousal.

Further direction the viva could take

Most examiners will not wish to dwell in detail on receptor subtypes, other than to discover whether you know the sites of action of anaesthetic-related drugs. You may then be asked about clinical disorders of 5-HT function.

- Disorders include migraine (often treated with 5-HT$_{1D}$ agonists), depression (commonly treated with SSRIs) and anxiety (sometimes treated with a 5-HT$_{1A}$ agonist). Excessive doses of tramadol may manifest with extreme serotoninergic effects (the 'serotonin syndrome') (page 253).

Nitric oxide

Commentary

There are at least 5000 research publications on this ubiquitous molecule, whose importance has been recognized only since the 1980s. Much as you might wish to share your exploration of this enormous body of work, the 8 minutes of the viva will not allow it, and a broad overview is all that can reasonably be expected. Although it appears to mediate such a large number of functions, its direct implications for anaesthesia are disappointingly modest. You will, however, need to know some of the basic details of its synthesis and chemistry, as well as those areas of anaesthetic practice and pharmacology for which nitric oxide (NO) does have relevance.

The viva

You may be asked to describe NO and its functions.

- **NO** is a free radical gas which is formed in a reaction between molecular oxygen and L-arginine. The reaction is catalysed by nitric oxide synthetase (NOS) and leads to the formation of NO and citrulline.

- **NOS isoforms (iNOS, eNOS and nNOS):** there are three NOS isoforms. The single inducible form, iNOS, is expressed in response to pathological stimulation in a variety of cells, including macrophages, neutrophils and endothelial cells. It is induced by several chemical mediators, such as interleukins, β-interferon and TNF. The two constitutive forms are eNOS, which is present in endothelium (and some other cells such as cardiac myocytes and platelets), and nNOS, which is present in neurons. The activity of the constitutive isoforms of NOS is governed by intracellular calcium-calmodulin, whereas iNOS is calcium-independent. The quantity of NO generated by iNOS exceeds by about 1000 times that which is formed by the constitutive enzymes.

- **Actions:** NO appears to be a central signalling molecule which modulates many aspects of physiological function. As endothelium-derived relaxing factor (EDRF), it regulates blood pressure and regional blood flow, as well as limiting platelet aggregation. As a neurotransmitter, NO may have a role centrally in memory, consciousness and CNS plasticity. Its peripheral roles include gastric emptying. An absence of nNOS is characteristic of infants with hypertrophic pulmonary stenosis. It has a non-specific role in the immune system, and by mechanisms such as the inactivation of haem-containing enzymes and nitrosylation of nucleic acids can destroy pathogens and tumour cells.

- **Cardiovascular effects:** it is a small lipophilic molecule which diffuses rapidly across cell membranes to combine with thiol groups to form nitrosothiol compounds. It binds to the iron moiety to activate soluble guanylyl cyclase. This enzyme catalyses the formation of cyclic guanosine monophosphate (cGMP) with the activation of protein kinases, protein phosphorylation and finally the relaxation of vascular smooth muscle.

- **Inactivation:** as a free radical gas, NO has a half-life measured in seconds (variously quoted as 0.50–1.0 s, up to 5 s). It is inactivated after forming complexes with haemoglobin, and with other haem-containing molecules. The affinity of haem for nitric oxide is more than 10 000 times greater than its affinity for O_2. It is also inactivated by a series of oxidation reactions that produce nitrate. This is then excreted renally.

Direction the viva may take

You are likely to be asked about the anaesthetic relevance of this molecule.

- **Vasodilators:** the nitrovasodilators such as glyceryl trinitrate (GTN) and sodium nitroprusside (SNP) act by producing exogenous NO in a reaction mediated by glutathione-S-transferase and cytochrome P450. Vascular smooth muscle is constantly in a state of NO-mediated vasodilatation, the compound being formed in response to shear stresses in the vessel wall. The venous circulation has a lower basal release. This is the reason why drugs such as GTN and SNP are more effective dilators of the venous rather than the arterial circulation. NO deficiency may contribute to hypertension or organ ischaemia.

- **Interactions with volatile anaesthetics:** volatile agents inhibit NOS and so reduce production from endothelial cells. The end effect of volatile administration is not vasoconstriction however, because NO inhibition is offset by direct mechanisms which influence vascular smooth muscle tone. It has been argued, although not universally accepted, that NOS inhibition by volatiles may decrease MAC, that NO influences conscious level, and that it may have a role as one of the mediators of general anaesthesia.

- **Inhaled NO:** its half-life is very short and so when the gas is inhaled it acts to reduce pulmonary vascular resistance without exerting any systemic effects. It may therefore be of use in patients with intrapulmonary shunts typical of conditions such as ARDS. Systemic administration causes indiscriminate pulmonary vasodilatation, which can only worsen the ventilation–perfusion mismatch. Inhaled NO, in contrast, is delivered to better-recruited alveoli where it dilates the associated pulmonary vessels and reduces shunt fraction. It is also a bronchodilator. In theory, its use should benefit patients with impaired right heart function and those with pulmonary hypertension. Clinical experience is probably greatest in the treatment of neonates with respiratory distress syndrome. Although NO has also been used to treat ARDS there is no evidence that it is superior to other strategies such as prone ventilation, and difficulties with safe delivery systems have also limited its use.

- **Delivery:** this can be problematic because, at concentrations greater than around 100 parts per million (ppm), the free radical gas is highly reactive and toxic. It is stored in nitrogen in a concentration of 1000 ppm, and has been given in doses that range from 250 parts per billion up to 80 parts per million.

Plasma proteins

Commentary

This is a rather non-specific topic which could branch off into unpredictable directions for which you may not be prepared. A reliable strategy may be to dwell on the core subject in as much descriptive detail as you can muster, so as to avoid being asked, say, about the functions of one of the many hormones that are transported by plasma proteins or about the immunology of γ-globulins.

The viva

You will be asked about the proteins that are normally present in plasma.

- Plasma is the non-cellular component of the intravascular space and comprises around 3500 ml in a 70-kg adult man, accounting for about 5% of total body weight.
- Amongst the considerable quantity of ions, inorganic and organic molecules (including electrolytes, urea, creatinine, fats, amino acids, sugars, metals, vitamins and enzymes) are a large number of plasma proteins. These comprise albumin, the globulins and fibrinogen.
- **Albumin:** albumin has a molecular weight of around 69 000 and is quantitatively the most important, with a plasma concentration of 5 $g\,dl^{-1}$ (35 $g\,l^{-1}$ in blood). Albumin makes the greatest contribution (20 mmHg) to the plasma oncotic pressure, and is a versatile carrier protein for numerous substances, including bilirubin, calcium, metals, fatty acids, amino acids, enzymes, hormones and drugs. It is synthesized in the liver at a rate of 0.2 $g\,kg^{-1}\,day^{-1}$.
- **Globulins:** the globulin fraction is divided further into α_1, α_2, β_1, β_2 and γ subtypes. Their molecular weights average around 200 000 but they are quantitatively less

significant with a plasma concentration of $1.5\,\mathrm{g\,dl^{-1}}$ ($10\,\mathrm{g\,l^{-1}}$ in blood). They contribute about $5\,\mathrm{mmHg}$ to plasma oncotic pressure. The α and β fractions are synthesized in the liver and include coagulation factors, transport proteins such as α_1-acid glycoprotein (which binds bupivacaine, for example) and precursors such as angiotensinogen. They also include steroid and thyroid hormone binding globulin, as well as acute phase proteins, such as C-reactive protein. Complement is a series of plasma proteins which are also produced in the liver.

- γ-**globulins:** the γ-globulins are antibodies which are synthesized in plasma cells. There are five different classes: immunoglobulin ($\mathrm{I_g}$) G, which is the most abundant and which, together with IgM, is responsible for complement fixation; IgA, which is a secretory antibody; IgD, which mediates the recognition of antigens by lymphocytes; and IgE, which is found on the cell membranes of mast cells and which mediates the classic anaphylactic type 1 hypersensitivity reaction (page 397).
- **Fibrinogen:** this is a large molecule of molecular weight variously quoted as between 340 000 and 500 000, which has a plasma concentration of $0.5\,\mathrm{g\,dl^{-1}}$ ($3.5\,\mathrm{g\,l^{-1}}$ in blood), contributing about $1\,\mathrm{mmHg}$ to plasma oncotic pressure. It is a crucial part of the final coagulation common pathway. (It is Factor I.)
- **Other functions:** plasma proteins are weakly ionized because of their carboxyl (-COOH) and amino (-NH) groups, which dissociate to form anions at body pH. This gives them a buffering capacity which amounts to about 5% of the total. (Some texts quote 15%.)

Direction the viva may take

The examiner may choose one or more aspects and relate them to anaesthesia or intensive care. This means that the viva ceases to be as tightly structured, and the fact that one examiner might question you about immunological function while another might choose coagulation will undermine their ability to mark you as rigorously on this section of the viva. You should, none the less, be prepared to say something sensible about the following topics.

- Coagulation (page 260), immunological function (page 395), oncotic pressure (page 352), buffers and disease states that are associated with abnormalities of plasma proteins (liver dysfunction causing hypoalbuminaemia, multiple myeloma).

Thyroid function

Commentary

This viva may include a discussion of the anaesthetic implications of thyroid disease, but will also cover the basic physiology of thyroid function. Even if details of the biochemistry elude you, at least ensure that you can outline the effects of thyroxine.

The viva

You may be asked about the anaesthetic implications of thyroid disease. Overt thyrotoxicosis and myxoedema are rare, but anaesthetic mismanagement of either condition may be disastrous. You cannot answer this convincingly without discussing thyroid hormone, and so you will probably have the opportunity to give only a brief outline of the diseases before moving on.

- **Airway problems:** all forms of thyroid disease may be associated with large goitres, which may extend retrosternally and cause airway problems.
- **Hyperthyroidism:** the well known clinical features are predictable from knowledge of the actions of the hormone. Excess thyroid hormone hyperstimulates almost all metabolically active tissue. Severe cases may have cardiac arrhythmias and heart failure. The cardinal principle underlying the anaesthetic management of thyrotoxic patients is to render them euthyroid prior to surgery.
- **Hypothyroidism:** in contrast, hypothyroid patients need much smaller doses of anaesthetic drugs. The BMR is greatly reduced, and with it cardiac reserve. Uncorrected myxoedema may be associated with amyloidosis, with consequent cardiac and renal impairment.

You will then be asked about the normal functions of the thyroid gland and thyroid hormone.

- **The thyroid gland** produces thyroid hormone, which is an iodine-containing amino acid that is central to metabolism. In essence it maintains the metabolic rate that is optimal for normal cellular function.
- **Production:** the production of thyroxine first involves iodide trapping within the gland by a process of active transport. Iodide is rapidly oxidized to iodine prior to the iodination of tyrosine with the formation of diiodotyrosine (DIT). Two molecules of DIT condense to form T_4. Thyroxine is then stored in the colloid of the thyroid bound in a peptide linkage as part of the large thyroglobulin molecule. It then undergoes proteolysis and release into the circulation. Most of the hormone is released in the form of T_4 with only about 5% secreted as T_3. Once in the circulation about one-third of T_4 is converted to T_3.
- **Secretion:** secretion is controlled by the thyroid-stimulating hormone (TSH) of the anterior pituitary, which in turn is regulated by thyrotropin-releasing hormone (TRH) from the hypothalamus. The process is subject to negative feedback control by thyroid hormones which act both at the pituitary and hypothalamus. The proteolysis of stored thyroid hormone is inhibited by iodide.
- **Binding:** carriage in the circulation is via binding to albumin and thyroxine-binding globulin (TBG). TBG has very high affinity and so most circulating T_4 is bound. T_3 is bound equally by TBG and by albumin. Free T_3 and T_4 concentrations in plasma are very low.
- **Functions:** in summary, thyroid hormones stimulate oxygen consumption, act as a regulator of carbohydrate and lipid metabolism, and have an important role in normal growth and maturation. The hormones enter cells and T_3 binds to thyroid receptors in the nuclei. T_3 acts more rapidly and is three to five times more potent than T_4. The hormone–receptor complex then binds to DNA and changes the

expression of a variety of different genes that code for enzymes that regulate cell function. Thyroxine is calorigenic, increasing the oxygen consumption of almost all metabolically active tissues. (Exceptions include the brain, anterior pituitary, testes, uterus, lymph nodes and spleen.) T_4 actually depresses pituitary oxygen consumption, presumably via a negative feedback mechanism. It increases the force and rate of myocardial contraction, increases the number and affinity of β-adrenergic receptors and enhances its response to circulating catecholamines. As a catabolic hormone it increase lipolysis and stimulates the formation of low-density lipoprotein receptors. It increases protein breakdown in muscle and enhances carbohydrate absorption from the gut.

Direction the viva may take

You may finally be asked about the medical management of thyroid disease.

- **Hyperthyroidism:** these patients should be rendered euthyroid before surgery. One approach is to achieve this over 2–3 months using propylthiouracil, which decreases thyroid synthesis and inhibits the peripheral conversion of T_4 to T_3. Carbimazole can be used as an alternative. This also decreases synthesis of thyroid hormone, possibly by inhibiting iodination of tyrosine residues in thyroglobulin. For 10 days or so prior to surgery patients are also given potassium iodide to reduce the vascularity of the gland. An alternative and less time-consuming option is to control the manifestations of thyroid overstimulation using β-adrenoceptor blockers for 2–3 weeks preoperatively, together with potassium iodide as above. Emergency surgery in hyperthyroid patients carries the risk of a thyrotoxic crisis, also known as 'thyroid storm', in which there is a sudden further extreme surge of metabolic stimulation, with hyperpyrexia, diaphoresis, tachycardia and arrhythmias. Intravenous β-blockade using propranolol (or esmolol if there is concern that the patient is in cardiac failure), together with intravenous potassium iodide, should allow adequate control. Larger doses of anaesthetic agents may be required to compensate for their more rapid distribution and metabolism.
- **Hypothyroidism:** the opposite of thyroid storm is myxoedema coma, which is characterized by obtunded cerebration, marked hypothermia, alveolar hypoventilation and bradycardia. Correction of hypothyroidism is usually undertaken slowly, giving oral thyroxine, although intravenous T_3 can be used in emergency situations. This risks provoking myocardial ischaemia and should be avoided if possible. T_4 can be given, but its conversion to T_3 under these circumstances is greatly depressed.

Further direction the viva could take

You may be asked, almost as an aside, why patients with thyrotoxicosis develop proptosis, and why hypothyroidism is known as myxoedema. It will have (almost) no bearing on whether you pass or fail, but there is no point in becoming unnecessarily dejected by not knowing the answer to the final question of the section.

- Skin contains various proteins combined with polysaccharides, hyaluronic acid and chondroitin sulphuric acid. In hypothyroidism these complexes accumulate, and so promote water retention along with a characteristic coarsening of the skin, which becomes puffy. When treated with thyroid hormone these complexes are metabolized with resolution of the 'myx'-oedema.

- Exophthalmos is a characteristic of autoimmune Graves' disease and is caused by swelling of the muscles and connective tissues of the orbit, which leads to proptosis. This effect is due not to thyroid hormone but to autoimmune attack on the tissues by cytotoxic antibodies. These are formed in response to antigens that are common to the eye muscles and to the thyroid.

Nutrition

Commentary

Nutrition has become a separate science, and in many hospitals there are specific teams which manage the needs both of the perioperative surgical patient as well as the critically ill. You will nevertheless be expected to know something about it because nutrition is a topic that reappears in the exam. You will not have to know specific details of trace element or vitamin concentrations, but you can anticipate a broad discussion of the effects of starvation, of the indications for nutritional support, of the major components of feeds, and the place of enteral and parenteral routes of administration.

The viva

You may be asked about the indications for nutritional support in the surgical or the critically ill patient, and the physiological changes that are associated with starvation.

- **Indications for nutritional support:** cachectic patients with a preoperative weight loss of 15% or more, or who have effectively been starved for over 10 days (for example, because of dysphagia), have improved outcomes if they receive nutritional support before surgery. There are numerous other indications, including malabsorption owing to small bowel resection, small bowel fistulas, radiation enteritis, intractable diarrhoea and vomiting, and hyperemesis gravidarum.
- **Starvation:** hepatic glycogen stores are depleted within 24–48 hours, after which adipose tissue is the source of fatty acids for use as an energy substrate. A small number of cell types, amongst which are erythrocytes and cells in the renal medulla, can utilize only glucose, and this has to be provided via amino acids that are produced from protein breakdown. The CNS normally depends on glucose, but can function using ketones as an energy substrate. During prolonged fasting there is an obligatory protein loss of at least 20 g daily. (Catabolism is a form of accelerated starvation with glycogenolysis, lipolysis and proteolysis.)

You may then be asked to outline normal nutritional requirements.

- **Nutritional requirements – energy:** basal expenditure can be judged from the Harris–Benedict equation (which links weight, height and age) or from nomograms.

Kilocalorie needs range from around 30 kcal kg^{-1} in the non-stressed ambulatory state to 60 kcal kg^{-1} in sepsis or following major trauma. After severe thermal injury, which exemplifies an accelerated catabolic state, patients may require 80 kcal kg^{-1}.

- **Nutritional requirements – protein:** this can be estimated empirically. Demands may range from 0.5–1.0 g kg^{-1} in the non-stressed state to 2.5 g kg^{-1} under conditions of extreme stress.
- **Assessment of nitrogen balance:** each gram of nitrogen is equivalent to 6.2 g of protein or 30 g of muscle. In catabolic states patients are in negative balance. Losses can be determined over each 24-hour period by measuring urinary urea and incorporating the value into a formula, a typical example of which is: 24-hour nitrogen loss $=$ (Urinary urea mmol 24hr^{-1} $\times$ 0.028) $+$ 4. 0.028 is a factor that converts urea in mmoles to grams of nitrogen, and 4 grams is the approximate total lost daily in faeces, skin, hair and urine as non-urea nitrogen.
- **Nutritional requirements – fluids:** a simple formula for basal requirements in a temperate climate is 100 ml kg^{-1} for the first 10 kg body weight, 50 ml kg^{-1} for the next 10 kg, and then 20 ml kg^{-1} thereafter. To this total must be added the various losses as appropriate. (This formula can also be used to approximate normal kilocalorie requirements.)

Direction the viva may take

You will then be asked about nutritional sources, the routes by which they may be given, and the potential complications.

- **Calorie sources:** carbohydrate (glucose) and protein (amino acids) provide 4 kcal of energy per gram, fat provides 9 kcal g^{-1}. (Alcohol provides 7 kcal g^{-1}.) Glucose-rich solutions are associated with hyerglycaemia and fatty infiltration of the liver, with excess CO_2 production which increases the respiratory quotient (RQ) to unity, with hyperinsulinaemia and fluid retention, hypophosphataemia causing reduced tissue oxygenation, and with decreased immune function. Lipid administration (10 or 20% emulsion) reduces reliance on glucose as a calorie source with its attendant problems and provides essential fatty acids. Hyperlipidaemia can complicate its administration. Protein is given in the form of crystalline amino acids.
- **Additives:** these include extra electrolytes, where appropriate, together with phosphate and magnesium, trace elements, including zinc, copper, manganese, chromium and selenium, and the full range of fat-soluble and water-soluble vitamins.
- **Other supplements:** glutamine appears to improve energy utilization and protein synthesis in skeletal muscle as well as enhancing both gut immunity and lymphocyte function. Arginine also improves lymphocyte function, as well as influencing wound healing. Omega-3 fatty acids may modulate the inflammatory response to trauma and in sepsis.
- **Parenteral nutrition:** total parenteral nutrition (TPN) may be necessary in specific cases such as short bowel syndrome, but under most circumstances enteral feeding is preferred. Complications associated with the parenteral route include all those associated with central venous catheterization, as well as the problems of impaired gastrointestinal structure and function; a loss of normal bowel flora with increased

bacterial translocation; hepatic steatosis and acalculous cholecystitis. Infection is a significant risk and TPN has the added disadvantage of high cost.

- **Enteral nutrition:** in contrast, enteral feeding improves splanchnic blood flow, maintains better gastrointestinal tract integrity, and is associated with greater nitrogen retention and enhanced weight gain. It also improves immune defences by increasing the secretion of IgA.
- **Complications:** many of these have been covered above. In summary, they include the complications of central venous access, hyperglycaemia, fatty infiltration of the liver, increased CO_2 production with implications for weaning from mechanical ventilation, hyperlipidaemia, bacterial translocation and cholecystitis.

Pharmacology

Chirality

Commentary

The science of chirality is somewhat indigestible, and you might feel aggrieved were this to be the only pharmacology that you were given the opportunity to discuss in the exam. The introduction of levobupivacaine and ropicaine, however, has given this subject some topical relevance and, so even if you cannot unravel the nomenclature convincingly, you will have to be prepared to talk about drugs which can be presented as pure enantiomers. (If you are struggling for facts it may help if you remember that in the case of the newer drugs, 'R' stands for 'risky' and 'S' stands for 'safe'.)

The viva

The subject may be introduced by a discussion of drugs that are chiral, in particular local anaesthetics. Drugs such as bupivacaine and prilocaine are racemic mixtures which contain equal numbers of isomers or enantiomers (see below). The improved safety profile of single enantiomer preparations has given chirality more immediate anaesthetic relevance.

- **Bupivacaine:** the S(−) enantiomer has less affinity for, and dissociates quicker from, myocardial sodium channels. The risk of cardiovascular and CNS toxicity is reduced. The S(−) enantiomer also exerts some vasoconstrictor activity.
- **Ropivacaine:** this is the pure S(−) enantiomer of propivacaine. It also has a safer cardiovascular profile in overdose.
- **Prilocaine:** the S(+) enantiomer is a stronger vasoconstrictor and is metabolized more slowly than the R(−) form which therefore produces higher concentrations of *o*-toluidine and a greater risk of methaemoglobinaemia.
- **Lidocaine (lignocaine):** this is achiral.

You will then be asked in more detail about chirality and isomerism.

- 'Chirality' is derived from the Greek, means 'having handedness', and defines a particular type of stereoisomerism. Right and left hands are mirror images of each other but cannot be superimposed when the palms are facing in the same direction. There are many drugs which exist as right- and left-handed forms that are mirror images but which cannot be superimposed. These particular isomers are known as 'enantiomers' ('substances of opposite shape'), and this form of stereoisomerism is dependent on the presence of one more chiral centre; typically a carbon atom with four groups attached. These enantiomers have the capacity to rotate polarized light, and so are also known as optical isomers. Their physicochemical properties are otherwise identical. Confusion can arise because of the differing nomenclature that has been used to describe chiral substances.

- One convention describes optical activity: enantiomers that rotate plane polarized light to the right are described as (+). This is the same as (dextro) or (d). Enantiomers that rotate plane polarized light to the left are described as (−), which is the same as (laevo or levo) or (l).

- Another convention, which is largely historical, is based on the configuration of a molecule in relation to (+) glutaraldehyde, which was arbitrarily assigned a 'D' (not 'd') configuration. Compounds were denoted 'D' or 'L' according to comparison with the model substance, and the optical direction added where appropriate. This method of description is limited to stereoisomers of amino acids and carbohydrates.

- The currently accepted convention is that which assigns a sequence of priority to the four atoms or groups attached to the chiral centre. The molecule is described as though it were being viewed from the front with the smallest group extending away from the viewer. If the arrangement of the largest to the smallest groups is clockwise, then the enantiomer is designated 'R' for rectus. If the arrangement is anticlockwise it is designated 'S' for sinister. The optical direction is then added to complete the description. This gives, for example, S(+) prilocaine, and R(+) tramadol. Drug manufacturers have contributed to residual confusion about nomenclature by calling S(−) bupivacaine 'levobupivacaine', whereas logic (but not commercial interest) dictates that it should have been called 'sinister bupivacaine'.

Direction the viva may take

You may be asked about the relevance of chirality for other anaesthetic drugs.

- Chiral drugs that are found in nature are usually single enantiomers, because they are synthesized enzymatically in reactions that are stereospecific. Such drugs include adrenaline, atropine, cocaine, ephedrine, hyoscine, morphine and noradrenaline. All are levorotatory and still have the designation (l).

- Most synthetic chiral drugs are racemic mixtures, and in the case of the examples above, are less potent than the pure enantiomers because the d-forms are much less active. This is not surprising, because drug receptor sites are likely to contain chiral amino acids which are stereoselective.

- The clinical behaviour of the enantiomers, and in particular their toxicity, is related to the chiral form, which is of particular relevance to a number of anaesthetic-related compounds.
- **Local anaesthetics:** as above.
- **Ketamine:** the S(+) enantiomer has a greater affinity for its main binding site (the NMDA receptor) and is up to four times as potent as the R(−) form. Its administration is also associated with fewer emergence and psychotomimetic phenomena, and it is now available (in Germany only) as a commercial preparation.
- **Etomidate:** this presented as the pure R(+) enantiomer ('R' in this case standing for 'required effect' rather than 'risk').
- **Isoflurane, enflurane, desflurane, halothane:** these are all chiral compounds that show some stereoselectivity in action. This selectivity is too modest to warrant their production as pure enantiomers. **Sevoflurane** is achiral.
- **Tramadol:** tramadol is a racemic mixture of R(+) and S(−) enantiomers. The (+) enantiomer appears to have relatively low activity at μ receptors, but the higher affinity of its main M1 metabolite results in a sixfold increase in analgesic potency. (The μ effects in humans are unimpressive.) The S(−) enantiomer inhibits the CNS re-uptake of noradrenaline and 5-HT.

Propofol

Commentary

Propofol is the most commonly used agent for induction of anaesthesia in the UK. It is also used in total intravenous anaesthesia (TIVA) and for sedation in intensive care. This makes it a core drug and so you will not be surprised that detailed knowledge will be expected. However, the structured nature of the viva will constrain the examiners from concentrating in excessive detail on any one aspect of the topic. Alternatively, you may be asked to compare it either against the 'ideal' or against the other main intravenous hypnotics.

The viva

This may start with an introductory question about the advantages and disadvantages of TIVA. Many of the advantages arise from the avoidance of other agents and so the list could be a long one. You will not therefore spend very long on this section before moving on to the basic pharmacology.

- **Advantages:** many of these are based on opinion rather than evidence, but include good recovery characteristics, avoidance of inhalational agents and their pollution, less nausea, and cardiostability.
- **Disadvantages:** perceived problems include the risk of awareness, linked to the wide variability between subjects, the complexity and cost of equipment, and the importance of secure intravenous access.

You may then be asked why propofol is a suitable agent for TIVA.

- It is a highly lipophilic hypnotic that distributes rapidly from blood to the effector site. It then undergoes further rapid redistribution to muscle and fat before being metabolized.
- The initial distribution half-life, α, of propofol is short (2–3 minutes) while intermediate distribution, β_1, takes 30–60 minutes. The terminal phase decline, β_2, is less steep and takes 3–8 hours. The immediate volume of distribution is 228 ml kg^{-1}, but the steady state volume of distribution in healthy young adults is around 800 litres.
- **Context-sensitive half-life (half-time):** this is the time taken for the plasma concentration to halve after an infusion designed to maintain constant blood levels is stopped. This is different not only for dissimilar drugs but also for the same drug depending on the duration of infusion. The context-sensitive half-life for propofol is 16 minutes after 2 hours of infusion, and 41 minutes after 8 hours. Although this compares less well with remifentanil (4.5 minutes and 9.0 minutes) it means nonetheless that accumulation is modest when the drug is infused for moderate periods.
- **Clearance:** the whole body clearance of propofol is 2500 ml min^{-1}.

You may then be asked in more detail about aspects of propofol, sufficient to satisfy the examiner that your underlying knowledge is sound. You will not cover every system.

- **Chemistry:** propofol is a substituted stable phenolic compound: 2,6-di-isopropyl-phenol. It is highly lipid-soluble and water-insoluble and is presented as either a 1% or 2% emulsion in soya bean oil. Other constituents include egg phosphatide and glycerol. It is a weak organic acid with a pKa of 11. It is not contraindicated in patients who are allergic to eggs. Egg albumin is antigenic, whereas egg phosphatide, which is derived from the yolk, is not.
- **Mechanisms:** it enhances inhibitory synaptic transmission by activation of the Cl$^-$ channel on the β_1 subunit of the GABA$_A$ receptor. It also inhibits the N-methyl-D-aspaftate (NMDA) subtype of the glutamate receptor (page 360).
- **Clinical uses:** these include induction and maintenance of anaesthesia in adults and children, sedation in intensive care, and sedation during procedures under local or regional anaesthesia. Its anti-emetic effects can benefit chemotherapy patients when given by low-dose infusion.
- **Dose and routes of administration:** the drug is used only intravenously. A dose of 1–2 mg kg^{-1} will usually induce anaesthesia in adults. Children may require twice this dose. TIVA infusion rates vary greatly, but would typically range between 4 and 12 mg kg^{-1} h^{-1}. Propofol is an effective anti-emetic when given at a rate of 1 mg kg^{-1} h^{-1}.
- **Onset and duration of action:** an induction dose of propofol will lead to rapid loss of consciousness (within a minute). Rapid redistribution to peripheral tissues (distribution half-life is 1–2 minutes) leads to rapid awakening.

Main effects and side effects

- **CNS:** propofol causes CNS depression and induction of anaesthesia. It may be associated with excitatory effects and dystonic movements, particularly in children.

The EEG displays initial activation followed by dose-related depression. The data sheet states that it is contraindicated in patients with epilepsy, although this is disputed and many anaesthetists disregard the injunction.

- **Cardiovascular system:** systemic vascular resistance falls yet it is unusual to see compensatory tachycardia. A relative bradycardia is common and the blood pressure will fall. Propofol is a myocardial depressant.
- **Respiratory system:** propofol is a respiratory depressant which also suppresses laryngeal reflexes. (Without this attribute it is unlikely that the use of the laryngeal mask airway would have become so well established.)
- **Gastrointestinal system:** the drug is anti-emetic.
- **Other side effects:** propofol causes pain on injection. Preparations which include medium-chain triglycerides in the formulation have reduced this problem. There is a risk of hyperlipidaemia in intensive care patients who have received prolonged infusions. Its data sheet states that it should not be used in pregnancy.
- **Pharmacokinetics:** propofol is highly protein-bound (98%) and has a large volume of distribution ($4 \, l \, kg^{-1}$). Distribution half-life is 1–2 minutes and the elimination half-life is 5–12 hours. Its metabolism is mainly hepatic with the production of inactive metabolites and conjugates which are excreted in urine.
- **Miscellaneous:** propofol is not a trigger for malignant hyperpyrexia and it may also be used safely in patients with porphyria. It does not release histamine and adverse reactions are very rare.

Ketamine

Commentary

Ketamine is unique amongst anaesthetic agents in that, by causing 'dissociative anaesthesia', a single dose can produce profound analgesia, amnesia and anaesthesia. It finds its way into the exam more frequently than its clinical use might deserve, but investigation of the S(+) isomer as an agent with fewer side effects has renewed the drug's promise. Its dissimilarity from the other induction agents means that it may be the sole subject of the viva.

The viva

You may be asked what makes ketamine different from the other induction agents in common use.

- **Differences:** unlike other agents ketamine is both anaesthetic and analgesic, producing these effects by actions across a range of receptors. In contrast to propofol, thiopental and etomidate it is sympathomimetic, elevating levels of circulating catecholamines and increasing cardiac output and systemic vascular resistance. Ketamine is a respiratory stimulant which preserves laryngeal reflexes and tone in the upper airway. It antagonizes the effects of ACh and 5-HT on the bronchial tree and causes clinically useful bronchodilatation. It is also different in that it is not limited to the intravenous and rectal routes but can also be given intramuscularly, orally, nasally, extradurally and intrathecally. (This accounts for some of the anaesthetic interest in the drug.)

You may then be asked about its clinical uses and thereafter about its basic pharmacology.

- **Clinical uses:** ketamine can be used for the induction of anaesthesia in adults and children, for so-called 'field' anaesthesia as a single anaesthetic agent outside the hospital setting, for bronchodilatation in severe refractory asthma, and for sedoanalgesia during procedures performed under local or regional anaesthesia. Given extradurally or intrathecally it prolongs by three to four times the duration of analgesia provided by local anaesthetic alone. It is finding increasing use in the treatment of chronic regional pain syndromes (CRPS) and for depression that is associated with this condition.
- **Doses:** an intravenous dose of $1–2\,mg\,kg^{-1}$ will induce anaesthesia. The intramuscular dose is $5–10\,mg\,kg^{-1}$. Subhypnotic doses for sedoanalgesia are usually up to $0.5\,mg\,kg^{-1}$. The addition of $0.5\,mg\,kg^{-1}$ to a sacral extradural block in children with local anaesthetic will increase the duration of action fourfold. Nasal and oral doses are $6–10\,mg\,kg^{-1}$ and the rectal dose is $10\,mg\,kg^{-1}$. (Dose regimens for pain syndromes are varied and complex: patients with CRPS, for example, have been treated by an infusion of $0.1–0.2\,mg\,kg^{-1}\,h^{-1}$ over 5 days, but details are well beyond the scope of this viva.)
- **Chemistry:** ketamine is a cyclohexanone derivative of phencyclidine (PCP). This is an anaesthetic agent used in veterinary practice and which is also a drug of abuse ('Angel dust'). It is water-soluble and is presented in three different concentrations. The solution is acidic, at pH 3.5–5.5. Most formulations now contain preservative, which precludes its use in central neural blockade, although preservative-free preparations can be obtained. It is usually presented as a racemic mixture of two enantiomers, although the pure $S(+)$ enantiomer is available in (and from) Europe.
- **Mechanisms:** ketamine is an NMDA receptor antagonist. The NMDA receptor is an L-glutamate receptor in the CNS, glutamate being the major excitatory neurotransmitter in the brain. The receptor incorporates a cation channel to which ketamine binds. Ketamine also has effects on opioid receptors, acting as a partial μ (OP3) antagonist and as a partial agonist at κ (OP2) and δ (OP1) receptors. It may therefore exert its analgesic effects after intrathecal or extradural injection at spinal κ receptors.
- **Onset and duration of action:** an induction dose of ketamine does not lead to hypnosis within one arm–brain circulation time. Consciousness will be lost after 1–2 minutes, but the patient may continue to move and to make incoherent noises. Intramuscular administration will take 10–15 minutes to take effect. The duration of action is between 10 and 40 minutes.

Main effects and side effects

- **CNS:** ketamine induces dissociative anaesthesia. Afferent input is not affected but central processing at thalamocortical and limbic levels is distorted. Anecdotally, it is reported that ketamine is less effective in brain-damaged patients. The drug produces profound analgesia as well as amnesia. It increases ICP and $CMRO_2$.

- **Cardiovascular system:** ketamine is sympathomimetic and increases levels of circulating catecholamines. On isolated myocardium, however, it acts as a depressant. Indirect effects result in tachycardia, increases in cardiac output and blood pressure, and a rise in myocardial oxygen consumption.
- **Respiratory system:** it is a respiratory stimulant which is said to preserve laryngeal reflexes and tone in the upper airway (this is not always obvious at high doses). It is an effective bronchodilator.
- **Gastrointestinal system:** it causes salivation. As with most sympathomimetic anaesthetic agents, the incidence of nausea and vomiting is increased.
- **Other effects:** the use of ketamine has been limited by its CNS side effects. It is associated both with an emergence delirium and also with dysphoria and hallucinations. Emergence delirium is a state of disorientation in which patients may react violently to minor stimuli such as light and sound. The psychotomimetic effects are a separate phenomenon, which can become manifest many hours after apparent recovery from anaesthesia. Benzodiazepines may attenuate the problem.
- **Pharmacokinetics:** ketamine is weakly protein-bound (25%). Metabolism is hepatic: demethylation produces the active metabolite norketamine, which has one-third the potency of the parent compound. Further metabolism produces conjugates which are excreted in urine.
- **Miscellaneous:** there is increasing interest in the use of the S(+) enantiomer which is three to four times as potent as the R(−) enantiomer, and which is associated with shorter recovery times and with fewer psychotomimetic reactions. Consensus opinion has it that ketamine can probably (with caution) be used in patients with porphyria.

Thiopental and etomidate

Commentary

It may seem perverse to link thiopental (thiopentone) and etomidate in the same question, but it may happen because thiopental is no longer the core agent that it once was. Its use, like that of etomidate, has shrunk to the point where in many units it is used mainly for emergency anaesthesia. Etomidate is the only other mainstream drug that is used solely as an induction agent (unlike propofol and ketamine) and so it is logical to explore their differences.

The viva

You may be asked what factors might influence your choice between these two agents. The discussion will not be a very long one and the viva will then move on to their basic pharmacology.

- It can be argued that both thiopental and etomidate are now almost niche drugs that are used for very specific purposes. Both lead to rapid loss of consciousness in one arm–brain circulation time. Etomidate has the advantages of cardiostability, minimal histamine release and a low incidence of hypersensitivity reactions. It is used mainly in emergency cases in patients who may be hypovolaemic, in those in whom haemodynamic stability is of particular importance, and in those with limited cardiac reserve. (Some anaesthetists take the view that the same outcome can be accomplished with appropriately low doses of thiopental.) Thiopental is probably the default choice for rapid sequence induction of emergency anaesthesia. It is also a potent anticonvulsant and is the most effective treatment for refractory status epilepticus.

- **Disadvantages:** etomidate is painful on injection, causes myoclonus and in many patients is emetic. Another major drawback is its potent inhibition of steroidogenesis. Thiopental is a myocardial and haemodynamic depressant, does not suppress airway reflexes and is antanalgesic. It is highly irritant, and inadvertent intra-arterial injection is more dangerous than with other induction agents. Hypersensitivity reactions are rare (1 in 15–20 000) but when they occur are severe. Neither thiopental nor etomidate is safe in patients with porphyria.

You will then be asked to compare their pharmacology in more detail.

- **Chemistry:** etomidate is a carboxylated imidazole. It is water-soluble but has been formulated in propylene glycol 35% to improve the stability of the solution. This is a high osmolarity organic solvent which may be responsible for some of the adverse effects. A newer preparation presents etomidate in a lipid formulation containing medium chain triglycerides. It is a pure R(+) enantiomer. Thiopental is the sulphur analogue of the barbiturate pentobarbitone and in solution has a pH of 10.4. The ampoules contain nitrogen to prevent any reaction with atmospheric CO_2.
- **Mechanism of action:** both drugs appear to enhance inhibitory synaptic transmission by activation of the Cl^- channel on the β_1 subunit of the $GABA_A$ receptor.
- **Clinical uses:** both are used for the induction of general anaesthesia in adults and children. Etomidate cannot be used for maintenance of anaesthesia, nor for sedation in intensive care because of its effects on steroid metabolism (see below). Thiopental can be given by infusion, usually to control grand mal convulsions.
- **Dose and routes of administration:** both can be given by the intravenous and rectal routes. The intravenous dose of etomidate is 0.2–0.3 mg kg^{-1} (6 mg kg^{-1} pr); that of thiopental is 3–5 mg kg^{-1} (50 mg kg^{-1} pr).

Main effects and side effects

- **CNS:** both drugs are CNS depressants. Etomidate may be associated with marked myoclonus although the EEG displays no epileptiform activity. Thiopental is a potent anticonvulsant which decreases cerebral blood flow, ICP and CMRO$_2$. Etomidate also reduces these indices but does not significantly affect cerebral perfusion pressure.
- **Cardiovascular system:** etomidate is associated with negligible changes in arterial blood pressure or heart rate. It is said to maintain cardiac output and to

have minimal myocardial depressant effects. There are, however, some Doppler studies which have shown that cardiac index actually falls but systemic vascular resistance rises (mediated by a_{2B}-adrenoceptors in vascular smooth muscle). Etomidate produces the least alteration in the balance of myocardial oxygen supply and demand. It is these characteristics that make the drug popular for induction of anaesthesia in patients with limited circulatory or cardiac reserve. Thiopental causes dose-related myocardial depression and hypotension.

- **Respiratory system:** etomidate has some respiratory depressant effects, but these are transient and much less marked than is seen with barbiturates or propofol. Neither agent inhibits hypoxic pulmonary vasoconstriction.

- **Gastrointestinal system:** etomidate is emetic and is associated with a high incidence of nausea and vomiting. Thiopental is not.

- **Pharmacokinetics:** etomidate is 75% protein-bound and has a volume of distribution (V_d) of 2.0–4.5 $l\,kg^{-1}$. The distribution half-life ($t_{1/2\alpha}$) is 2–4 minutes and the elimination half-life ($t_{1/2\beta}$) is 1–4 hours. It is metabolized by ester hydrolysis and N-dealkylation in the liver to inactive compounds which are excreted renally. Thiopental is 85% protein-bound and has a similar V_d of 2.5 $l\,kg^{-1}$. The distribution half-life ($t_{1/2\alpha}$) is very short, at 1–2 minutes, and the elimination half-life ($t_{1/2\beta}$) is 10 hours. It undergoes hepatic oxidation to an inactive carboxylic acid derivative and to pentobarbital, an active oxybarbiturate which is metabolized slowly.

- **Miscellaneous:** etomidate does not release histamine and the incidence of hypersensitivity reactions is extremely low (fewer than 1 in 50 000). Thiopental is associated with histamine release and hypersensitivity reactions are more common (1 in 15–20 000). Neither drug triggers malignant hyperpyrexia. Etomidate increases levels of δ-ALA synthetase and is considered unsafe in porphyria. Thiopental as a barbiturate is contraindicated.

- **Adrenocortical suppression:** etomidate is an inhibitor of steroidogenesis in the adrenal cortex. Its imidazole structure (a ring comprising three carbon and two nitrogen atoms) allows it to combine with cytochrome P450 to prevent cortisol production. Specifically it blocks two enzymes, 17-α hydroxylase and 11-β hydroxylase, which catalyse at least six of the reactions in the biosynthetic pathways from cholesterol to hydrocortisone (cortisol). The mineralocorticoid and glucocorticoid pathways are linked, and etomidate inhibits both the formation of corticosterone, which is a precursor of aldosterone, as well as hydrocortisone. You will not be expected to know these pathways in any detail, but the enzyme inhibition does explain why etomidate is one of the most potent inhibitors of steroid production that has so far been synthesized. The immunosuppressant effects of etomidate were unmasked by studies in which mortality rates in intensive care patients were demonstrably higher in those who had been sedated with a continuous infusion. It has since been shown that impaired adrenocortical function will follow even a single induction dose, and that, although the enzyme inhibition is reversible, it may still persist for up to 8 hours. Thiopental has no such effects.

Inhalational agents: comparison with the ideal

Commentary

This is a standard introduction to a discussion of the agents that are available. After you have outlined the desirable characteristics of your ideal agent you will be asked how one or more of the drugs in current use compare. The way that this question is structured means that the subject tends to be discussed at a quite superficial level, although you will need to be prepared to explain some of the concepts in more detail. Much of the information is still relatively soft, so include numerical data where you can. Be aware of the important purported differences in their effects on systems, but recognize also that comparisons have been established via studies of dissimilar methodology which have sometimes yielded conflicting results. This means that you cannot be expected to discuss detailed comparative information.

The viva

You may be asked first to describe the properties of an ideal volatile anaesthetic agent. You will also be asked, either as you describe each property or subsequently, to compare one or more of the currently available agents against this ideal. (In the interests of completeness, xenon is mentioned intermittently in the account below. This is because there is much less information available. There are enough data, however, to indicate that of all the agents it is xenon that most closely approaches the ideal, and the examiners will be very interested if you have actually used it.)

Characteristics of the ideal inhalational agent might include the following.

- **Safety:** the ideal agent would be safe by virtue of its specificity for the nervous system. It would, in other words, allow a controlled state of insensibility in which all other physiological indices such as cerebral and myocardial blood flow remained unchanged. No such agent exists, and so patients receiving inhalational agents may be at potential risk from the secondary, undesirable effects of an agent, from direct toxic effects, or from toxic products of metabolism.
- **Respiratory:** the potential to cause airways irritation is discussed below. All the drugs are respiratory depressants, and cause a decrease in tidal volume with an increase in respiratory rate. They are effective bronchodilators.
- **Cardiovascular:** all the halogenated agents have cardiovascular effects, but none so marked as to preclude their clinical use.
  — Halothane is the most arrhythmogenic. It causes a dose-related fall in mean arterial pressure (MAP) and may also cause bradycardia, junctional rhythms and ventricular premature beats. It sensitizes the myocardium to catecholamines, particularly in the presence of acidosis and hypercapnia. Experience with this agent in the UK is fast disappearing.
  — Enflurane similarly causes dose-related cardiovascular depression, but is not arrhythmogenic.

— Isoflurane leads to a dose-dependent reduction in systemic vascular resistance (SVR) and coronary vascular vasodilatation. Heart rate increases and cardiac output and contractility are maintained. Isoflurane was believed to cause a coronary steal syndrome in which coronary vasodilatation diverted blood away from stenotic vessels. Controlled trials have suggested that it is no worse than any other volatile in this regard.

— Desflurane causes a similar fall in SVR and MAP, while heart rate rises and cardiac output are maintained.

— Sevoflurane also leads to dose-dependent cardiovascular depression, with decreases in MAP, SVR and contractility. The heart rate does not increase and the agent causes less coronary vasodilatation than isoflurane.

— Xenon is cardiostable.

- **CNS:** all the halogenated agents increase cerebral blood flow (CBF), which can cause a rise in ICP that in some circumstances may be deleterious.

  — Sevoflurane preserves cerebral autoregulation better than the other agents.

  — Desflurane, in contrast, abolishes autoregulation at 1.5 MAC. Alone amongst the agents it increases CSF production.

  — At 1.0 MAC, isoflurane and sevoflurane are associated with minimal changes in CBF and ICP.

  — Enflurane is associated with abnormal epileptiform activity in the EEG, particularly if its administration is accompanied by hypocapnia.

- **Uterus:** all the agents, apart from nitrous oxide and xenon, cause dose-related uterine relaxation.

- **Malignant hyperpyrexia:** halothane is the most dangerous, although all the halogenated agents are reported triggers for this condition.

- **Efficacy:** by definition, the agent has to be able to induce and maintain a state of anaesthesia, and all the halogenated agents produce dose-dependent narcosis. Some are more 'potent' than others in the sense that their effects are produced at lower concentrations, but clinically this is of little relevance. According to this criterion, for example, halothane is almost nine times as potent as desflurane. A much more significant property is the blood solubility, as quantified by the blood–gas partition coefficient. The less soluble the agent the lower the amount required to produce a given partial pressure and the more rapid the onset of action. In ascending order, therefore, the agents can be ranked: xenon, whose blood–gas partition coefficient is only 0.17, desflurane (0.42), nitrous oxide (0.47), sevoflurane (0.68), isoflurane (1.4), enflurane (1.9) and halothane (2.3). 'Potency' in respect of inhalational agents is in effect defined by the MAC at which 50% of the population will not display reflex movement in response to a standard surgical stimulus. This is the MAC^{50}, but the MAC^{95} (the prevention of movement in 95% of subjects) is more useful. MAC^{50}s are: halothane (0.75), isoflurane (1.17), enflurane (1.63), sevoflurane (1.8), desflurane (6.6) xenon (60–70) and nitrous oxide (105).

- **Airways irritation:**

  — Sevoflurane is non-irritant to the upper airway and bronchi, and inhalational induction can be swift and effective in the most testing of circumstances.

  — Halothane shares the same characteristics, but is slightly more pungent.

— Enflurane is not dissimilar, although inhalation induction is more prolonged.
— Isoflurane is more irritant to airways and is associated with a higher incidence of coughing and breath holding.
— Desflurane is the most inferior agent in this respect, its other benefits being offset by its effective capacity to provoke laryngospasm, excessive secretions and apnoea.

• **Toxicity**
— Nitrous oxide depresses bone marrow function via its oxidation of the cobalt atom in the vitamin B12 complex (page 208).
— Sevoflurane may produce the potentially but not demonstrably toxic compound A (see below), as well as free fluoride ions.
— Enflurane also produces fluoride ions, while halothane is implicated in post-exposure hepatic dysfunction (see below).

• **Metabolism:** inhaled agents are eliminated through the lungs, but metabolism still occurs, principally by cytochrome P450 oxidation in the liver. None of the agents has active metabolites, but clearly the greater the proportion that undergoes hepatic metabolism the greater is the excretory load.
— Xenon is an inert gas which undergoes no biotransformation.
— Nitrous oxide undergoes minimal metabolism (0.004%), mainly by gut micro-organisms.
— Desflurane is resistant to metabolism (0.02%) and serum fluoride levels do not rise even after prolonged administration.
— Isoflurane metabolism is around 0.2%, which can lead to a small rise in fluoride concentrations.
— Enflurane metabolism is higher, at around 3%, and serum fluoride levels may reach 25 μmol l^{-1}, which may be of theoretical importance in patients with pre-existing renal impairment. (Fluoride is nephrotoxic at levels of 50 μmol l^{-1} and above.)
— Sevoflurane undergoes 3–5% metabolism and produces more fluoride ions than enflurane. Serum fluoride concentrations may reach 15–25 μmol l^{-1} after 1 MAC hour of administration. In theory, it should be used with caution in patients with renal dysfunction, but this is not regarded universally as a contraindication for its use. The chemical structure of sevoflurane is such that it cannot undergo biotransformation to an acyl halide, and so, unlike halothane, enflurane, isoflurane and desflurane, its metabolism does not result in the formation of trifluoroacetylated liver proteins and subsequent production of anti-trifluoroacetylated protein antibodies.
— Halothane is the most extensively metabolized of the inhalational agents, with 20–40% being degraded by both reductive and oxidative pathways. A trifluoroacetylated compound produced by oxidation can bind to liver proteins, triggering in susceptible patients an immune reaction which may precipitate hepatic necrosis. This is a separate problem from the transient postoperative rise in liver enzymes, which may be seen in up to 20% of patients.

• **Stability:** this refers to the molecular stability of the compound when exposed to the normal range of environmental conditions, and to the specific circumstances of its use in an anaesthetic breathing system. Ideally, it should be stable to light and to temperature, it should undergo no spontaneous degradation and require no preservatives, it should be non-flammable and non-corrosive and should be safe in the presence of soda lime and alkali. Most of the agents perform well against these criteria: some specific exceptions include the following.

— Nitrous oxide supports combustion.

— Desflurane has a low boiling point that is close to room temperature (23.5°C).

— Sevoflurane reacts with strong monovalent hydroxide bases, such as those which are used in soda lime and barium lime CO_2 absorbers, to produce a number of substances, including compound A. (The reaction with barium lime is about five times more rapid than with soda lime.) Of the degradation products (compounds A, B, D, E and G), only A, which is a vinyl ether, has been shown to have any toxicity, but the dose-dependent renal damage noted in rats has never been seen in humans despite many millions of administrations.

— Halothane may degrade when exposed to light and so is presented in amber bottles in thymol 0.01% as a preservative. Accumulated thymol can affect vaporizer function.

- **Xenon:** this gas most closely approaches the ideal agent. It provides effective hypnosis and analgesia together with some muscle relaxation. It is non-irritant and, although it depresses respiration to the point of apnoea, it is cardiostable. It undergoes no metabolism, is not toxic and does not cause allergic reactions. It is stable in storage, is non-flammable and is environmentally neutral. However, when it is used in a semi-closed breathing system it costs £1200 an hour, falling to £180 an hour when used with ultra-low flows of $0.3 \, l \, min^{-1}$, so, until a highly efficient xenon recycling system can be developed, this almost ideal inhalational agent will never find widespread use.

Nitrous oxide

Commentary

Not that long ago there were some candidates for the then equivalent of the Final FRCA who were thoroughly discomfited by a written question on the 'pharmacology of nitrous oxide' (N_2O). This was hardly surprising, because few anaesthetists then had much interest in the drug and it was ignored largely as being simply a carrier gas with modest analgesic properties. This perception did the complex pharmacology of the drug a disservice, and there followed an upsurge of interest, both in its potential toxicity as well as in its mechanisms of action. This interest appears now to be waning but, given the continued and ubiquitous use of N_2O, it remains a core anaesthetic agent about which detailed knowledge will be expected. Some anaesthetists never use the drug and it polarizes opinion. Your assessment should therefore be dispassionate, unless it becomes clear that your examiner shares your own views.

The viva

The pharmacology and toxicology is complex and so the topic may be introduced via a question about the place of N_2O in modern anaesthetic practice. This is more likely following the large multicentre study that appeared in *Anesthesiology* in 2007 (Myles *et al.*, 2007).

Advantages

- It is a useful carrier gas for more potent anaesthetic agents.
- It has a rapid onset and equilibration because of its very low blood–gas partition coefficient (0.47).
- The induction of anaesthesia is accelerated via the second gas effect, in which the rapid uptake of N_2O from the alveoli increases the alveolar concentration of other agents.
- It is a potent analgesic whose effects are usually underestimated. The drug acts partly at opioid receptors and transiently has the potency of morphine. This is not surprising given data showing that entonox (N_2O/O_2) affords better pain relief during labour (effective analgesia in around 50% of mothers) than pethidine (effective analgesia in about 35%).
- It is a weak anaesthetic (MAC^{50} is 105%) but, in combination with its analgesic actions, it decreases the MAC of other inhalational agents.

Disadvantages

- **Outcome after major surgery:** the Australian paper referred to above recruited over 2000 patients who were undergoing major surgery expected to last over 2 hours. Its authors asserted that major complications were greater in the group that received N_2O than in the group that received 80% O_2 in air, and concluded that the routine use of the agent should be questioned. However, no patients received 30% O_2 in air and so it was not possible to determine whether the purported beneficial effects were caused by a high FiO_2, the avoidance of N_2O, or both. (The arguments continue.)
- **Effect on air-filled spaces:** the diffusing capacity of N_2O relative to nitrogen is high ($\times 25$).
  — In non-compliant air-filled spaces, pressure increases (in the middle ear, in nasal sinuses, and in the eye if it has been filled with gas such as SF_6 after vitreoretinal surgery). The pressure change is related arithmetically to the alveolar partial pressure of N_2O, so that administration of 50% N_2O leads to a pressure increase of 0.5 atmospheres.
  — In compliant air-filled spaces, volume increases (significant for pneumothoraces, bullae, bowel, air embolus, cuffs of tracheal tubes). After 4 hours of 66% N_2O the volume of the bowel increases by 200%. The volume change is related geometrically to alveolar partial pressure of N_2O; the percentage increase is given by the % N_2O divided by ($1.0 - FiN_2O$). So, at 50% the final percentage volume increase is $50/0.5 = 100\%$. At 75%, a pneumothorax will triple in size after 30 minutes of N_2O administration.

Myles PS *et al.* (2007). Avoidance of nitrous oxide for patients undergoing major surgery: a randomized controlled trial. *Anesthesiology*, **107**(2), 221–31.

- **Bone marrow toxicity and neurotoxicity:** see below.
- **Emesis:** this is probably caused by a combination of its sympathomimetic and opioid effects, together with the effects of bowel distension.
- **Second gas effect:** this results in diffusion hypoxia (which is of modest clinical relevance; it lasts less than 10 minutes and can be overcome with supplemental oxygen).
- **Respiratory depression:** there is an increase in respiratory rate to offset decreased tidal volume; this is common to all volatile agents.
- **Cardiovascular system:** N_2O is a direct negative inotrope and chronotrope. Cardiac contractility is decreased if cardiac function is already impaired; its use exacerbating ischaemic change in any situation in which myocardial O_2 supply is exceeded by demand. It is an indirect stimulant (via its sympathomimetic action). It increases pulmonary vascular resistance in the presence of pre-existing pulmonary hypertension.
- **Greenhouse effect:** N_2O is a greenhouse gas; anaesthesia contributes about 1% of the global total.

Direction the viva may take

You may then be asked about mechanisms of action and its potential toxicity.

Anaesthesia

- **GABA$_A$ (mainly inhibitory) and NMDA (mainly excitatory) receptors in the CNS:** N_2O appears to have no effect on GABA$_A$ receptors but strongly inhibits NMDA-activated currents. There is concern that NMDA antagonists can be neurotoxic, which is a potential problem if N_2O is used alone under hyperbaric conditions. If GABA$_A$ agonist agents or facilitators (such as benzodiazepines) are used in addition, they may exert a protective effect to offset this damage.
- **Dopamine receptors.** N_2O stimulates some dopaminergic neurons; this may mediate release of endogenous opioid peptides and explains why the effects of N_2O are partly antagonized by naloxone.

Analgesia

- **Opioid peptide release:** this occurs in the peri-aqueductal grey matter of the midbrain, and stimulates descending noradrenergic pathways which modulate pain processing via noradrenaline release. Noradrenaline acts at a_2-receptors in the dorsal horn.
- **Other theories:** N_2O may activate a supraspinal descending pain inhibition system with an increase in encephalinergic interneurons in the substantia gelatinosa of the cord. These endogenous encephalins inhibit transmission via substance P-dependent synapses.

Toxicity

- **Bone marrow toxicity and neurotoxicity.**
  — A biochemical lesion in the liver (methionine synthetase inhibition) is demonstrable after only 40 minutes of N_2O administration.

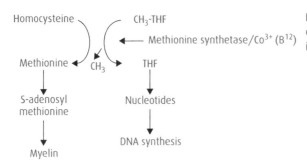

Fig. 4.1 Nitrous oxide toxicity; effect of methionine synthetase inhibition. THF, tetrahydrofolate.

— N_2O oxidizes the cobalt atom in vitamin B^{12} (cyanocobalamin) from Co^+ to Co^{3+} in a very simple reaction; vitamin B^{12}, however, is a co-factor for the enzyme methionine synthetase.
— Methionine synthetase catalyses the transfer of a methyl group in a linked methyltransferase reaction. The methylation of homocysteine forms methionine, while the demethylation of CH_3-tetrahydrofolate leads to the formation of tetrahydrofolate (Figure 4.1).
— Inhibition of methionine synthesis, therefore, prevents the production of methionine and tetrahydrofolate. Methionine is a precursor of S-adenosyl methionine (SAM). SAM is incorporated into myelin, and its absence leads to subacute combined systems degeneration of the cord in chronic B^{12} deficiency, and acutely to dorsal column function impairment (from experimental data after 48 hours of 20% N_2O administration). Tetrahydrofolate is an important substrate involved in nucleotide and DNA synthesis (hence the development of megaloblastic anaemia in folate and B^{12} deficiency).
— The administration of methionine and folinic acid will provide substrates to allow biosynthesis to continue below the level of the enzyme block.
• **Teratogenicity**
— The mechanisms above plus its other actions are believed to contribute to possible teratogenicity: a_1-adrenoceptor agonism is associated with disorders of left/right body axis development (such as situs inversus). The association is not strong; almost 25 million administrations of the drug take place in the US annually without obvious sequelae.

If you have exhausted the information above, then you will be heading for a '2 +', and so you might as well be equipped with a few final miscellaneous facts.

• Malignant hyperpyrexia: there is one definite case report, so N_2O is a weak trigger.
• Hyperbaric N_2O is excitatory, leading to a threefold increase in respiratory rate, diaphoresis and cardiovascular a-adrenergic stimulation. At increased pressure, N_2O becomes an anaesthetic (MAC is 105%), but it also causes CNS-mediated muscle rigidity and catatonic jerking.

Neuromuscular blocking drugs

Commentary

Questions on neuromuscular blockers can be unpredictable. A single agent may form the basis of a viva, or you may be asked about one or more of the drugs during discussion of another subject such as the neuromuscular junction. What follows below is not intended to provide a comprehensive monograph on each of the drugs. It aims simply to identify those particular aspects on which an examiner might concentrate, such as aspects of pharmacodynamics or pharmacokinetics that are of specific interest.

The viva

Topics may include depolarizing relaxants and their problems, the newer non-depolarizing agents, and the means whereby their action is terminated.

- **Classification:** depolarizing relaxants act as agonists at the ACh receptor, and, having induced the conformational change that allows the ionophore to open, remain bound to the receptor for some minutes. Non-depolarizing relaxants, in contrast, are competitive inhibitors of ACh at the post-junctional nicotinic receptors. They bind to one or both of the a units to prevent ACh access, but induce no conformational change in the receptor. The a subunits are separated by a distance of 1.4 nm, but it is not necessary for quaternary nitrogen radicals to have the same spatial separation for the drugs to exert their effect.
- **Depolarizing muscle relaxants:** see page 211.
- **Non-depolarizing relaxants:** all are quaternary amines, whose potency is increased if the molecule contains two quaternary ammonium radicals. There are two main groups: the benzylisoquinoliniums (drugs ending in –*urium*), and the aminoster-oids (drugs ending in -*uronium*). The aminosteroids in general show greater cardiovascular stability and cause less histamine release.
- **Established agents:** (the duration of action that is quoted below is the time following an intubating dose at which there is 25% recovery and pharmacological reversal can be used.)
  - *Atracurium:* this is a bisquaternary amine, a benzylisoquinolinium mixture of 16 potential isomers. It has a medium duration of action which is reversible pharmacologically at 25 minutes. It may cause histamine release.
  - *Cisatracurium:* this is one of the isomers of atracurium, which has a slightly longer duration of action (45 minutes), and has greater cardiovascular stability because it is less likely to provoke histamine release.
  - *Mivacurium:* this is a benzylisoquinolinium diester, with a short duration of action reversible at 15 minutes. Its capacity to cause histamine release is similar to that of atracurium.
  - *Pancuronium:* this is a bisquaternary aminosteroid whose vagolytic and sympathomimetic actions made its use traditionally popular in haemodynamically

compromised patients. It is long acting (75 minutes), and its metabolism is primarily renal, with 60% being excreted unchanged.

— *Vecuronium:* this is the monoquaternary homologue of pancuronium, which was developed in an attempt to create a 'clean' version of the older drug. It has minimal cardiovascular effects, and a short duration of action (30–35 minutes).

— *Rocuronium:* this is another monoquaternary aminosteroid which is very similar to vecuronium when used in equipotent doses. It provokes minimal histamine release and is cardiostable apart from modest vagolytic effects after large doses. When given in high doses ($0.9\,\text{mg}\,\text{kg}^{-1}$) it provides good conditions for tracheal intubation within 60–75 seconds (hence its name: '*R*apid *O*nset ve*curonium*') and lasts for around 45 minutes. Lower doses ($2 \times ED^{95}$, as is typical for muscle relaxants) last for around 35 minutes. It has a specific anatagonist: *suggamadex* (Org 25969). This is an α-cyclodextrin (a ring of six linked sugar molecules) which chelates rocuronium molecules and removes them from the receptors. This specific action appears to reverse the effect of rocuronium from any depth of neuromuscular block.

- **Other agents:** drugs such as rapacuronium, pipecuronium and doxacurium have either been withdrawn from use because of adverse effects or have faded from the market.
- **Metabolism and elimination:** most are eliminated by more than one mechanism.
  — *Suxamethonium:* this predominantly undergoes ester hydrolysis (by plasma cholinesterase); a small amount is hydrolysed by non-specific plasma esterases, and 10% is excreted unchanged through the kidney.
  — *Mivacurium:* this is also metabolized by plasma cholinesterase at a slightly slower rate (88%) than suxamethonium. Abnormal cholinesterases will therefore increase its effective action more than suxamethonium. In E_uE_a heterozygotes (page 212) it will last for 2 hours, and in E_aE_a homozygotes its action will be prolonged for 8 hours or more.
  — *Atracurium:* about 10% is excreted renally, about 40–45% is hydrolysed by hepatic esters, and a further 45% undergoes Hofmann degradation at body temperature and pH (this reaction was first identified in industrial processes). The cleavage occurs at the linkage between the carbon chain and the quaternary nitrogen. Ester hydrolysis takes place at the site of the double carbon bond. Hofmann degradation produces laudanosine, a potentially epileptogenic metabolite which has not been shown to cause problems in humans.
  — *Cisatracurium:* metabolism is similar to atracurium, except a greater proportion (60–70%) undergoes Hofmann elimination.
  — *Pancuronium:* 60% is excreted renally, unchanged. The remainder is deacetylated in the liver (with the formation of some 3-desacetyl active metabolites) and rendered water-soluble by glucuronidation.
  — *Vecuronium:* about 30% is excreted renally, while the remainder undergoes hepatic deacetylation. Like pancuronium it produces an active 3-desacetyl metabolite.
  — *Rocuronium:* its elimination is mainly hepatic, and it does not form an active 3-desacetyl metabolite.

Direction the viva may take
You may be asked about the site of action of neuromuscular blockers and how you can assess their effects. See page 155.

Suxamethonium

Commentary
Suxamethonium is arguably the only drug used in anaesthesia for which there is as yet no real alternative, although some might make the case for high-dose rocuronium as a substitute. It is a very familiar drug and so you will not be invited simply to give an account of its actions. Instead, you might be asked to justify its role in modern anaesthesia, which will inevitably involve a discussion of the significant potential problems associated with its use.

The viva
You might be asked by way of introduction whether you believe that suxamethonium has a future in clinical practice. (The question is prompted by the imminent availability of sugammadex, which is the specific reversal agent for rocuronium.) If you hold strong views that you can justify, then share them with the examiners; otherwise it is prudent to take a balanced approach to the evidence.

- Suxamethonium provides the quickest means of achieving tracheal intubation. In severe laryngospasm in a patient without intravenous access it can also be given intramuscularly or intra-lingually (in a dose of $4\,mg\,kg^{-1}$). At least one meta-analysis has asserted that, despite its many adverse effects (see below), it is still the first line agent in rapid sequence induction.
- Rocuronium has a much more benign side effect profile and in a high dose of $1.0\,mg\,kg^{-1}$ it provides intubation conditions equivalent to those provided by suxamethonium, albeit up to 35 seconds slower. The problem of the prolonged paralysis that would follow such a dose may disappear with the availability of suggamadex, whose theoretical promise may or may not be confirmed when more widespread clinical experience follows its introduction in 2008.
- **Actions:** depolarizing muscle relaxants (of which suxamethonium is the only currently available example) act as agonists at the ACh receptor, but, unlike acetylcholine, once having induced the conformational change that allows the ionophore to open, they remain bound to the receptor for some minutes.
- **Structure:** in common with all muscle relaxants, suxamethonium is a quaternary amine, which is the dicholine ester of succinic acid. This compound is almost identical to two molecules of ACh. It is bisquaternary and each of its ammonium radicals, $N^{+}(CH_3)_3$, bind to the a units of the ACh receptor.
- **Indications:** it is an ultra-short-acting agent whose prime use is to allow rapid tracheal intubation in patients who are at risk of pulmonary aspiration of gastric

contents. It can be used intermittently (with the problems of bradycardia with subsequent doses) and also by infusion. The maximum quoted total dose is $10 \, \text{mg} \, \text{kg}^{-1}$. Larger doses risk inducing phase II block.

- **Problems:**

  — *Myalgia:* this should not be underestimated because it can be very severe. Its mechanism is unclear; although suxamethonium causes fasciculations and an increase in muscle creatine phosphokinase (CPK), neither of these is directly related to post-administration pain. Myoglobin can also be detected in urine. Early ambulation, female gender, middle age, and, it is said, lack of muscular fitness, are all associated with a higher incidence, as are rapid injection and repeated smaller doses. Techniques used to attenuate the problem include pre-treatment with a non-depolarizing relaxant, dantrolene, lignocaine and phenytoin.

  — *Hyperkalaemia:* serum potassium may rise about $0.5 \, \text{mmol} \, \text{l}^{-1}$ in the normal patient, but this increase can be dangerously high in patients in whom muscle cells are damaged or in whom muscles are denervated. Damaged muscle leaks potassium, while denervated muscle demonstrates an increase in extrajunctional ACh receptors. Conditions in which suxamethonium should be avoided, therefore, include renal failure, burns, spinal cord damage, polyneuropathies and crush injury. Dangerous rises can also occur in the critically ill, and the drug must be used with caution in intensive care patients.

  — *Prolonged action owing to decreased enzyme activity:* suxamethonium undergoes ester hydrolysis in a reaction that is catalysed by plasma cholinesterase. Qualitative and quantitative changes in this enzyme have a substantial effect on the drug's duration of action. Enzyme activity is reduced by decreased enzyme synthesis due to liver disease, starvation, carcinomatosis, pregnancy, renal disease and myxoedema (hypothyroidism). Such reduction may increase by several times its normal duration of action of 3–5 minutes. Prolongation may also result from competition by other drugs metabolized by esterases, such as diamorphine, ester-linked local anaesthetics, esmolol, and monoamine oxidase inhibitors. Anticholinesterases inhibit both plasma cholinesterase as well as acetylcholinesterase.

  — *Prolonged action owing to abnormal enzyme:* qualitative differences result from inherited deficiencies of plasma cholinesterase. Its synthesis is controlled by autosomal recessive genes, of which 14 different mutations have so far been identified. The normal gene is characterized as E_u, and the commonest atypical gene as E_a (others include the fluoride gene, E_f, and the silent gene, E_s). The action of suxamethonium in a heterozygote, $E_u E_a$, will be prolonged by around 30 minutes, whereas in a homozygote, $E_a E_a$, this will extend to several hours, and will be longer still in the case of $E_a E_s$ and $E_s E_s$ variations. Testing using inhibition by dibucaine and fluoride has been superseded by direct assay of cholinesterase activity. Suxamethonium apnoea is not life-threatening, but it is important to maintain anaesthesia in any patient who is receiving supportive ventilation.

  — *Malignant hyperpyrexia and anaphylaxis:* it is a trigger for malignant hyperpyrexia, and, although allergic reactions are rare, anaphylaxis is more commonly seen with suxamethonium than with any other muscle relaxant, accounting for almost 50% of reactions. (There were two fatal cases described in the 1991–1993 report of the *Confidential Enquiry into Maternal Mortality*.)

- **Metabolism and elimination:** the primary metabolic route is ester hydrolysis in the presence of plasma cholinesterase. A small amount is hydrolysed by non-specific plasma esterases, and 10% is excreted unchanged through the kidney.

- **Assessment of neuromuscular block:** (page 155). Using a nerve stimulator, a single twitch will elicit a diminished or absent response. If a train-of-four stimulus is applied, there will be no decrement in the height of successive twitches. Tetanic stimulation may evoke a small sustained response but without any post-tetanic facilitation.

Opiates/opioids

Commentary

This may not appear as a question on its own, although it might be linked to the subject of patient-controlled analgesia (PCA) or aspects of postoperative pain relief. Opiates are central to anaesthetic practice and so you will be expected to have a comprehensive grasp of their pharmacology. There is some confusion over the terms 'opiate' and 'opioid'. The word 'opiate', strictly defined, is any drug that is derived from the opium poppy, *Papaver somniferum*. However, according to this definition, morphine and codeine phosphate are classed as opiates, whereas diamorphine (which is diacetylated morphine) is not. It is more logical, therefore, to use 'opiate' as the noun, and 'opioid' as the adjective, or alternatively, to use the term 'opioid' to mean any drug that acts at the opioid receptor. It would be more logical still to abandon the word 'opiate' altogether, but in the meantime the residual uncertainty means that you will not be disadvantaged if you tend to use the terms interchangeably.

The viva

As the rational use of opioids does depend on an understanding of their basic pharmacology, this is a reasonable place for the viva to start.

All the pure μ-agonists have similar pharmacodynamic effects; their differences are primarily pharmacokinetic. This means that you are likely to be asked in some detail about the underlying mechanisms of action of opioids as a whole, and in less detail about the individual drugs. You will probably be familiar with most of them so have confidence in your clinical experience of their use.

- **Opioid receptors:** there are three main opioid receptor subtypes: μ (mu), κ (kappa) and δ (delta), which are also referred to respectively as OP3, OP2 and OP1 receptors. Their natural ligands are endomorphins (μ), dynorphins (κ) and enkephalins (δ). Opioids have a number of effects at the cellular level: they inhibit intracellular adenyl cyclase via G protein-coupling; they hyperpolarize cell membranes by facilitating the opening of post-synaptic potassium channels; and they inhibit neurotransmitter release by decreasing the function of voltage-gated calcium channels. μ-receptors are believed to mediate not only analgesic effects, but also respiratory depression. κ-receptors have more spinal and peripheral than central analgesic effects, as do the δ-receptors. (The σ (sigma)-receptor is not considered to be a true opioid receptor, but mediates psychotomimetic effects both of opiates and of other types of psychoactive agents.) There is a further receptor, known as the 'opioid receptor-like type 1' (ORL1), which also inhibits calcium channels and increases cellular potassium efflux. Its natural ligand is orphanin FQ. No exogenous agonists are yet available.

- **Opioid actions:** these are almost too well known to repeat but, to summarize, opioids have a mixture of inhibitory and excitatory effects. Inhibitory actions mediate sedation, anxiolysis, analgesia, respiratory depression (including inhibition of the respiratory response to hypoxia), inhibition of cough, and loss of vascular smooth muscle tone. Excitatory effects explain miosis (stimulation of the Edinger–Westphal nucleus), nausea and vomiting via direct actions at the chemoreceptor trigger zone, ADH release from the posterior pituitary, urinary retention owing to enhanced detrusor muscle tone, bronchoconstriction caused by an increase in smooth muscle tone, and constipation owing to increased activity in the circular muscle of the bowel which prevents effective peristalsis. Other effects include histamine release, pruritus (which may not be mediated by μ-receptors, as it is not reliably reversed by naloxone) and chest wall rigidity. This is associated with rapid injection of the more potent opioids, but its mechanism has not been elucidated.

Direction the viva may take

You might be asked about postoperative analgesia or about PCA. The discussion below concentrates on the latter, but you should be able to adapt the information should the questioning come from a different angle. You may therefore be asked to outline the advantages and disadvantages of PCA. These are fairly generalized and lack strong evidence, so the questioning will soon move on to the basic pharmacology.

- **Advantages:** PCA is popular with patients because of the autonomy and control that it gives them, and so is particularly useful in those who might otherwise be reluctant to request analgesia and for who dislike intramuscular injections. It is popular with nurses for the same reasons, and because it can save nursing time. It is popular with doctors because most PCA regimens by and large can cope with the very wide variability that characterizes patients' requirements for postoperative opioids. As a generalization, it is efficacious and safe.
- **Disadvantages:** it is important that a PCA does not lessen the direct personal contact between the patient and nursing staff. Electronic pumps can limit mobility, while disposable devices lack the facility to track demand and the total analgesic dose delivered. Security can also be a problem. PCA is still a system that delivers bolus doses, which results in peaks and troughs of effect. This can be overcome by adding a background infusion, but potentially this is at the expense of safety.

You will then be asked which drugs are suitable for this purpose. (Questioning will concentrate on the differences between the drugs, which are mainly pharmacokinetic, rather than their similarities.)

- **Morphine:** it is accepted that this is the most successful drug for PCA because it offers the best compromise between combination of efficacy and duration of action. A bolus dose has its peak effect at around 15 minutes and lasts 2–3 hours. It is metabolized in the liver to morphine-6-glucuronide (5–15%), which is more potent than the parent compound (its precise relative potency has not been quantified because studies have looked at different aspects of opioid effect rather than at analgesia alone), and to morphine-3-glucuronide (50%) which has no analgesic effects. In fact, there is a suggestion that in high concentrations the compound is antalgesic. This may explain why increasing the dose of morphine to patients with cancer can sometimes exacerbate their pain. A typical PCA regimen involves giving bolus doses of 1.0 mg with a lockout time of 5 minutes.

- **Diamorphine:** this is a semisynthetic derivative of morphine, diacetylmorphine, which consists of two molecules of morphine. The compound has no activity at μ-receptors until it is metabolized to 6-monoacetylmorphine and thence to morphine (both are active). It is thus a prodrug with the same properties as morphine. Some clinicans claim nonetheless that anecdotally it is less emetic and more euphoriant than morphine. (When given intrathecally its much higher lipid solubility does appear to confer some advantages.) It can be used in a PCA system at half the morphine dose (being twice as potent) with the same lock-out time.

- **Pethidine:** the side effect profile is very similar to that of morphine, but pethidine is still regarded as an alternative opioid in patients who are intolerant of morphine. It has a rapid onset of action but its effects are shorter. It differs in some other material respects. One of its metabolites is norpethidine, which is a convulsant. Prolonged or high-dose administration should therefore be avoided. The drug is related structurally to atropine and so also has anticholinergic actions. It relaxes bronchial and vascular smooth muscle and is antispasmodic. It is a membrane stabilizer and has a local anaesthetic effect. It can be used for PCA (bolus doses of 10–20 mg with a 5-minute lockout). One of its useful indications is for the treatment of anaesthesia-induced postoperative shivering (25 mg by slow iv injection).

- **Fentanyl:** this is a phenylpiperidine like pethidine and which itself is the parent compound of alfentanil and remifentanil. Onset of effect is at 1–2 minutes, with a peak action at 4–5 minutes and an effective duration of action after a single bolus of up to 30 minutes. It is highly lipid-soluble and its metabolites are inactive. It is a drug that accumulates when given by infusion (or by repeated bolus injection); its context-sensitive half-time (CSHT) after 2 hours of constant infusion is 48 minutes, which, after 8 hours of infusion, extends to 282 minutes. It can be used for PCA with bolus doses of 10–20 μg and a lockout time of 5–10 minutes.

- **Alfentanil:** this is also a phenylpiperidine compound but with a shorter duration of action than fentanyl. After peaking at 1 minute after iv injection, its effects last for only 5–10 minutes. The drug accumulates when given by infusion, its CSHT being 50 minutes after 2 hours.

- **Remifentanil:** this is a phenylpiperidine ester whose action is terminated by non-specific tissue esterases. Its main product of metabolism has minimal potency (<0.5%). This gives it a short and predictable duration of action which is confirmed by its CSHT. It is effectively context-insensitive because the CSHT is 4.5 minutes after 2 hours of infusion, and only 9.0 minutes after 8 hours. Its very rapid offset of action makes it unsuitable for PCA for postoperative pain, but it has been used for labour analgesia. (Bolus doses 20–40 μg with a 2-minute lockout.)
- **Other pure μ-agonists:** these include codeine phosphate (which is metabolized to morphine), its semisynthetic derivative dihydrocodeine, hydromorphone (which is a potent morphine derivative used mainly in the treatment of severe cancer pain), and oxycodone (which has high oral bioavailability (up to 75%) and which is becoming more popular for the treatment of postoperative pain). Oxycodone has one weakly active metabolite, oxymorphone. (The usual oral dose of oxycodone is 5–10 mg given 4–6-hourly.)
- **Tramadol:** tramadol is a racemic mixture of R(+) and S(−) enantiomers, of which the R(+) enantiomer has low initial activity at μ-receptors; however, the higher affinity of its main metabolite (*o*-desmethyltramadol) results in a sixfold increase in analgesic potency. Nevertheless, the μ effects in humans are not impressive, although opioid side effects such as nausea, constipation and dysphoria are still apparent. The S(−) enantiomer inhibits the re-uptake of noradrenaline and 5-HT within the CNS. Tramadol has been used in PCA with 10–20 mg boluses and a 5-minute lockout. It causes less nausea than morphine but at the cost of inferior analgesia.

Local anaesthetics: actions

Commentary
Questions about local anaesthesia are popular because the subject can switch readily between basic science and its clinical implications. Mechanisms of action may not be a topic on their own but may form part of questions on the agents themselves and their toxicity, or as a supplement to a discussion of nerve blocks.

The viva
You may be asked about the mechanism of action of local anaesthetics.

- **Definition:** a local anaesthetic agent is defined as a compound which produces temporary blockade of neuronal transmission when applied to a nerve axon.
- **Drugs:** numerous drugs share this characteristic with conventional local anaesthetics. They include anticonvulsants, many antiarrhythmics, including bretylium and β-adrenoceptor blockers, some phenothiazines and some antihistamines, as well as drugs such as pethidine. None is used as a local anaesthetic, but all have a similar mechanism of action. The range of local anaesthetic agents used in the UK is small and is restricted largely to lidocaine (lignocaine), bupivacaine, prilocaine and, to a lesser extent, ropivacaine.

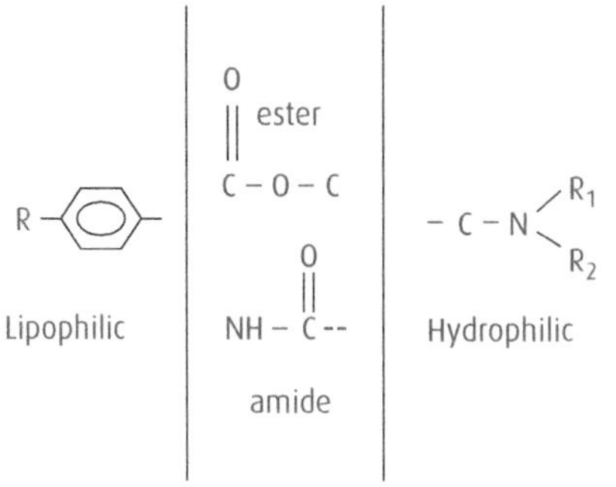

Fig. 4.2 Structure of local anaesthetics.

$$R - \bigcirc - \overset{\begin{array}{c} O \\ \| \\ C - O - C \end{array}}{\underset{\begin{array}{c} O \\ \| \\ NH - C -- \end{array}}{}} \quad - C - N \overset{R_1}{\underset{R_2}{\diagdown}}$$

Lipophilic   ester

amide   Hydrophilic

- **Basic structure:** all local anaesthetics are chemical descendants of cocaine and comprise a lipophilic aromatic portion, which is joined via an ester or amide linkage to a hydrophilic tertiary amine chain (Figure 4.2).
- **Normal action potential:** local anaesthetic action is best described in the context of a normal nerve action potential. The axon maintains a voltage differential of 60–90 mV across the nerve membrane. At rest the membrane is relatively impermeable to the influx of sodium (Na^+) ions, and is selectively permeable to potassium (K^+) ions. In the resting cell membrane this selective permeability allows a small net efflux of K^+ ions, which leaves the axoplasm electrically negative (polarized). At rest, Na^+ ions tend to flow into the axon, both because the inside is electrically negative and because of the concentration gradient. This resting membrane potential is maintained by the Na^+/K^+ pump which continually extrudes Na^+ from within the cell in exchange for K^+, using ATP as an energy source. When specific sodium channels in the axonal membrane are opened, there is a selective permeability to Na^+ ions, and the membrane depolarizes. Repolarization takes place when voltage-dependent K^+ channels open to permit a large efflux of K^+. As the membrane becomes less negative, more Na^+ channels open, and open more rapidly; more Na^+ ions enter the cell and depolarization is further accelerated.
- **Impulse propagation:** the impulse is propagated by the spread of inward current through the conducting medium of the axoplasm to adjacent inactive regions. Inward currents from all the active nodes integrate as they spread, ensuring that impulse propagation will continue.
- **Local anaesthetic action:** these mainly block the function of the sodium channels, which exist in 'open', 'resting' and 'inactivated' conformational states. Local anaesthetic affinity is higher when the channel is in the open or inactivated state. The drugs exert no effect on cellular integrity or metabolism, but when a sufficient concentration is reached in the perfusing solution, depolarization does not occur in response to an electrical stimulus. Na^+ influx is blocked, although repolarization associated with K^+ efflux is unaffected. The agents in their cationic ionized form block the sodium channels on the inside of the axoplasm. External perfusion has no effect; the uncharged form must penetrate the cell wall before dissociating. The nerve blockade is concentration-dependent and ends when the local anaesthetic concentration falls below a critical minimum level. Local anaesthetics work by stabilizing the axonal membrane, and will stabilize all

excitable membranes, including those of skeletal, smooth and cardiac muscle. Local anaesthetics also block some potassium ion channels, broaden the action potential and enhance binding by maintaining the sodium channel in the open or inactivated state.

Direction the viva may take

It is almost inevitable that you will be asked about pKa.

- **pKa:** local anaesthetics exist in equilibrium between ionized and non-ionized forms. The ratio of the two states is given by the Henderson–Hasselbalch equation (originally derived to describe the pH changes resulting from the addition of H^+ or OH^- ions to any buffer system). The Ka is the dissociation constant which governs the position of equilibrium between the charged and uncharged forms. By analogy to pH, the pKa is the negative logarithm of that constant. Rearranging the equation pH $=$ pKa $+$ log $[HCO_3^-]$ / $[H_2CO_3]$ gives: pKa $=$ pH $-$ log [base] / [conjugate acid]. This is the same as saying [base] / [conjugate acid] $= 1.0$, so the dissociation constant, or pKa, is the pH at which equal amounts of drug are present in the charged and uncharged state.
- **Clinical implications:** a pKa of 7.4 indicates that, at body pH, there are equal numbers of molecules in the charged and uncharged forms. Most local anaesthetics have pKa values higher than body pH, and the more distant the dissociation constant from body pH the more molecules that exist in the ionized form. The pH scale is logarithmic; hence if a drug has a pKa of 8.4 it is 1 pH unit (i.e. a tenfold H^+ concentration) away from body pH. At 7.4 there is a 10:1 ratio, i.e. the drug is 90% ionized and 10% non-ionized. At pKa 9.4 the difference is 100-fold, so at body pH of 7.4, 99% of the drug will be charged. Uncharged base is necessary for tissue penetration and so drugs with lower pKa usually have a more rapid onset of action. Thus, lidocaine and prilocaine (pKa 7.7) have a shorter latency than bupivacaine (pKa 8.1). This dominance of the non-diffusible cation also explains the reason why local anaesthetics are much less effective in the presence of inflamed and acidotic tissue. Note, however, that pKa is not the only factor involved. Concentration and intrinsic potency are also important. Drugs also have to penetrate a perineural membrane of connective tissue, and this property has not been well quantified, thus chloroprocaine (popular in the USA) has one of the fastest onsets of action of all local anaesthetics, despite having a pKa of 9.1.
- **Barriers to drug passage:** peripheral nerves contain both afferent and efferent axons which are enclosed in a fine matrix of connective tissue which embeds the axons – the *endoneurium*. The fascicles of axons are enclosed within a squamous cellular layer, the *perineurium*, which is an effective semi-permeable barrier to local anaesthetics. The whole structure is surrounded by a sheath of collagen fibres, the *epineurium*, which permits easy diffusion of local anaesthetic. So, in the case of a myelinated sensory nerve, the local anaesthetic molecule may have to traverse four or five connective tissue and lipid membrane barriers. The most important of these is the perineurium, and this squamous cell layer, connected by tight junctions, is one of the main reasons why, under clinical conditions, only about 5% of the injected anaesthetic dose will actually penetrate the nerve.

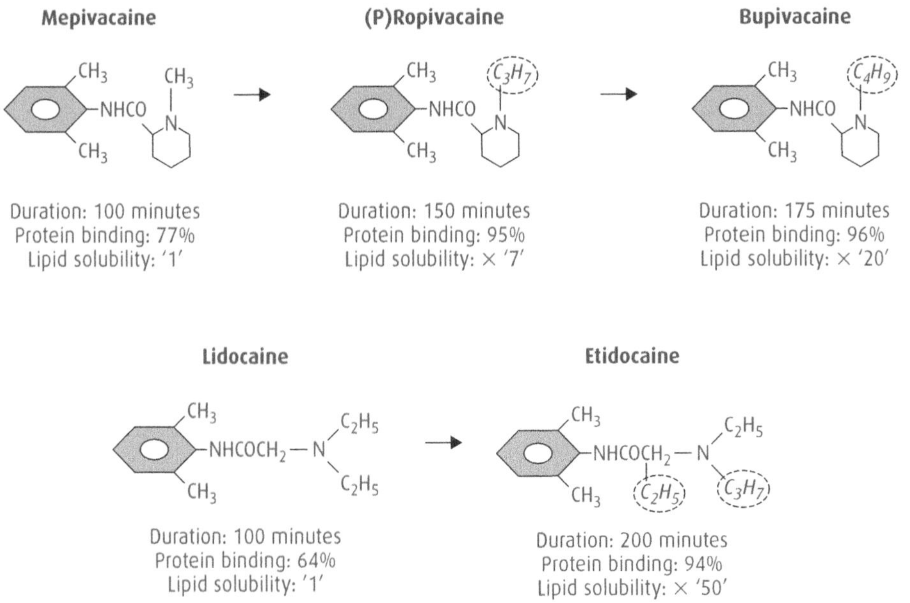

Fig. 4.3 Structure–activity relationship of local anaesthetics.

Further direction the viva could take

You may be asked about other factors that may influence local anaesthetic action.

- **Structure–activity relationships of local anaesthetics:** the site of local anaesthetic action is a protein structure in the Na^+ channel. The affinity of the drug to the channel, which determines its duration of action, is related to the length of the aliphatic (open carbon) chains on the compound. Small structural changes also influence factors such as lipid solubility and protein binding. These are summarized in Figure 4.3.
- **Lipid solubility:** this is a prime determinant of potency, which is increased by the substitution of longer side chains. The parent compound of ropivacaine and bupivacaine is mepivacaine, which has a single methyl group attached to the tertiary amine. Ropivacaine and bupivacaine are identical apart from propyl (C_3H_7) and butyl (C_4H_9) side chain substituents, respectively. These small structural changes mean that bupivacaine has three times the lipid solubility of ropivacaine and twenty times that of mepivacaine. Etidocaine (a drug whose capacity to cause a preferential motor block has rather restricted its popularity) has a structure very similar to that of lidocaine; however, the addition of an ethyl (C_2H_5) group to the intermediate linking chain and substitution of a propyl group for the ethyl on the amide portion increases lipid solubility by 50 times. (This also doubles its duration of action; highly lipid-soluble agents are highly concentrated in tissue and dislodge slowly.) From least to most lipid-soluble, therefore, the local anaesthetics are ranked: prilocaine, lidocaine, ropivacaine, bupivacaine and etidocaine. The relationship between lipid solubility and potency is not linear and above a fourfold increase in

partition coefficient there is a ceiling beyond which there is little observed increase in potency. (The esters procaine and chloroprocaine have low lipid solubility, and so are delivered in high 2–3% concentrations. Amethocaine and bupivacaine have high lipid solubility and produce effective anaesthesia at 0.25%.)

- **Protein binding:** this is also affected by structural differences in the molecule. Longer aliphatic substituents increase affinity for the sodium channel and prolong the duration of action. Bupivacaine and ropivacaine are both ~96% protein-bound. Lidocaine and prilocaine are much more weakly protein-bound (65% and 55%, respectively), with actions lasting for around 100 minutes. High protein binding decreases toxicity by reducing the proportion of free drug in the plasma.
- **Frequency dependence:** you will be doing well if you get as far as discussing this phenomenon, which is discussed in more detail on page 228.

Local anaesthetics: toxicity

Commentary

Local anaesthetic techniques such as combined sciatic, femoral and obturator nerve blocks for knee surgery are popular. The use of large drug doses for these nerve and other plexus blocks means that local anaesthetic toxicity is not merely an academic possibility. In this viva you need to reassure the examiners that your practice is safe.

The viva

You will be asked first about the symptoms and signs and then about the immediate management of local anaesthetic toxicity.

- **Clinical features:** the patient may complain of circumoral tingling and paraesthesia, light-headedness and dizziness. They may have visual and auditory disturbance manifested by difficulty in focusing and tinnitus. They may be disorientated. The objective signs are usually excitatory, with shivering, twitching, tremors in the face and extremities preceding full grand mal convulsions. Cardiac arrhythmias may be obvious on ECG monitoring, but these do not usually supervene until blood levels exceed by several times the convulsant dose.
- **Generic management:** the generic supportive ABC approach includes ventilation and inotropes as indicated.
- **Specific management**
  — *Cardiac arrhythmias:* if bupivacaine has been used, then resuscitation may be prolonged. Amiodarone ($5 \, \mathrm{mg \, kg^{-1}}$) is the drug of choice for most induced arrhythmias, apart from ventricular fibrillation (VF). Historically, refractory VF was treated with bretylium ($5 \, \mathrm{mg \, kg^{-1}}$), which is no longer available in the UK. Recent recommendations support the infusion of lipid emulsion. Cardiac toxicity may be related to the local anaesthetic inhibition of a carrier, carnitine acylcarnitine translocase, which transports AcylCoA moieties (derived from FFAs, from ketones and indirectly from lactate) for utilization by myocyte

mitochondria. There is some evidence suggesting that lipid may reverse this toxicity, perhaps by providing an energy substrate, although the mechanism is not clear. A typical regimen is intravenous Intralipid 20%, $1\,ml\,kg^{-1}$ stat, repeated at 3–5-minute intervals, with the remainder of a 500 ml bag infused over 15 minutes.

— *Grand mal convulsions:* phenytoin (usually given in a starting dose of $15\,mg\,kg^{-1}$) has a membrane-stabilizing local anaesthetic action. A better choice might be thiopental. It is a very effective anticonvulsant which, in small bolus doses of 50 mg, should suppress a fit that has been induced by local anaesthetic toxicity, but if necessary can be given as an infusion of 1–$3\,mg\,kg^{-1}\,h^{-1}$. Diazemuls, midazolam or lorazepam can also be used to abort convulsive activity.

You may then be asked about the factors that predispose a patient to local anaesthetic toxicity.

- **Site of injection:** the primary influences are the vascularity of the anatomical site of injection, and the presence locally of tissue such as fat, which may bind local anaesthetics. There is a spectrum of absorption, which is greatest after intercostal and paracervical block, and thereafter, in descending order, sacral extradural (caudal) block, lumbar and thoracic extradural block, brachial plexus block, sciatic and femoral nerve block and subcutaneous infiltration. Absorption from this last site is so delayed that some authors have described using doses that far exceed recommended maxima. Lidocaine $35\,mg\,kg^{-1}$, for example, has been used during tumescent liposuction.

- **Drug dosage and concentration:** it is not only the peak level, but also the rate of rise that may contribute to local anaesthetic toxicity. The total mass of drug may also be less important than its concentration: a dilute solution of the same dose is associated with lower peak levels. You may be asked the maximum doses that can be used. Because factors such as the rate of injection and the site of administration have such a substantial influence on blood levels, there is little logic to the maximum doses of local anaesthetics that are usually cited. If you are asked this question then feel free to preface your answer with a comment to that effect. The commonly quoted maximum doses are: lidocaine $3.0\,mg\,kg^{-1}$, $7.0\,mg\,kg^{-1}$ with adrenaline; bupivacaine $2.0\,mg\,kg^{-1}$; prilocaine 400 mg total dose (600 mg with adrenaline); and ropivacaine 150 mg total dose, with or without adrenaline.

- **Vasoconstrictors:** the use of vasoconstrictors lowers the maximum blood concentrations, but does not prolong the time to peak. There is also a complex interrelation with the inherent vasoactivity of local anaesthetics, all of which (apart from cocaine, which is a potent vasoconstrictor) demonstrate biphasic activity. At very low concentrations all enhance vascular smooth muscle activity and cause vasoconstriction. At clinical doses they demonstrate vasodilator activity that is dose-dependent and which varies for each drug. Racemic bupivacaine is a vasoconstrictor at low concentrations and is a less effective vasodilator than levobupivacaine 0.75%. Lidocaine also constricts at low concentrations but dilates at clinical levels. Increased blood flow increases vascular uptake and decreases duration of action.

- **Binding:** local anaesthetics bind mainly to a_1-acid glycoprotein, which is a high-affinity low-capacity site and, to a lesser extent, to low-affinity high-capacity sites on albumin. The binding decreases as pH decreases, and so toxicity is increased by hypoxia and acidosis. A decrease in intracellular pH will lead to increased ionization within the axoplasm and ion trapping. The convulsive threshold is inversely related to arterial PCO_2.

- **Pulmonary sequestration:** high blood levels may be attenuated by temporary sequestration of local anaesthetic within the lung. A high lung:blood partition coefficient encourages some uptake by the lung, and because the extravascular pH of lung is lower than that of plasma this encourages ion trapping. Prilocaine is sequestered more effectively than bupivacaine, whose uptake in turn is greater than that of lidocaine.

- **Allergic reactions:** genuine allergy to amides is extremely rare, but is commoner with esters. Allergic reactions are due mainly to para-aminobenzoic acid (PABA), which is a product of the metabolism of ester local anaesthetics such as procaine, benzocaine, chloroprocaine and amethocaine.

- **Toxicity:** the cardivascular and CNS toxicities that may be seen are common to all local anaesthetic agents, and are predictable in light of the known mechanism of action of these drugs. Local anaesthetics work by stabilizing the axonal membrane, and will stabilize all excitable membranes, including those of skeletal, smooth and cardiac muscle (page 217).

- **CNS:** as the blood concentrations increase, an initial excitation gives way to generalized CNS depression with respiratory depression and arrest. The excitatory phase is caused by the selective blockade of inhibitory pathways in the cortex. Convulsive activity supervenes when bupivacaine concentrations reach 2–4 μg ml^{-1} and lidocaine levels reach 10–12 μg ml^{-1}.

- **Cardiovascular effects:** these are complex and vary between the agents. Lidocaine can be used as a primary treatment for ventricular arrhythmias. It decreases the maximum rate of depolarization, but does not alter the resting membrane potential. In cardiac tissue, depolarization is related to sodium influx through fast channels and calcium influx through slow channels. The slow channels are responsible for the spontaneous depolarization of the sinoatrial node (SAN). Cardiac conduction slows with increasing blood levels, and this is manifest by an increased PR interval and duration of the QRS complex (ventricular depolarization). High doses depress SAN pacemaker activity, perhaps by inhibiting the slow calcium channels, and they also depress atrioventricular nodal conduction. In addition, local anaesthetics exert a dose-dependent negatively inotropic action on the myocardium. This effect relates directly to the potency of the agents. Bupivacaine is more dangerous than lidocaine in overdose by predisposing patients to arrhythmias and VF. The underlying mechanism for this effect is not known, but it appears to cause a unidirectional block with re-entrant tachyarrhythmias. Bupivacaine markedly reduces the rapid phase of depolarization, and recovery from this block is much slower than with lidocaine. The drug binds avidly to myocardial cells; there is a decrease in the rate of depolarization and action potential duration, with subsequent conduction block and electrical inexcitability. Local anaesthetics inhibit carnitine acylcarnitine translocase as described above.

- **Myotoxicity:** local anaesthetics will damage muscle into which they are injected directly. Skeletal muscle is a regenerating tissue and so this is not usually a clinical problem, although persistent diplopia has been reported following the use of bupivacaine 0.75% concentrations for retrobulbar ophthalmic block.

- **Prilocaine toxicity:** prilocaine is held to be one of the safest local anaesthetics. Its use in high doses may lead to methaemoglobinaemia (page 227).

Local anaesthetics: alkalinization

Commentary

This technique is of clinical interest because it shortens the onset time of effective anaesthesia, and is particularly useful in the context of extending an epidural block for urgent operative delivery. It is of interest to FRCA examiners because it allows candidates to demonstrate their understanding of the basic mechanisms of local anaesthetic action and to explain concepts such as pKa.

The viva

You might be asked how you would extend an epidural block for Caesarean section.

- **Top-up solutions:** assuming that your starting point is a standard low-dose local anaesthetic/opiate epidural that has been established for labour, there are a number of options. These vary according to local preference but typical regimens include: levobupivacaine 0.5% × 20 ml; lidocaine 2% × 20 ml; and levobupivacaine 0.5% × 10 ml plus lidocaine 2% × 10 ml. It is common to add adrenaline 100 μg (5 μg ml^{-1} is 1 in 200 000), and many anaesthetists add an opiate such as fentanyl or diamorphine. Some also alkalinize the solutions by adding sodium bicarbonate 8.4%, 1.0 ml per 10 ml.

If you have not suggested adding adrenaline or NaHCO$_3$, the examiner is likely to prompt you, because part of the purpose of this question is to explore your understanding of the mechanisms of local anaesthetic action. You may be asked, therefore, how you could shorten the onset time of the block.

- **Adrenaline:** the addition of adrenaline increases both the duration of block and its efficacy. Its effect on onset time (or 'latency') is less straightforward. Pre-mixed solutions have a lower pH than plain solutions and so the onset of block may actually be delayed. If the adrenaline is mixed with lidocaine immediately before epidural injection, then the latency is decreased, whereas if mixed with bupivacaine it appears to make little difference. Local vasoconstriction certainly increases the effective concentration in the epidural space, and it is also possible that a_2-mediated analgesia may result from intrathecal spread. Presumably bupivacaine/adrenaline mixtures have a lower pH which offsets these effects.
- **Bicarbonate:** the addition of NaHCO$_3$ significantly reduces the latency of lidocaine, although its effect on bupivacaine is less impressive, with some studies reporting only a 2–3-minute improvement.

You may then be asked why the addition of alkali should shorten the onset time.

- **Basic chemistry:** as described above, local anaesthetics are chemical descendants of cocaine and comprise a lipophilic aromatic portion, which is joined via an ester or amide linkage to a hydrophilic tertiary amine chain (see Figure 4.2). The presence of the amino group means that they are weak bases, existing in solution partly as the free base, and partly as the cation, as the conjugate acid. (They are usually presented as aqueous solutions of the hydrochloride salts of the tertiary amine. The tertiary amine is the base. They are therefore prepared as the water-soluble salt of an acid, usually the hydrochloride, which is stable in solution.) When the acid HA dissociates to H^+ and A^-, the anion A^- is a base because it serves as a proton receptor in the reverse reaction. The special relationship of base A^- to the acid HA is acknowledged by calling it the conjugate base of the acid.
- **Drug action:** the axoplasmic part of the sodium channel is blocked by the ionized part of the local anaesthetic molecule, but a charged moiety will not traverse the lipid and connective tissue membranes. It is only when existing in the uncharged form that the drug can gain access to the axoplasm.
- **Equilibrium and pKa:** drugs exist in rapid equilibrium between the non-ionized (N:) and the ionized species (NH^+). Both ionized and non-ionized drug forms can inhibit Na^+ channels, but access to the axoplasm is via the uncharged species. Once within the axoplasm the local anaesthetic becomes protonated. Local anaesthetics have pKa values higher than body pH, and the further away the dissociation constant is from body pH the more molecules that exist in the ionized form. (For fuller details see page 218.)
- **Alkalinization:** the addition of bicarbonate will raise the pH of the weakly acidic solution nearer the pKa. Addition of 1.0 ml $NaHCO_3$ 8.4% to 10.0 ml of lidocaine 2% will raise its pH from 6.5 to 7.2. (With bupivacaine 0.5% the pH rise is only to 6.6.) More drug will exist in the non-ionized form and so penetration will be more rapid.
- **Carbonation:** this is a variation on alkalinization, and is based on a similar principle but with a different site of action. Most local anaesthetics are marketed as hydrochloride salts; it is, however, possible to combine the base form with carbonic acid to form the carbonate salt rather than the hydrochloric acid. The H_2CO_3 is in equilibrium with dissolved CO_2. After infiltration of the drug, it is believed that the increased amount of CO_2 moves into the axoplasm, where it increases the levels of the weak carbonic acid. This lowers the intracellular pH and thereby favours cation production. In clinical practice this theoretical promise has not been realized.

Direction that the viva may take

If you have exhausted the core material above then you will have to be prepared for the viva to take a potentially variable course. Further aspects of local anaesthesia about which you could be asked include:

- **Inflammatory modulation:** the inflammatory response is initiated partly by G-coupled receptor proteins. Local anaesthetics have been shown to interact with some of these proteins to modify the physiological response.

- **Protein binding and lipid solubility:** protein binding influences the duration of action of a compound, and lipid solubility is a prime determinant of intrinsic anaesthetic potency. Lidocaine has low lipid solubility, whereas that of bupivacaine is high (page 219).
- **Newer preparations:** the duration of action may be prolonged by the use of lipid emulsions (which increase non-ionized proportion and release active drug more slowly), suspensions, liposomes (which are amphipathic lipid molecules encapsulating local anaesthetic), and polymer microspheres. You will not be expected to know about these in any detail.
- **Adjuncts:** you may be asked what adjuvant drugs may be added to local anaesthetics to enhance their action (page 228).

Bupivacaine, ropivacaine, lidocaine and prilocaine

Commentary
It is hard to predict exactly how a question about local anaesthetics will be constructed, and it may be that the information below may arise as part of a discussion about local anaesthetic techniques or local anaesthetic toxicity. Conceivably the examiner might take a conventional approach and ask you about the 'ideal local anaesthetic agent' and how the available drugs compare against this standard. It can be difficult not to answer this question with a list of negatives which has been known to extend to the absurd: 'the ideal agent should not transmit variant CJD or other prion diseases'. True enough, but scarcely relevant. It is preferable to concentrate on aspects about which you have some comparator knowledge, such as onset time, duration, clinical efficacy and toxicity. You will only spend time discussing agents that are in mainstream use in the UK, namely bupivacaine, ropivacaine, lidocaine (lignocaine) and prilocaine. You are unlikely to be asked about niche drugs such as amethocaine and articaine.

The viva
You may be asked about the factors which make you choose a particular local anaesthetic. This will be a prelude to a more detailed discussion about the basic pharmacology.

- In general, the choice is influenced by considerations such as onset time, duration and toxicity. Potency is less of a practical issue; what is important is the behaviour of local anaesthetics at equipotent doses. Lidocaine and prilocaine have more rapid onset of action (shorter latencies) than bupivacaine and ropivacaine. Bupivacaine is more potent and has a longer duration of action than ropivacaine. The judgement that ropivacaine is associated with motor sparing is discussed below. Levobupivacaine and ropivacaine have a similar toxicity profile; both are more hazardous in overdose than either lidocaine or prilocaine, which is the safest of all the amides, and which is the agent of choice for intravenous regional anaesthesia (IVRA).

Other amides

Prilocaine

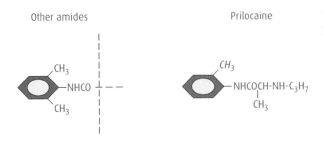

Fig. 4.4 Toluidine ring: prilocaine and other amides.

You will then be asked about the physicochemical differences which are responsible for the variations in clinical behaviour. (In the interests of clarity these are separated out in the account below, although there is frequently some overlap. Duration of action, for example, is related both to lipid solubility and to protein binding.)

- **Definitions:** all four are local anaesthetics which produce a reversible block of neuronal transmission, and which are synthetic derivatives of cocaine. They each possess the same three essential functional units, namely a hydrophilic chain joined by an amide linkage to a lipophilic aromatic moiety (see Figure 4.2). Simple modifications to any of the three parts of this basic structure can have marked effect on the pharmacology of the drugs.
- **Structures:** The parent compound of ropivacaine and bupivacaine is **me**pivacaine, which has a single **me**thyl group attached to the tertiary amine. **Bu**pivacaine is identical apart from a **bu**tyl (C_4H_9) side chain. The structure of ropivacaine (which is effectively a derivative of bupivacaine and which is prepared as the pure S enantiomer of **pro**pivacaine) differs only in its shorter **pro**pyl (C_3H_7) substituent on the piperidine nitrogen atom. Prilocaine has a different structure in the lipophilic moiety with a single methyl group on the aromatic ring (unlike the 2,6-xylidine ring in the other amides). This makes this aromatic toluidine ring less stable and more rapidly metabolized (Figure 4.4). Lidocaine and prilocaine both have a tertiary amine rather than a piperidine ring at the hydrophilic end of the structure.
- **Onset time:** as discussed above (page 218), the latency of local anaesthetics is related to their pKa and the ease with which drugs reach neural tissue. Drugs with a lower pKa usually have a more rapid onset of action, so lidocaine and prilocaine (pKa 7.7) work more quickly than bupivacaine and ropivacaine (pKa 8.1). (This may be only part of the explanation: chloroprocaine has a swifter onset despite its pKa of 9.1.)
- **Potency:** this is determined primarily by lipid solubility, which is increased by the substitution of longer side chains. Bupivacaine's longer butyl (C_4H_9) side chain increases at least threefold its lipid solubility in comparison with ropivicane with its shorter propyl (C_3H_7) substituent.
- **Protein binding:** this is also affected by structural differences in the molecule. The affinity of local anaesthetics for the sodium channel is related to the length of the aliphatic chains. Affinity determines duration of action: hence ropivacaine, with its shorter propyl chain, has a duration of action of 150 minutes as compared with 175 minutes for bupivacaine. Both drugs are around 96% protein-bound. Lidocaine and prilocaine are much more weakly protein-bound (65% and 55%, respectively), with

actions lasting for around 100 minutes. High protein binding decreases toxicity by reducing the proportion of free drug in the plasma.

- **Toxicity:** ropivacaine was developed as a safer alternative to bupivacaine. Its myocardial and CNS toxicity has been quoted as being 25% less than racemic bupivacaine. The cardiovascular and CNS toxicity of bupivacaine, however, is a function of the R(+) enantiomer. The S(−) enantiomer has less affinity for, and dissociates faster from, myocardial sodium channels. Animal studies confirm a fourfold decrease in the incidence of ventricular arrhythmias and VF. Symptoms of CNS toxicity in human volunteers such as tinnitus, circumoral numbness, apprehension and agitation are also less with infusions of the S(−) enantiomer. This is now available as levobupivacaine (Chirocaine), and would appear to be no more dangerous than ropivacaine. However, both these drugs are more toxic than lidocaine and prilocaine. Prilocaine is both less lipid-soluble and more weakly protein-bound than lidocaine, yet plasma concentrations are lower even when the same dose is given by the same route, and it is some 40% less toxic. The less stable toluidine ring is more rapidly metabolized to ortho(o)-toluidine. This would be a positive safety feature were it not for the fact that the o-toluidine metabolite causes methaemoglobinaemia by oxidizing the ferrous iron in haemoglobin to the ferric state. The loss of oxygen-carrying capacity shifts the oxygen–haemoglobin dissociation curve to the left. (SpO_2 readings are usually around 85%.) As methaemoglobin crosses the placenta, this further compromises oxygen delivery to the fetus. Prilocaine is generally avoided in pregnancy. (The S(+) enantiomer of prilocaine is a stronger vasoconstrictor than the R(−) form, is metabolized more slowly and therefore produces lower concentrations of o-toluidine.) Normal methaemoglobin concentrations are <1%; toxicity is evident when this rises to >10%. It can be treated with the reducing agent methylene blue, $1 \, mg \, kg^{-1}$.

- **Vasoactivity:** all local anaesthetics apart from the potent vasoconstrictor cocaine show biphasic activity, being vasodilators at high concentrations and vasoconstrictors at low. The vasoconstriction at low concentrations appears to be associated particularly with the S enantiomers. Ropivacaine probably exerts greater vasoconstrictor activity than bupivacaine, but it is no less toxic and has a shorter duration of action, so this vasoconstrictor activity probably confers little benefit. Prilocaine causes significantly less vasodilatation than lidocaine (so lasts longer despite being less lipid-soluble). At clinical doses the drugs have variable vasodilator activity. Bupivacaine dilates arterioles only at supraclinical levels, whereas lidocaine does so at clinical doses.

- **Sensory–motor dissociation:** this refers to the capacity of a local anaesthetic to block sensory nerves preferentially while sparing motor nerves. It is of particular advantage when the drugs are used in continuous epidurals for labour and for surgical analgesia. Selective block is a genuine phenomenon; etidocaine, for example, demonstrates more potent motor than sensory block. It is highly lipid-soluble and penetrates better than bupivacaine into the large myelinated A-α motor fibres. It also penetrates into the cord itself to provide long tract anaesthesia. But what of the claim that ropivacaine exhibits greater sensory–motor dissociation than other local anaesthetics? This has been based largely on studies that have used doses that are supramaximal for sensory block, at which the greater motor blocking effect of bupivacaine is obvious. If the doses are reduced, then little motor block will be evident with either drug, but the differences in sensory block will be revealed. It is well known that this group of local anaesthetics demonstrates preferential sensory block; the purported superiority of ropivacaine is illusory and is based on the fact that it is simply a less potent drug.

- **Frequency dependence:** this is another factor which helps to explain true sensory–motor dissociation. Drug entry into the sodium channels occurs when the channel is open during the period of membrane depolarization. Nerves conduct at different frequencies; pain and sensory fibres conduct at high frequency whereas motor impulses are at a lower frequency. This means that the sodium channels are open more times per second. Lidocaine, prilocaine, bupivacaine and ropivacaine all produce a more rapid and denser block in these sensory nerves of higher frequency. This is not true of drugs such as etidocaine, which is associated with a much more profound motor block.
- **Metabolism:** amide local anaesthetics bind mainly to α_1-acid glycoprotein (high-affinity low-capacity binding site), and to albumin (low-affinity high-capacity). They undergo aromatic hydroxylation, amide hydrolysis and N-dealkylation (phase 1 reactions) in the liver. There is some suggestion of extrahepatic pulmonary metabolism (uptake and sequestration is greatest with prilocaine).

Spinal adjuncts to local anaesthetics

Commentary

This is a question about the drugs that can be added to epidural or intrathecal solutions of local anaesthetics as a means of prolonging or enhancing their action. You may not have direct experience of non-opiate adjuncts, and so this part of the discussion is likely to be purely theoretical. If, however, you have ever worked with an anaesthetist who is an enthusiast for the use of subarachnoid ketamine, then feel free to say so, because most examiners will be interested to learn of your experiences. There can be some confusion about the term 'spinal' in the context of drug administration. Texts refer to 'spinal' opioids because that describes not their route of administration, but their site of action.

The viva

You will be asked how you might prolong the analgesic effect of a neuraxial block.

- **Spinal opioids:** the successful use of epidural morphine was first reported in 1979, and since that time several different opioids have been administered via the epidural and intrathecal routes. In the UK these include diamorphine, morphine, fentanyl, pethidine and methadone. Both onset and duration of action are related to the lipid solubility of the drug. Morphine has low lipid solubility, whereas that of fentanyl is high, and this is reflected in durations of action of 18 hours and 2–4 hours, respectively. The lipophilic drugs cross rapidly into the cord, while hydrophilic agents remain partly within the CSF, in which they may be carried rostrally to act on higher centres. This is the mechanism by which delayed respiratory depression may be caused. It is thus more common with morphine than with other drugs, and is better monitored by sedation scoring rather than respiratory rate. Pulse oximetry may be misleading because a high inspired oxygen concentration may mask ventilatory failure. Other complications of spinal opiates include nausea, vomiting, urinary retention and pruritus. Naloxone as a specific μ-antagonist will reverse some of these symptoms, but it may also reverse the analgesia. A logical alternative treatment, which can be useful for pruritus, is intravenous nalbuphine. This drug antagonizes μ-receptor-mediated effects while maintaining analgesia via κ-receptor agonism. (This is despite the fact that pruritus may not be mediated via μ-receptors as it is not reliably reversed by naloxone.)

- **Opioid receptors:** opioid receptors were identified in the dorsal horn of the grey matter of the spinal cord in the mid-1970s, with early work confirming that epidural morphine was associated with prolonged analgesia. The site of action appears to be the specific receptors that are located in the dorsal horn of the spinal cord. They are most densely concentrated in the substantia gelatinosa, which comprises lamina II and part of lamina III of the laminae of Rexed. At least 75% of the receptors are presynaptic, and they mediate inhibition of the release of nociceptive transmitters such as substance P, following stimulation of the primary afferents.

- **Vasoconstrictors:** these have long been used to prolong the duration of anaesthesia provided by both intrathecal and epidural local anaesthetics, although the practice is much less common in the UK than in the USA. There is evidence from controlled trials which suggests that the practice is safe, in that it does not lead to spinal cord ischaemia and neurological damage. There is also evidence that the addition of vasoconstrictors does not have a consistent action; the addition of adrenaline prolongs the action of intrathecal amethocaine but has little effect when added to bupivacaine or lignocaine. The reasons for this disparity are unknown. Vasoconstrictors that have been used include adrenaline, phenylephrine and octapressin.

- **α_2-agonists:** it was discovered over 50 years ago that intrathecal adrenaline had a significant analgesic effect, which has since been shown to be due to its α_2-agonist actions at presynaptic and postsynaptic receptors in the spinal cord. Presynaptic activation inhibits noradrenaline release from the nerve terminal and thereby influences descending pathways, but this alone is insufficient to explain all the analgesic effects. Clonidine doubles the duration of action of intrathecal bupivacaine, prolonging both sensory and motor block. Its complications include hypotension, dry mouth and sedation. The dose–response curve for hypotension is complex because larger doses (as high as $450\,\mu g$) are associated with the smallest effects on blood pressure. Dexmedetomidine is both more potent and more α_2-selective.

- **NMDA receptor antagonists:** there are N-methyl-D-aspartate receptors in the dorsal horn of the spinal cord. Ketamine is effective by both extradural and intrathecal routes, and has been shown (in a preservative-free formulation) to quadruple the duration of effective analgesia in children when added in a dose of $0.5\,\mathrm{mg\,kg^{-1}}$ to sacral extradural (caudal) bupivacaine. Magnesium sulphate is also a physiological NMDA receptor antagonist which has been used as an effective adjunct for postoperative analgesia.

Direction the viva may take

You may not have time to discuss more than the commonly used adjuncts. If you have done well then the viva may move on to other agents that have been used. The underlying receptor theory is both complex and incompletely understood, and so you will do well simply to provide a broad overview.

- **Anticholinesterases:** part of the effect of a_2-agonists is mediated via the release of Ach from the dorsal horn, which indicates that cholinergic receptors are involved in endogenous modulation of pain sensations. The logic of this hypothesis means that the injection of an intrathecal anticholinesterase should have analgesic effects. So it has proved with neostigmine. The technique did not pass into clinical practice because doses sufficient to permit the use of neostigmine as the sole anaesthetic agent were accompanied by severe nausea and vomiting. Sub-analgesic doses do exert an opiate-sparing effect with minimal nausea, and it may be that cholinomimetic drugs will be developed to exploit this mechanism further.
- **GABA agonists:** intrathecal midazolam produces analgesia which is antagonized by flumazenil, and it is assumed that it enhances the action of GABA on GABA$_A$ receptors. The effects of a single dose can be prolonged, which raises the suspicion that it may be neurotoxic. Intrathecal baclofen, which is another GABA agonist, is licensed in the USA for the treatment of spasticity, but it can also produce effective analgesia without any evidence of toxicity.
- **Non-steroidal anti-inflammatory drugs (NSAIDs):** spinal NSAIDs may inhibit presynaptic adenyl cyclase in the dorsal horn and decrease neurotransmitter release. (This is an oversimplification of a process that may also involve postsynaptic NMDA-stimulated gene expression.) Clinical experience is limited to sporadic case reports.
- **Monoamine uptake inhibitors:** Amitriptyline enhances noradrenergic and serotonergic inhibition at spinal level after intrathecal administration.

Induced hypotension

Commentary

This question has been around since before the current examiners were themselves examined, and it is seen as a predictable and standard topic. You should be aware of the applied pharmacology, of the indications for the technique and of its potential complications.

The viva

You may be asked about the indications for induced hypotension.

- **Indications:** an old adage avows that induced hypotension should be used only to make the impossible possible, and not the possible easy. There was a time when surgeons were largely oblivious to that injunction, and induced hypotension had many indications, particularly for neurosurgical and head and neck procedures. Occasional surgeons will still insist that hypotension is essential, in cosmetic procedures such as rhinoplasty, for instance, but in reality the genuine indications have now shrunk to the point at which the technique is confined to a very few, very specialized surgical procedures, one example of which is the removal of choroidal tumours of the eye.

You will be asked about the intravenous drugs that can be used to induce hypotension.

- The subject lends itself readily to a structured approach. You can, for example, talk either about their physiological sites of action or organize your answer according to the groups of drugs that are available. This is almost, but not quite, the same thing: labetalol, for instance, is a hypotensive drug with more than one site of action.
- The prime determinants of arterial BP are CO (HR and SV) and SVR. Drugs used to induce hypotension can affect one or more of these variables.

Drugs which affect SVR
α-adrenoceptor blockers
- **Phentolamine:** this is a non-selective α antagonist (the ratio of $\alpha_1:\alpha_2$ effects is 3:1), which also has weak β-sympathomimetic action. It decreases BP by reducing peripheral resistance owing to its peripheral α_1-vasoconstrictor blockade and mild β-sympathomimetic vasodilatation. The α_2-blockade increases noradrenaline release. The dose is 1–5 mg, titrated against response and repeated as necessary. The drug has a rapid onset of 1–2 minutes, and has an effective duration of action of around 15–20 minutes.

Peripheral vasodilators
- **Glyceryl trinitrate (GTN) nitroglycerine:** its hypotensive action is mediated via nitric oxide (NO). NO activates guanylate cyclase, which increases cyclic GMP (from guanosine triphosphate) within cells. This in turn decreases available intracellular Ca^{2+}. The drug causes more venous than arteriolar dilatation, and hence it decreases venous return and preload. Myocardial oxygen demand is reduced because of the decrease in ventricular wall tension. GTN has a rapid onset (1–2 minutes) and offset (3–5 minutes), which can allow precise control of BP. A typical infusion regimen would be to start at around 0.5 $\mu g\,kg^{-1}\,min^{-1}$, titrated against response. There is no rebound hypertension when the infusion is discontinued. The drug increases cerebral blood flow (CBF) and ICP. Tolerance to the effects of GTN may develop, which may partially be prevented by intermittent dosing.
- **Sodium nitroprusside (SNP):** SNP is another nitrovasodilator which mediates hypotension via NO. In contrast to GTN, it causes both arterial and venous dilatation, leading to hypotension and a compensatory reflex tachycardia. The drug has a complex metabolism that results in the production of free cyanide (CN^-), which, by binding irreversibly to cytochrome oxidase in mitochondria, is highly toxic, causing tissue hypoxia and acidosis. Toxicity is manifest when blood levels exceed 8 $\mu g\,ml^{-1}$. The maximum infusion rate is 1.5 $\mu g\,kg^{-1}\,min^{-1}$, and the total dose must not exceed 1.5 $mg\,kg^{-1}$. Treatment of toxicity is with sodium thiosulphate 50%

(20–25 ml intravenously over 5 minutes) and/or cobalt edetate 1.5% (20 ml rapidly). SNP also increases CBF and ICP. Coronary blood flow is increased. The rapid onset (1–2 minutes) and offset (3–5 minutes) of effect allows good control of BP, although patients may demonstrate rebound hypertension when the infusion is stopped. Tachyphylaxis may be seen in some patients; the mechanism is uncertain. The solution is unstable and so the giving set must be protected from light.

Ganglion blockers

- **Trimetaphan:** this is an antagonist at the nicotinic receptors of both sympathetic and parasympathetic autonomic ganglia, but it has no effect at the nicotinic receptors of the neuromuscular junction. It has some a-blocking actions and is a direct vasodilator of peripheral vessels. It is a potent releaser of histamine, which contributes to its hypotensive action. Reflex tachycardia is common, and this may present a problem during surgery which mandates a quiet circulation. Trimetaphan also antagonizes hypoxic pulmonary vasoconstriction. The drug is given by infusion at a rate of 20–50 $\mu g\,kg^{-1}\,min^{-1}$.

Direct vasodilators

- **Hydralazine:** this produces hypotension by direct vasodilatation together with a weak a-antagonist action. This is mediated via an increase in cyclic GMP and decrease in available intracellular Ca^{2+}. The tone of arterioles is affected more than venules. Reflex tachycardia is common. It is less easy to titrate the dose against effect and the drug finds its main use in the control of hypertension in pregnancy. The maximum infusion rate is 10 $mg\,h^{-1}$.

Drugs which affect cardiac output (CO)

- **β-adrenoceptor blockers:** there are many examples – all are competitive antagonists, but their selectivity for receptors is variable. Selective β_1-antagonism is clearly a useful characteristic. Their influence on BP is probably because of decreased CO via a decreased HR, together with some inhibition of the renin–angiotensin system. Unopposed a_1-vasoconstriction may compromise the peripheral circulation without causing hypertension.
- **Atenolol:** this is a selective β_1-antagonist except in high doses. It is long acting with a $t_{1/2}$ of around 7 hours. Its use as a bolus (150 $\mu g\,kg^{-1}$ over 20 minutes) is usually to treat cardiac arrhythmias rather than to induce hypotension.
- **Esmolol:** this is a relatively selective β_1-antagonist. It is ultra-short-acting, with a $t_{1/2}$ of around 9 minutes. It is rapidly metabolized by non-specific ester hydrolysis. Its infusion dose is 50–200 $\mu g\,kg^{-1}\,min^{-1}$.
- **Labetalol:** this acts both as a- and β-antagonist (in a ratio that is quoted variously as 1:5 and 1:7), which mediates a decrease in SVR without reflex tachycardia. It is a popular drug in anaesthetic, obstetric anaesthetic and intensive therapy use. Its elimination $t_{1/2}$ is 4–6 hours. It can be given as a bolus of 50 mg intravenously, or at a rate of 1–2 $mg\,kg^{-1}\,h^{-1}$.
- **Propanolol:** this is a non-selective β-antagonist which is usually given as a bolus of 1.0 mg, repeated to a maximum of 5.0 mg (in a patient who is anaesthetized).

a_2-adrenoceptor agonists

- **Clonidine:** this is an a-agonist with affinity for a_2-receptors some 200 times greater than that for a_1. Its hypotensive effects are mediated via a reduction in central sympathetic outflow and by stimulation of presynaptic a_2-receptors which inhibit noradrenaline release into the synaptic cleft. It also possesses analgesic and sedative actions. Its elimination $t_{1/2}$ is too long at around 14 hours to allow its use for fine control of acutely raised BP, but it can be a useful adjunct in low doses.

Direction the viva may take

You will probably be asked finally to discuss the complications of induced hypotension.

- **Dangers and complications:** these relate predictably to the consequences of hypoperfusion in key parts of the circulation. Precipitate falls in BP may lead to CVA and to myocardial ischaemia. Drug-induced hypotension usually shifts the autoregulatory curve to the left, and thereby confers thereby a degree of protection. In patients who are previously hypertensive, however, the curve is shifted to the right, making them more vulnerable to catastrophic drops in perfusion of essential areas. (You may be asked to draw the curve of cerebral autoregulation to demonstrate these shifts. See Figure 3.9.)
- **Exacerbating influences:** the effects of induced hypotension will be enhanced by factors such as hypovolaemia, the use of other drugs with hypotensive actions such as volatile anaesthetic agents, the reduction in venous return associated with IPPV, and drugs which release histamine. The head-up position may also further diminish effective cerebral perfusion.

Clonidine

Commentary

Clonidine is an old drug, which has been used in the treatment of hypertension and of migraine, in angina, as an anxiolytic, as a treatment for glaucoma and as a nasal decongestant. It has also been used in conditions as diverse as neuropathic pain and attention deficit hyperactivity disorder (ADHD). Anaesthesia has found new uses for this agent, whose actions cannot totally be explained in terms of agonism at a_2-adrenoceptors. It is an interesting compound.

The viva

The question is likely to be open-ended, but most of the relevant information should be found below.

- Clonidine is an agonist at a_2-adrenoceptors. It has some minor activity at a_1-receptors (the ratio of $a_1:a_2$ is 1:200) and, because it is an imidazoline derivative, also acts at imidazole receptors. Two subtypes have so far been identified, the I_1 and

I_2 receptors, which are located centrally and appear to mediate sedation and hypnosis. Clonidine is associated with a decrease in intracellular cyclic AMP via a Gi-protein receptor.

- It acts at presynaptic α_2-receptors, both centrally and peripherally, to inhibit the release of noradrenaline. α_2-receptors in the hypothalamus are inhibitory to the vasomotor outflow. Clonidine also acts postsynaptically in the adrenal medulla.
- At peripheral postjunctional α_2-receptors it mediates slow-onset vasoconstriction of long duration, to which its activity at α_1-receptors may contribute. This may explain why an intravenous dose may be associated with a transient rise in arterial BP.

Direction the viva may take

You are likely to be asked about the anaesthetic uses of clonidine in anaesthesia. Medical uses are included for completeness as they could form part of a supplementary question.

- **Stress and pressor responses:** clonidine can be used (in a dose of $5\,\mu g\,kg^{-1}$) to attenuate both the endocrine stress response to surgery and the pressor responses to laryngoscopy and tracheal intubation.
- **Adjunct to anaesthesia and analgesia:** a dose of $1-2\,\mu g\,kg^{-1}$ intravenously reduces the MAC of inhaled volatile agents and decreases the requirement for systemic analgesics.
- **Hypotensive anaesthesia:** $1-2\,\mu g\,kg^{-1}$ intravenously can produce modest and sustained hypotension which may improve operating conditions during which bleeding would otherwise mask the surgical field.
- **Antisialogogue effect:** a side effect of clonidine administration is reduced salivary secretion; this property can be used in the perioperative period.
- **Alcohol withdrawal:** clonidine inhibits the exaggerated release of sympathomimetic neurotransmitters during acute alcohol withdrawal. It has also been used to attenuate the symptoms of opiate withdrawal.
- **Sedation and anxiolyis:** it has both sedative and anxiolytic actions.
- **Neuropathic pain:** clonidine can attenuate symptoms in some patients.
- **Shivering:** a low dose (up to $0.5\,\mu g\,kg^{-1}$) may ameliorate postanaesthetic shivering.
- **Medical uses:** it has long been used as an anti-hypertensive agent whose usefulness is limited by the severe rebound hypertension that can follow discontinuation of treatment. In a smaller dose it has a place in the prophylaxis of migraine. Some patients with ADHD respond well, and clonidine has also been used in the management of Tourette's syndrome.
- **Adjuvant use in regional anaesthesia:** there appear to be no α_2-receptors on the axons of peripheral nerves, although the addition of clonidine to local anaesthetic does increase (modestly) the duration of action of most blocks. It produces a small decrement of nerve conduction at high concentrations, acting preferentially on C-fibres. In contrast, neuraxial clonidine does extend the block. The addition of $2\,\mu g\,kg^{-1}$ to local anaesthetic solutions for sacral extradural (caudal) block doubles the duration of effective analgesia. The same is true of clonidine given intrathecally. The side effects are those of sedation, dry mouth, and, it is said, refractory hypotension, although this is not always an obvious problem in clinical practice.

Intrathecal a_2-agonists achieve analgesia partly through cholinergic activation, hence the brief interest in using spinal neostigmine as an adjunct.

- (**Dexmedetomidine:** the drugs act in a similar way. Dexmedetomidine, which is the R isomer of medetomidine, has the advantage of being a more selective a_2-agonist than clonidine, and it has more pronounced effects on central a-receptors. It awaits a licence for human use in the UK.)

Anti-arrhythmic drugs

Commentary

You will still find statements in textbooks to the effect that some form of arrhythmia (defined as the absence of normal sinus rhythm) complicates between 60 and 90% of all anaesthetics. The figures are based on studies which are now two or three decades old and which largely pre-date modern anaesthetic drugs and techniques. Yet, although the incidence seems high it remains true that transient disturbances of cardiac rhythm are common. Some of these are innocuous but others have the potential to evolve into more malignant rhythms that may threaten cardiovascular stability and which require urgent treatment. The rational management of arrhythmias is helped by some knowledge of cardiac electrophysiology and it is this, more than the individual drugs themselves, which will probably be the scientific focus of the viva. The varying receptors, ion channels and ion pumps, many of which differ throughout parts of the conducting system and myocardium, contain vastly more detail than you will be expected to convey. A broad understanding of the principles of ion fluxes should be enough.

The viva

The viva could begin with a clinical discussion of the common acute arrhythmias that are encountered during anaesthesia, but at some stage you are going to be asked about anti-arrhythmic drugs and their mechanism of action. Many of them have an action on sodium, calcium and potassium channels, and so this is probably the logical place to start.

The cardiac action potential

- **Phase 4** – the 'pacemaker potential': in *non-conducting tissue* (atrial and ventricular myocytes, and Purkinje tissue), the negative resting membrane potential (RMP) of around $-90\,\text{mV}$ is maintained by high outward conductance of K^+ (gK^+) through open K^+ channels. During this time, fast Na^+ channels and slow (L-type) Ca^{2+} channels are closed. The membrane-bound ATP-dependent Na^+/K^+ exchange pump continues to extrude three Na^+ ions in exhange for two K^+ ions. In non-conducting tissue, therefore, the pacemaker potential is unimportant. In nodal and conducting tissue, however, there occurs a gradual depolarization owing to greater inward Na^+ (gNa^+) and Ca^{2+} (gCa^{2+}) conductance during late diastole. The negative membrane potential in early diastole also activates a cation channel that is permeable to both

Na^+ and K^+ and which generates the inward I_f current (the i_f or 'funny' current is an inward pacemaker current which is activated by membrane hyperpolarization).

- **Phase 0** – rapid depolarization: at the threshold level of around $-65\,mV$ the fast sodium channels open with a large transient increase in gNa^+. (This is triggered in non-conducting tissue by an action potential (AP) in an adjacent cell.) The sudden influx in Na^+ generates a fast-response AP (meanwhile, the potassium channels close and K^+ efflux ceases).
- **Phase 1** – this is the period of rapid partial repolarization mediated by a short-lived hyperpolarizing efflux of K^+: the sodium channels close and inward gNa^+ drops.
- **Phase 2** – this is the plateau phase which lengthens the cardiac AP (in contrast to the much shorter APs generated in nerves and skeletal muscle) and which is produced mainly by the large influx of Ca^{2+} ions through slow (longlasting L-type) calcium channels which open at a membrane potential of around $-40\,mV$. During phase 2, cardiac fibres are absolutely refractory to repeated depolarization. (This is the effective refractory period (ERP), which protects the heart from multiple compounded APs.)
- **Phase 3** – repolarization: this is caused by a large increase in gK^+ (efflux) and the inactivation of the Ca^{2+} channels (influx). The Na^+/K^+ pump re-establishes the resting membrane potential. Phase 3 is a relative refractory period during which a stimulus may generate an AP large enough to be propagated, but it will be conducted more slowly than usual.

Direction the viva will take

In the light of the previous information, you may then be asked about classifications of anti-arrhythmic drugs.

- **Vaughan–Williams:** the traditional Vaughan–Williams classification (1970) is convenient, is still in use, and is an oversimplification. It does not account for drugs that have more than one site of action (such as amiodarone); it fails to find a satisfactory classification for compounds such as adenosine and digoxin; and it is based on the assumption that all the agents are channel blockers, whereas some drugs activate either receptors or ion channels.
  — *Class I:* these drugs block sodium channels by binding to sites in the a-subunit, and reduce the maximum rate of depolarization during phase 0 of the cardiac AP. All share the same underlying mechanism of action but are further subdivided into classes Ia, Ib and Ic according to the specific characteristics of the Na^+ channel block that they produce. The electrophysiological differences are subtle and relate amongst other complexities to the different affinity of drugs to channels in the resting, open and refractory state. You are not likely to have to explain this in detail. Examples of the drugs include: Ia, disopyramide; Ib, lidocaine; and Ic, flecainide.
  — *Class II:* includes (some) ß-adrenoceptor antagonists, including propranolol, atenolol, metoprolol and esmolol. These drugs increase the refractory period of the atrioventricular node and so may prevent recurrent supraventricular tachycardia, including paroxysmal atrial fibrillation (AF).
  — *Class III:* this group includes drugs such as amiodarone and sotalol, which are now known to have more than one action. (The original definition encompassed drugs

that prolonged the cardiac AP.) Their main mechanism of action is outward K^+ channel blockade which prolongs repolarization. This extends the Q–T interval and, rarely, these drugs can precipitate torsade de pointes. Amiodarone ($5\,mg\,kg^{-1}$ iv) is useful both for supraventricular and ventricular arrhythmias. Sotalol is racemic; the S-enantiomer is a ß-blocker, and both R and S forms prolong the AP. Other class III agents include ibutilide and dofetilide (used to convert AF).

— *Class IV:* these drugs block voltage-sensitive Ca^{2+} channels, thereby slowing conduction through the SA and AV nodes. Examples include verapamil, which is preferentially selective for cardiac tissues, and diltiazem. The drugs are ineffective in treating ventricular tachycardias, and verapamil given intravenously for this purpose has been fatal. $MgSO_4$ is a natural Ca^{2+} antagonist (an increase in intracellular Mg^{2+} inhibits Ca^{2+} influx through Ca^{2+} channels). It is effective at abolishing ventricular tachyarrhythmias, particularly torsade de pointes, and those induced by adrenaline, digitalis and bupivacaine.

- **Adenosine** acts at the A^1 receptor (which is linked to the muscarinic K^+ channel). By enhancing K^+ efflux adenosine hyperpolarizes cells and slows AV conduction. It has a very short duration of action (20–30 seconds) and, in a dose of 3–6 mg iv (repeated prn), provides effective chemical cardioversion of SVT.

- **Digoxin** and other cardiac glycosides increase contractile force and decrease AV node conduction, mainly via their inhibitory effect on the membrane Na^+/K^+-ATPase, and an increase in intracellular Ca^{2+}. Digoxin's long term effect may be caused mainly by the increase in vagal tone.

- **The 'Sicilian gambit' classification:** this represented an attempt in 1990 by a European Society of Cardiology working group to rationalize the actions of drugs according to the ion channels and the receptors on which they act. (It was described as a 'gambit', somewhat pretentiously, because it was viewed as an opening move rather than as a complete explanation.) The classification so far extends to blockers of Na^+ channels, Ca^{2+} channels, K^+ channels, the I_f current, α-adrenoceptors, ß-adrenoceptors and muscarinic receptors, to activators of the adenosine receptor, and to suppressors of the Na^+/K^+ pump.

Further direction the viva may take

You could be asked about the electrophysiological basis of common arrhythmias.

- **Sinus bradycardia:** the commonest acute cause is an increase in vagal tone, either unmasked by anaesthetic agents with no intrinsic vagolytic activity, or provoked by surgical stimuli such as traction on the peritoneum or the extraocular muscles. Vagal activation at the SA node increases gK^+ (outwards) and reduces slow channel gNa^+ and gCa^{2+} (inwards), decreases the slope of the pacemaker potential, and suppresses the I_f current. Hyperkalaemia may stop pacemaker activity by increasing gK^+ (outward).

  - **Drug effects:** calcium-channel blockers, as their name suggests, inhibit slow inward Ca^{2+} currents during phases 4 and 0, and some, such as diltiazem, can slow the heart rate. Digoxin enhances parasympathetic activity (and slows conduction through the AV node). ß-adrenoceptor antagonists prevent the normal inhibition of vagal tone mediated by sympathetic activity (which normally increases heart rate by decreasing gK^+ outwards and increasing slow gCa^{2+} and gNa^+ inwards, thereby increasing the slope of the pacemaker potential during phase 4).

— *Hyperkalaemia:* this hyperpolarizes the cell, induces bradycardia and can even stop SA nodal firing.

— **Hypoxia:** this is the most ominous cause of bradycardia. It can cause complete cessation of pacemaker activity because of lack of cellular oxygen.

- **Sinus tachycardia:** this is not an arrhythmia, but is included for completeness. Sympathetic stimulation increases heart rate by decreasing gK^+. It also increases slow inward gCa^{2+} and gNa^+ and enhances the I_f current.

- **Ectopic pacemaker activity (ventricular premature beats):** non-conducting cells do not usually depolarize until activated by the pacemaker impulses. Under some circumstances, however, they do have a rising phase 4 which means that they can generate an AP spontaneously and themselves act as pacemakers. This occurs because of an increased inward movement of Ca^{2+} which reduces the membrane potential to threshold ($-65\,mV$). Increased intracellular Ca^{2+} results particularly from myocardial ischaemia, but is also associated with adrenergic stress and high dose cardiac glycosides. Ischaemia also closes fast Na^+ channels and inhibits the Na^+/K^+ pump (which requires ATP (and oxygen) to maintain a low intracellular Na^+ against its concentration gradient).

— **Hypokalaemia:** this increases the rate of phase 4 depolarization by decreasing gK^+ and thereby increases the heart rate.

- **Re-entry (pre-excitation) tachycardia:** these pre-excitation rhythms arise when a wave of depolarization that can travel down different conducting pathways encounters a block. The impulse continues down the normal path but should the paths then rejoin, the depolarization can travel retrogradely up the blocked segment only to depolarize the normal conducting pathway prematurely. The cycle repeats itself and thus gives rise to a tachyarrhythmia (typically supraventricular). Re-entrant circuits can be congenital (as in the accessory pathways of the Wolff–Parkinson–White syndrome) or acquired, following myocardial damage.

- **Atrial fibrillation:** this is the commonest arrhythmia in clinical, although not anaesthetic, practice. It has multiple causes including myocardial ischaemia, sepsis and autonomic stimulation. It appears mainly to be a re-entry abnormality in which multiple propagating waves of depolarization are initiated by ectopic foci (which may originate from the pulmonary veins).

ß-adrenoceptor blockers

Commentary

ß-adrenoceptor blockers may form the subject matter for a whole viva, or they may be part of a more general discussion of anti-hypertensive drugs and anaesthesia. Their use in hospital is of continued interest, and some vascular surgeons have even started to prescribe perioperative atenolol. This has implications for anaesthetic management. There are a large number of β-blockers and you will not be expected to know about subtle pharmacological differences between them. You will need to know enough about the receptors on which they act to be able to address the question from first principles but, as this is straightforward, much of the questioning will be clinically orientated.

The viva

You may be asked about the clinical uses of β-blockers and how they exert their effects.

- **β-adrenoceptors**: the actions of β-blockers are predictable from what is known about β-adrenoceptors. The important effects (from an anaesthetic perspective) that they mediate include increases in heart rate (β_1), myocardial contractility (β_1), conduction velocity ($\beta_2 > \beta_1$), and cardiac glycogenolysis ($\beta_1 > \beta_2$). β_2-receptors are responsible for relaxation of bronchial and vascular smooth muscle.

Cardiovascular uses

- **Angina pectoris:** the drugs are myocardial depressants which reduce cardiac work by blocking the effects of sympathetic stimulation. They decrease left ventricular wall tension, heart rate and resting contractility, and thereby reduce myocardial oxygen consumption. β-blockers do not lead to coronary vasodilatation. Patients with myocardial ischaemia may benefit from long-term therapy, and survival following myocardial infarction (MI) is increased.
- **Arrhythmias:** β-blockers lead to a decrease in automaticity, an increase in the duration of the cardiac AP and an increase in the effective refractory period at the AV node. They are useful in treating cardiac arrhythmias that are dependent on sympathetic activity, particularly SVTs. It is not advisable to use them to manage abnormalities of rhythm that have been induced by acute MI. β-blockers may worsen these arrhythmias and precipitate heart failure. (They are Vaughan–Williams class II anti-arrhythmics (page 236).
- **Hypertension:** the anti-hypertensive actions of β-blockers are not fully explained; peripheral resistance may remain unchanged, although cardiac output usually drops. There is no consistent relationship between treatments or with alterations in renin levels. The drugs may also inhibit 5-HT both centrally and peripherally.
- **Perioperative ischaemia:** a study by Mangano that was published in the *New England Journal of Medicine* in 1996 concluded that the administration of atenolol to patients undergoing non-cardiac surgery and who were known to be at risk of ischaemic cardiac events halved the incidence of silent postoperative myocardial ischaemia, halved mortality and cardiac complication rates for up to 2 years, and reduced the incidence of perioperative infarction. The evidence was based on only 200 patients but, in conjunction with some other published work, was enough to convince a number of anaesthetists to adopt the practice. Others have been more sceptical, commenting that it is rare for cardiovascular therapies to demonstrate relative risk reductions of greater than about 35% because they target only some of

Mangano DT *et al.* (1996). Effect of atenolol on mortality and cardiovascular morbidity after noncardiac surgery. *New England Journal of Medicine*, **335**, 1713–20.

the many pathogenic mechanisms that underlie cardiovascular disease. Mangano's study pre-dated the widespread use of perioperative epidural analgesia and it has also been pointed out that initial small trials that claim improbably large benefits are frequently superseded by much larger trials which typically show more modest or even no treatment effects. The Perioperative Ischaemic Evaluation (POISE) trial investigated the benefit of perioperative metoprolol and reported in late 2007. To the surprise of many, this suggested that although it reduced the risk of MI, it increased the risks both of serious stroke and overall death. For every 1000 patients treated, metoprolol would prevent 15 MIs but at the cost of an excess of 5 disabling CVAs and 8 deaths.

- **Hypertrophic cardiomyopathy:** propranolol reduces the encroachment of the hypertrophic septum into the left ventricular outflow tract under influence of sympathetic activity.
- **Pressor responses:** β-adrenoceptor blockers, particularly the ultra-short-acting esmolol, can be used to attenuate the pressor response to laryngoscopy.
- **Thyroid disease:** β-blockers are used to reduce the manifestations of a raised metabolic rate in thyrotoxic patients requiring curative thyroid surgery.

Direction the viva may take

You may be asked about adverse effects.

- Propranolol was the first of many β-blockers to be synthesized. The clinical differences between them are probably less significant than is claimed. Some of the drugs are relatively cardioselective, but none is cardiospecific. This means that they will antagonize β_1-receptors at non-cardiac sites, and in higher doses will also affect β_2-receptors. All have the potential to provoke bronchoconstriction in asthmatics, and may worsen pulmonary function in patients with other forms of obstructive airway disease. These patients will then not respond to β_2-sympathomimetic treatment. Selective β_1-antagonists include atenolol, acebutolol, esmolol and metoprolol.
- Most of the other adverse effects are also related to their primary pharmacological actions. They may precipitate peripheral vascular ischaemia owing to unopposed α_1-vasoconstriction, and may mask the symptoms of hypoglycaemia. They may, in addition, contribute to hypoglycaemia by interfering with β_2-mediated glycogenolysis, carbohydrate and fat metabolism. Reduced exercise tolerance, dyspnoea and fatigue are other generic side effects. Drugs with membrane-stabilizing actions (MSA) such as propranolol and metoprolol are more likely to induce significant bradycardia or worsen pre-existing conduction abnormalities. Sotalol, which is a class III anti-arrhythmic drug, unlike other β-blockers, delays the slow outward potassium flux and extends the effective refractory period of the cardiac AP. This prolongation of the Q–T interval is associated (rarely) with torsade de pointes. In patients in whom cardiac decompensation is being prevented by sympathetic drive, β-blockers may precipitate cardiac failure, unless a drug is used which possesses intrinsic sympathomimetic activity (ISA) such as oxprenolol or pindolol. Fat-soluble drugs, particularly propranolol, are much more likely to penetrate the CNS and cause symptoms such as nightmares and sleep disturbance. This is less of a problem with the water-soluble compounds (such as atenolol and nadolol).

Further direction the viva could take

You may be asked about particular implications for anaesthesia and about specific anaesthetic uses for ß-blockers.

- The main problem is that a ß-blocked patient is one in whom sympathetic reflexes are blunted. This means that compensatory responses to actual or effective hypovolaemia (such as may accompany central neuraxial blockade) can be inadequate.
- Anaesthetists use the drugs for the urgent control of hypertension, including the pressor response to laryngoscopy. Esmolol is a cardioselective drug whose very short duration of action (the elimination half-life is 10 minutes or less) is terminated by non-specific plasma esterases. Labetalol can be used to provide control over a longer period. It has combined α- and ß-adrenoceptor blocking actions (in a ratio that is quoted variously as 1:5 and 1:7), but of differing durations of effect. The α block lasts for 30 minutes, whereas the ß block persists for 90 minutes.

Anti-hypertensive drugs and anaesthesia

Commentary

Hypertension is common and is treated by a wide range of drugs, often in combination. Most anti-hypertensive therapy has implications for anaesthesia. There is no unequivocal guidance as to whether patients should discontinue taking some of these agents (such as ACE inhibitors) prior to surgery, so be prepared to demonstrate to the examiners that you can make your own judgements based on an understanding of how the various drugs work.

The viva

You will be asked to discuss the implications for anaesthetic management of a patient who is receiving treatment for hypertension. The examiner may concentrate on only one or two classes of drugs, depending on how the question is structured.

- **ß-adrenoceptor blockers:** patients should continue taking these drugs and in some cases may be prescribed them *de novo* (page 239).
- **Diuretics:** the commonest diuretics are the thiazides, such as bendrofluazide, chlorthalidone and indapamide, which act on the distal tubule; and loop diuretics, typically furosemide, which act on the loop of Henle. These drugs decrease the active reabsorption of sodium and chloride, by binding to the chloride site of the electroneutral Na^+/Cl^- co-transport system to inhibit its action.
  - *Anaesthetic implications:* potassium loss can be significant, particularly in the elderly. Electrolytes should be checked prior to anaesthesia, and consideration should be given to withholding the drugs on the day of surgery.
- **Calcium channel antagonists:** therapeutically important calcium antagonists act on L-type calcium channels, and are of three main classes: phenylalkylamines (verapamil), dihydropyridines, (nifedipine, amlodipine) and benzothiazepines

(diltiazem). All three groups bind to the a_1-subunit of the calcium channel, and inhibit the slow inward calcium current in cardiac and smooth muscle cells. Verapamil has primarily cardiac effects, and acts as a negative inotrope and chronotrope. Nifedipine and related drugs are more selective for vascular smooth muscle and so are usually used to treat hypertension. They are primarily arterial and arteriolar dilators and have minimal influence on the venous system. The effects of diltiazem are intermediate but it, along with verapamil, is a class IV anti-arrhythmic. Both slow conduction through the SA and AV nodes where propagation of the AP is dependent on slow inward calcium flux. Verapamil terminates SVTs by causing partial AV block. Nifedipine may cause reflex tachycardia. Ca^{2+} channel blockers are all negative inotropes, but because they offload the myocardium by vasodilatation, cardiac output is usually maintained.

— *Anaesthetic implications:* there may be some synergistic action with volatile anaesthetic agents, which also affect slow Ca^{2+} channels in the myocardium and elsewhere. Nifedipine and verapamil may also potentiate the actions of non-depolarizing muscle relaxants.

- **Angiotensin-converting enzyme (ACE) inhibitors:** these drugs affect the renin–angiotensin system. Renin is a proteolytic enzyme secreted by the juxtaglomerular apparatus, which acts on angiotensinogen (a plasma globulin synthesized in the liver) to form angiotensin I. This inactive substance is converted to the potent vasoconstrictor angiotensin II by ACE. (Angiotensin II is then broken down further to angiotensin III and IV.) ACE is a membrane-bound enzyme on the surface of endothelial cells, and is particularly abundant in lung with its huge area of vascular endothelium. The local formation of angiotensin II can occur in numerous different vascular beds. ACE inactivates bradykinin and several other peptides. Bradykinin is an inflammatory mediator and vasoactive peptide which causes vasodilatation and increased vascular permeability. It may also cause bronchial and other smooth muscle constriction. Angiotensin acts on receptors to mediate vasoconstriction (its pressor activity is 40 times as powerful as that of noradrenaline), as well as noradrenaline release from sympathetic nerve terminals, sodium reabsorption from proximal tubules, and aldosterone secretion from the adrenal cortex. ACE inhibitors include captopril, enalapril, lisinopril and perindopril. These drugs mediate a significant fall in BP in hypertensive subjects, and reduce cardiac load by affecting both capacitance and resistance vessels. They have no influence on cardiac contractility, although they do act preferentially on angiotensin-sensitive vascular beds in the myocardium, brain and kidney. Cough is a common side effect of their use, due probably to bradykinin accumulation.

  — *Anaesthetic implications:* intraoperative hypotension has been reported following the concomitant administration of a general or regional anaesthetic. ACE inhibitors should be discontinued 24–48 hours prior to anaesthesia. If they have not been omitted then volume loading and vasopressors may be needed to maintain normal BP.

- **Angiotensin antagonists:** pure antagonists of the angiotensin I receptor (examples include losartan, valsartan) should in theory have a similar spectrum of benefit as ACE inhibitors. They have a better side effect profile and do not cause persistent cough, although they are less effective in the treatment of heart failure.

— *Anaesthetic implications:* these are broadly similar to those that apply to ACE inhibitors although, if not discontinued prior to surgery, they are even more likely to cause profound and refractory intraoperative hypotension.

Hypotension and its management

Commentary

This may end up largely as a viva about drugs to treat hypotension, but it will be introduced from first principles. Vasopressors are the logical treatment for falls in BP that have been induced pharmacologically, but they also find deployment in a variety of clinical scenarios in which patients are hypotensive. You will be expected to know about this class of drugs and to be able to demonstrate judgement in their use.

The viva

You might be asked to give some causes of hypotension.

A logical way of organizing your answer is to start by describing the prime determinants of arterial BP.

- Systemic BP is determined by cardiac output(CO), which is the product of heart rate(HR) and stroke volume(SV), multiplied by systemic vascular resistance(SVP) (i.e. $BP = CO \times SVR$).
- CO is a function of **HR** and SV.
- Hypotension may result from an inadequately compensated decrease in any one or more of these variables.

Reduction in HR ($BP = \mathbf{HR} \times SV \times SVR$)

- **Causes**
    - *Hypoxia:* pre-terminal hypoxia leads to bradycardia.
    - *Vagal stimulation:* profound bradycardia may follow traction on extraocular muscles, anal or cervical dilatation, visceral traction, and, sometimes, instrumentation of the airway.
    - *Drugs:* medication with drugs such as ß-adrenoceptor blockers and digoxin may be responsible. Anaesthetic drugs may also contribute. Volatile agents in high concentrations, halothane in normal concentrations, suxamethonium, opioids and anticholinesterases can all be associated with bradycardia. Low doses of atropine may provoke a paradoxical bradycardia (the Bezold–Jarisch reflex).
    - *Cardiac disease:* the commonest cause is ischaemic change affecting the conducting system.
    - *Metabolic:* acute hyperkalaemia may hyperpolarize the myocardial cell membrane with a resulting fall in HR.
    - *Spinal anaesthesia:* in theory, the block of the cardiac accelerator fibres from T_1 to T_4 should be associated with bradycardia. In practice, this is not often seen.

- **Management**
  - First of all diagnose the cause, and if it is amenable to treatment then act accordingly. Is it hypoxia? Treat immediately. Is it surgical stimulus? If so, then stop traction on the extraocular muscles or the mesentery. If drug treatment is required, the most effective immediate first line drug is an anticholinergic agent, usually atropine or glycopyrrolate. Neither is a treatment for hypoxia.

Reduction in SV (BP $= HR \times$ **SV** $\times$ SVR)

- **Causes**
  - The commonest cause is reduced venous return. This may be due to an actual reduction in circulating volume because of blood loss or dehydration or to an effective reduction in circulating volume caused by sympathetic block. SV may also be diminished because the ventricle is failing.

- **Management**
  - As before, it is important to diagnose the cause, and if it is amenable to treatment then act accordingly. Is it hypovolaemia? Resuscitate with the appropriate fluid. Is position contributing? Revert to recumbency or the head-down position; ensure lateral uterine displacement in the later stages of pregnancy. Beware aortocaval compression by the intra-abdominal mass that is not a gravid uterus. Is it a failing ventricle? Consider using inotropes to support ventricular function.

Reduction in SVR (BP $= HR \times SV \times$ **SVR**)

- **Causes**
  - The commonest cause of inadvertent profound hypotension is probably that which is induced by the sympathetic block associated with a spinal or epidural. In the context of critical care the commonest cause is sepsis.

- **Management**
  - The rational management of hypotension that has been induced pharmaco-logically is to treat it pharmacologically. The reduced SVR associated with sepsis is different, but it is still usually managed with a combination of vasopressor, fluids and inotropes.

Further direction the viva could take

You will be asked about the range of drugs available to treat hypotension.

Ephedrine

- **Pharmacology:** Ephedrine is a naturally occurring compound (from the Chinese plant *Ma Huang*), which is now synthesized for medical use. It is sympathomimetic and acts both directly and indirectly, possessing both α- and β-effects. It also inhibits the breakdown of noradrenaline (norepinephrine) by monoamine oxidase. This mixture of effects means that its main influence on BP is via an increase in CO. Its α_1-effects mediate peripheral vasoconstriction, while the β_1-effects are positive inotropy and chronotropy, and the β_2-effects are bronchodilatation (and vasodilatation). The bolus dose is 3–5 mg titrated against response and repeated as necessary. The drug has a rapid onset of action that is said to last for around 60 minutes, but which in practice appears to be less. Noradrenaline depletion owing to its indirect action leads to tachyphylaxis.

- **Clinical usage:** traditionally, it has been favoured in obstetric anaesthesia because it does not cause α_1-mediated vasoconstriction in the uteroplacental circulation. It has now been superseded by α_1-agonists because it is associated with a greater fetal acidosis (probably by increasing fetal metabolic demand). Ephedrine increases myocardial oxygen demand and so should be used in caution in patients with a pre-existing tachycardia or with cardiac disease. It is also arrhythmogenic. It is an effective bronchodilator.

Phenylephrine

- **Pharmacology:** phenylephrine is an α_1-agonist with mainly direct actions but with some weak β-activity. Its primary influence on BP is via α_1-vasoconstriction and an increase in peripheral resistance. The dose is 50–100 μg titrated against response and repeated as necessary. Onset is rapid but its duration of action is frequently less than the 60 minutes that is claimed.
- **Clinical usage:** it is an effective vasopressor which is especially popular in some cardiac units. It is also used more widely in obstetric anaesthesia despite traditional avoidance of all pressor drugs apart from ephedrine. Phenylephrine maintains maternal BP and neonatal cord pH better than ephedrine. It is not arrhythmogenic, but it can cause a reflex bradycardia which may require treatment with atropine or glycopyrrolate. It is useful in patients in whom a tachycardia should be avoided.

Metaraminol

- **Pharmacology:** metaraminol is a sympathomimetic with both direct and indirect actions and α- and β-effects (α-effects predominate). Its influence on BP is via α_1-vasoconstriction and increase in CO with increased coronary blood flow. The dose is 1–5 mg titrated against response and repeated as necessary. The onset of action is rapid (1–3 minutes) and the duration of action is around 20–25 minutes.
- **Clinical usage:** it is a potent and effective vasopressor, which is particularly useful for the treatment of hypotension due to sympathetic blockade.

Noradrenaline

- **Pharmacology:** noradrenaline is an exogenous and endogenous catecholamine. It is a powerful α_1-agonist with weaker β-effects. Its vasopressor effect is mediated via α_1-vasoconstriction and the increase in peripheral resistance. It is administered by intravenous infusion (0.05–0.2 μg kg^{-1} min^{-1}) and titrated against the desired level of arterial pressure. Its onset and offset of action are rapid.
- **Clinical usage:** noradrenaline is used more commonly in intensive care medicine than in anaesthesia, particularly to treat the low systemic vascular resistance associated with sepsis. Sudden discontinuation of an infusion may be accompanied by severe rebound hypotension. This explains the occasional requirement for the

drug following removal of a noradrenaline-secreting phaeochromocytoma. Reflex bradycardia is common.

Adrenaline

- **Pharmacology:** adrenaline is also an exogenous and endogenous catecholamine, which acts both as an α_1- and β-agonist. In low doses, β-mediated vasodilatation predominates, but the BP rises because of the increase in CO. In high doses, adrenaline causes α_1-vasoconstriction. It is given either as a bolus (in the case of circulatory arrest) or as an intravenous infusion in the same dose range as noradrenaline (0.05–$0.2\ \mu\mathrm{g\,kg}^{-1}\,\mathrm{min}^{-1}$).
- **Clinical usage:** the use of adrenaline as a vasopressor is effectively limited to catastrophic circulatory collapse and cardiac arrest.

Inotropes

Commentary

Anaesthetists need to know how to support a failing myocardium. The use of inotropes in critical care is routine and examiners will expect your knowledge of the applied clinical pharmacology to be sound. They will be aware that intensive care units have different preferred inotropes, and so you may well be given the opportunity to discuss the one with which you have had the most experience. You may also be asked to talk about a second line inotrope. You will add credibility to your account if you can make it evident that these are drugs with whose clinical use you are very familiar.

The viva

The subject may be introduced by setting it in a clinical context such as the circulatory failure associated with sepsis or the treatment of cardiogenic shock. Once it has been established that inotropes are central to management, the examiners will go on to develop the subject in some detail.

- The accurate definition of an inotrope is a substance that affects the force of muscular contraction, either positively or negatively. By common usage, however, the term 'inotrope' describes one of a range of drugs which increase myocardial contractility.
- Most inotropes act via a final common pathway to increase the availability of calcium within the myocyte. The activation of adenylyl cyclase leads to an increase in the production of cAMP from ATP, which in turn activates protein kinase A. This enzyme phosphorylates sites on the α_1-subunits of calcium channels, leading to an increase in open state probability, a rise in calcium flux and an increase in myocardial contractile force.
- The steps which lead to the activation of adenylyl cyclase are considerably more complex than this final pathway, there being at least 13 G protein-linked

myocardial cell membrane receptors. You will either be doing very well in the viva (or be very unlucky) should the examiner decide to dwell on these in any detail. β-adrenoceptors, 5-HT receptors, and histamine, prostaglandin and vasoactive intestinal peptide receptors interact with $G_{s(stimulatory)}$ proteins to activate ACh. Adenosine, ACh and somatostatin interact with $G_{i(inhibitory)}$ proteins to inhibit adenylyl cyclase activation, and α_1-adrenoceptors and endothelin receptors interact with G_q proteins to activate phospholipase C and thence protein kinases. (Unlike the 's' and 'i', the 'q' designation does not stand for anything specific but, essentially, was chosen arbitrarily from the later letters of the alphabet, the earlier ones having been reserved for classes of subunits that had already been identified.)

- Calcium leads to the final increase in contractility, and almost all the inotropes in common use have actions that are cAMP dependent. These include dobutamine, adrenaline, dopexamine, noradrenaline, dopamine, isoprenaline, enoximone, milrinone, ephedrine and glucagon. A much smaller group exerts its effects independently of cAMP. The most important are the cardiac glycosides digoxin and ouabain (no longer available in the UK).
- **Inflammatory response:** inotropes also appear to modulate the cytokine response. They inhibit secretion of TNF and alter the balance between pro-inflammatory cytokines, particularly IL-6; and anti-inflammatory molecules such as IL-10.

Direction the viva may take

You may then be asked about the inotrope(s) with which you are most familiar.

- **Dobutamine** is a synthetic catecholamine derivative of isoprenaline which is predominantly a β_1-adrenoceptor agonist. It also has dose-dependent effects at β_2- and α_1-receptors. It increases contractility, has minimal effects on heart rate and has little direct effect on vascular tone. It does not act at renal dopamine receptors, but may increase urine output by improving circulatory performance. The quoted dose range is $2.5–10.0 \ \mu g \, kg^{-1} \, min^{-1}$, titrated against response, but much higher rates may be needed in the critically ill.
- **Adrenaline** is an exogenous and endogenous catecholamine, which is both an α_1-and β-agonist. It causes an α_1-mediated increase in the force and rate of myocardial contraction, coupled with an increase in stroke volume secondary to enhanced venous return. In low doses, β_1-mediated vasodilatation is prominent, but the BP rises because of the increase in cardiac output. As the dose increases so both α- and β-effects are seen, while at high doses α_1-vasoconstriction predominates. In the context of critical care adrenaline is given by intravenous infusion at a rate of $0.05–0.20 \ \mu g \, kg^{-1} \, min^{-1}$.
- **Noradrenaline** is another exogenous and endogenous catecholamine. It is a powerful α_1-agonist with weaker β-effects which are most pronounced at low doses ($< 0.05 \ \mu g \, kg^{-1} \, min^{-1}$). Technically, it is more a vasopressor than a direct inotrope but it has become the first line agent in many critical care units. (Rises in SVR are associated with increases in cardiac contractility. This is the Anrep effect.)
- **Dopexamine** is a dopamine analogue which also acts both at dopaminergic and β_2-adrenergic receptors. It has no effect at α-receptors. It is an inodilator which

increases myocardial contractility while decreasing SVR. It also dilates the splanchnic circulation, which is the main property that finds favour amongst intensivists. The dose range is 0.5–6.0 $\mu g\,kg^{-1}\,min^{-1}$.

- **Dopamine** is an endogenous precursor of noradrenaline, which acts on dopaminergic DA_1 and DA_2 receptors as well as at adrenoceptors. Its effects are dose-dependent: at low doses (up to 5.0 $\mu g\,kg^{-1}\,min^{-1}$) it stimulates mainly dopamine receptors, and it was believed that, because this caused renal vasodilatation, it conferred a renal protective effect. (There is no evidence for this purported benefit.) At infusion rates of between 5 and 10 $\mu g\,kg^{-1}\,min^{-1}$ it causes β_1-mediated increases in myocardial contractility and cardiac output. As the dose rises further, α_1-vasoconstriction becomes more predominant, although it may still provoke tachycardia. Few now believe that dopamine is uniquely useful because of its renal dopaminergic effects and it is not a first line inotrope.

- **Isoprenaline** is a synthetic catecholamine with very potent β-adrenergic effects (both β_1 and β_2), but with no α-adrenergic activity. Given in a dose of 0.02–0.2 $\mu g\,kg^{-1}\,min^{-1}$ it leads both to an increase in myocardial contractility and heart rate. It is the drug of choice for pharmacological treatment of complete heart block and for overcoming overdose with β-blockers.

Further direction the viva could take

You may be asked to compare the inotrope(s) that you have been discussing with a second line drug or with one that has a different mechanism of action.

- **Enoximone and milrinone:** these also act via an increase in cAMP, which is mediated by inhibiting the action of phosphodiesterase-III (PDE-III). This enzyme is responsible for the intracellular degradation of cAMP. Both drugs increase contractility while causing peripheral vasodilatation. The dose of enoximone is 5–20 $\mu g\,kg^{-1}\,min^{-1}$ after a loading dose of 90 $\mu g\,kg^{-1}$; that of milrinone is 0.375–0.750 $\mu g\,kg^{-1}\,min^{-1}$ after a loading dose of 50 $\mu g\,kg^{-1}$. Because the effects of PDE-III inhibitors are not mediated via adrenoceptors these drugs can be useful if myocardial β-adrenoceptor downregulation has occurred and the receptors have become desensitized. This process may be associated with longstanding heart failure and prolonged exposure to circulating catecholamines, but it can also occur acutely (within minutes).

- **Digoxin** is one of the cardiac glycosides (another being ouabain from the African tree, *Ouabaio akokanthera*), which also acts ultimately via an increase in calcium in the sarcoplasmic reticulum. Unlike other inotropes, however, it inhibits Na^+/K^+ ATPase. It does so by binding to an extracellular α subunit. The resulting increase in sodium concentration reduces the inwardly directed gradient across the cell membrane. One of the mechanisms by which free intracellular calcium levels are kept low is the Na^+/Ca^{2+} exchange transporter. One calcium ion is extruded from the cell in exchange for three sodium ions. More calcium is therefore available for release from the sarcoplasmic reticulum with each AP.

- **Glucagon** exerts its positive inotropic effect via an increase in the synthesis of cAMP. It is rarely used for this specific purpose, but more commonly in the emergency treatment of hypoglycaemia. (It mobilizes hepatic glycogen.)

- **Ephedrine** is a sympathomimetic which has both direct and indirect a- and $ß$-effects, but which is used primarily as a vasopressor. It inhibits the breakdown of noradrenaline by monoamine oxidase, and this mixture of actions mean that its main influence on BP is via an increase in cardiac output. Its a_1-effects mediate peripheral vasoconstriction, while the $ß_1$-effects increase the force and rate of myocardial contraction. Tachyphylaxis limits its effectiveness.

Drugs used in the treatment of nausea and vomiting

Commentary

Postoperative nausea is a core problem. The effective prescription of anti-emetics requires some knowledge about their diverse sites of action. This viva may be combined with general questions about the physiology of vomiting (page 168).

The viva

You may be asked which patients are at particular risk of postoperative nausea and vomiting (PONV).

- **Patient factors:** those with a positive history of PONV (increases likelihood by a factor of three); female gender (incidence 2–4 × greater than in males); commoner during the second half of the menstrual cycle; greater in the obese, in the anxious, in the young and if postoperative ambulation is premature.
- **Surgical factors:** higher following intra-abdominal, intracranial, middle ear and squint surgery, and after laparoscopic and gynaecological procedures. Postoperative pain and anxiety are precipitants.
- **Anaesthetic factors:** opiates and all inhalational agents, including nitrous oxide, predispose patients to PONV. The same applies to agents with sympathomimetic actions such as ketamine. Hypoxaemia is a stimulus to vomiting.
- **Factors related to disease:** the list of potential causes is long and includes intestinal obstruction, hypoglycaemia, hypoxia, uraemia and hypotension.

You will then be asked about the applied pharmacology, with particular reference to the sites of action of the drugs that you cite.

- Nausea and vomiting are mediated by a number of sites with different receptors. This means that these symptoms can be treated by 'balanced anti-emesis' using drugs of differing actions. Although some drugs act at more than one receptor, their anti-emetic actions usually predominate at one.
- **Vestibular nuclei and the labyrinth:** these contain histamine (H_1) and muscarinic ACh (M_3) receptors. Drugs acting at this site include cyclizine, promethazine (H_1-antagonists), and hyoscine, atropine and glycopyrrolate (anticholinergic M_3-antagonists).

- **Visceral afferents:** these are mediated by serotonin (5-HT$_3$) receptors in the gut wall and myenteric plexus. Drugs acting at this site include ondansetron, granisetron and tropisetron (selective 5-HT$_3$ antagonists).
- **Vomiting centre (VC):** this contains primarily muscarinic ACh (M$_3$) and some histamine (H$_1$) receptors. It may also contain μ-opioid receptors. Drugs acting at this site are the same as those which affect the vestibular apparatus.
- **Chemoreceptor trigger zone (CTZ):** impulses from the CTZ to the VC appear to be mediated mainly via dopamine (D$_2$) and serotonin (5-HT$_3$) receptors. It may also contain δ-opioid receptors. In addition, substance P, which is a slow excitatory neurotransmitter, may have a role by acting at neurokinin-1 (NK$_1$) receptors. NK$_1$-receptors are abundant in the brain stem where emetic afferents converge. Drugs acting at this site include metoclopramide, domperidone, prochlorperazine, trifluoperazine, haloperidol, and, previously, droperidol, which is no longer available (D$_2$-antagonists); and vofopitant (this is an experimental NK$_1$-antagonist).
- **Drugs of uncertain sites of action**
  - *Cannabinoids:* synthetic derivatives such as nabilone appear to antagonize the emetic effects of drugs which stimulate the CTZ. Because the cannabinoid effects can themselves be antagonized by naloxone, it is postulated that opioid receptors are involved in their actions. An endogenous cannabinoid CB$_1$ receptor which modulates neurotransmitter release has been identified.
  - *Corticosteroids:* high-dose steroids such as dexamethasone or methyl prednisolone act as anti-emetics by mechanisms that are unclear.
  - *Propofol:* this has effective activity which has been used to treat cytotoxic-induced emesis. It would appear therefore to act at the CTZ.

Direction the viva may take

You may be asked about significant side effects of the anti-emetics that you prescribe.

- **Antimuscarinic drugs** (atropine, hyoscine, glycopyrrolate): all are potent antisialogogues, and so a dry mouth is almost invariable. Hyoscine is sedative.
- **Antidopaminergic drugs** (metoclopramide, prochlorperazine, haloperidol): these may cause acute extrapyramidal and dystonic effects which are caused by a preponderance of the antidopaminergic stimulatory actions over anticholinergic inhibitory actions in other parts of the CNS. This imbalance can be restored almost instantly with an intravenous anticholinergic agent such as benzatropine 1–2 mg. The phenothiazines may also cause sedation.
- **Antiserotoninergic drugs** (ondansetron, granisetron): their side effect profile is good, although headache has been reported as a complication of treatment in 3–5% of patients.
- **Cannabinoids** (nabilone, dronabinol): sedation is common, and the drugs may sometimes exert psychotomimetic effects similar to those induced by the parent compounds. Dry mouth and postural hypotension may also occur.
- **Corticosteroids** (methyl prednisolone, dexamethasone): the list of acute side effects includes steroid psychosis, which is related to a sudden increase in plasma levels of corticoids, and metabolic disturbance including hyperglycaemia, fluid retention and hypokalaemia. Short courses of high-dose steroids may cause peptic ulceration.

Drug overdose: prescribed and therapeutic drugs

Commentary

Patients take overdoses of numerous different drugs. The clinical features of drug poisoning may result from exaggeration of their normal effects or from the direct toxicity of the parent compound and its metabolites. Effective management of drug overdose in many cases of poisoning depends upon some understanding of the mechanism of action of the substances that have been ingested.

The viva

You will be asked first about the drugs that are most commonly taken in overdose. It is probable that you will also be asked to give a brief outline of your emergency management. The examiners will not be interested in a generic 'Airway, Breathing, Circulation' approach, but will want specific details where appropriate.

Antidepressants

The main classes of drugs are the tricyclic antidepressants (TCAs) such as amitriptyline and imipramine, and the selective serotonin re-uptake inhibitors (SSRIs) such as fluoxetine (Prozac) and paroxetine (Seroxat).

- **Mechanisms:** TCAs are tertiary amines and are related chemically to phenothiazines. They act by blocking the re-uptake of amines, primarily noradrenaline and 5-HT, by competitive inhibition of a transport protein binding site. They have minimal influence on dopaminergic synapses, but do affect muscarinic ACh and histamine receptors.

SSRIs are relatively selective for 5-HT uptake, have fewer anticholinergic side effects than TCAs and are safer in overdose. They can cause a 'serotonin syndrome' if used in combination with drugs such as monoamine oxidase inhibitors. Its features include hyperthermia, muscular rigidity and cardiovascular collapse.

- **Features of overdose:** the major problems are cardiovascular and neurological. Ventricular arrhythmias are common and are associated particularly with Q–T interval prolongation. In high doses they appear to block a specific cardiac potassium channel (the HERG channel). Ventricular fibrillation may supervene. Other potential arrhythmias include heart block and ventricular tachycardia. CNS effects include agitation and excitability, grand mal convulsions and coma. The muscarinic effects resemble those of atropine poisoning, with flushing, dry mouth, mydriasis and gastrointestinal stasis. Features of poisoning with SSRIs are analogous, but are generally less severe.
- **Management:** this is largely supportive. Benzodiazepines may abort convulsions. Cardiac arrhythmias should be treated only with extreme caution, if at all, because the combination of effects can be fatal. Magnesium is probably the least dangerous treatment, although intravenous lignocaine and amiodarone have been used. ECG monitoring is mandatory for at least 24 hours after ingestion. Induced alkalosis

(plasma pH >7.5) by the use of hyperventilation and intravenous $NaHCO_3$ may reduce the amount of free drug that is present.

Paracetamol

This is a ubiquitous simple analgesic.

- **Mechanisms:** paracetamol probably acts as an inhibitor of central prostaglandin synthesis, although its exact subcellular mechanism of action remains unclear. Evidence about any peripheral antiinflammatory action is conflicting. It is rapidly absorbed from the small intestine. Its therapeutic index is narrow because the liver enzymes which catalyse the normal conjugation pathways rapidly become saturated. The alternative metabolic pathway via mixed function oxidases produces a metabolite (N-acetyl-p-benzoquinine imine) which is toxic to cells both of the liver and of the renal tubules. This metabolite is normally conjugated with glutathione, but will accumulate when glutathione stores are depleted to cause centrilobular hepatic necrosis and renal tubular damage.
- **Features of overdose:** nausea and vomiting occur early, symptoms and signs of hepatic failure appear later.
- **Management:** definitive early treatment is with agents that will replenish glutathione stores and prevent hepatic damage. Methionine, which is a glutathione precursor, can be given orally, although the more common treatment is intravenous N-acetylcysteine. Fulminant hepatic failure can be treated only by hepatic transplantation.

Benzodiazepines

These anxiolytics and hypnotics, of which there are over 20 available for clinical use, are common prescription drugs. Typical examples are temazepam, diazepam and clonazepam. (Midazolam is a drug whose use is restricted largely to hospital.)

- **Mechanism of action:** benzodiazepines facilitate the opening of GABA-activated chloride channels and thereby enhance fast inhibitory synaptic transmission within the CNS. They bind to a separate receptor, which effects an allosteric change that increases the affinity of GABA for the $GABA_A$ receptor.
- **Features of overdose:** these drugs are relatively safe in overdose because, taken alone, they cause profound sedation but without respiratory depression, haemodynamic instability or secondary toxicity. In combination with other CNS depressants, however, they may be associated with marked respiratory depression.
- **Management:** flumazenil (Anexate) is a specific benzodiazepine antagonist which displaces benzodiazepines from the binding sites and reverses their effects. The effective duration of action of flumazenil is shorter than that of many of the drugs which it antagonizes, and so the dose (typically up to 500 µg intravenously) may need to be repeated. The incautious use of flumazenil may also unmask convulsions caused, for example, by TCAs, otherwise suppressed by the benzodiazepine overdose.

Tramadol

This is a synthetic piperidine analogue of codeine. It is an oral analgesic which is used for moderate pain, but which is not associated with drug dependence or abuse. It is not, therefore, a controlled substance.

- **Mechanisms:** for details see page 216. Tramadol has relatively low activity at μ-receptors, but also acts by inhibiting the re-uptake of noradrenaline and 5-HT within the CNS.
- **Features of overdose:** although activity at μ-opioid receptors is weak, after overdose patients may demonstrate typical features of sedation and respiratory depression. Of greater interest are the signs of a serotonin syndrome, which include agitation, tachycardia and hypertension, diaphoresis and muscular rigidity. Patients may also be hyperthermic and show other signs of deranged autonomic function. Disseminated intravascular coagulation has been reported, as has rhabdomyolysis and renal failure. Grand mal convulsions may supervene.
- **Management:** in general, the treatment of a tramadol overdose is supportive. Naloxone can be used to treat the opioid side effects, but the optimal management of a serotonin syndrome remains uncertain. The 5-HT$_{2A}$ antagonist cyproheptadine has been used, as have drugs such as dantrolene, propranolol and diazepam.

Alcohol

This is included because alcohol ingestion frequently complicates overdose with other drugs. TCAs, for example, can dangerously enhance the depressant effects of acute alcohol intake.

- **Mechanism of action:** ethanol facilitates the opening of GABA-activated chloride channels to increase fast inhibitory synaptic transmission within the CNS. It also acts to inhibit the NMDA receptor.
- **Features of overdose:** disinhibition is followed by CNS depression. The features of acute intoxication are too well known to warrant detailing. An important complication that must not be missed, however, is the effect of acute alcohol on glucose metabolism. Individuals who have recently ingested large volumes of alcohol are at risk of profound hypoglycaemia. The metabolism of alcohol to acetaldehyde is catalysed by alcohol dehydrogenase in a reaction which produces NADH from NAD^+. This effectively depletes NAD^+, which is an important co-factor in the gluconeogenetic conversion of lactate to pyruvate.
- **Management:** the metabolism of alcohol follows zero order kinetics and management is supportive.

Recreational drugs and drugs of abuse

Commentary

The abuse of recreational drugs is common, and patients may present either because of an adverse reaction or because, often unwittingly, they have taken or been given an overdose. It can be difficult to identify exactly what substances are involved because street drugs have no quality control, and because these adulterated compounds are often taken in combination. But, as is the case with prescribed drugs, an understanding of their mechanisms of action helps the rational management of overdose.

The viva

You are likely to be asked about the common drugs of abuse. There are some niche drugs, such as GHB (gamma-hydroxybutyrate) and Special K (ketamine), but the general pattern of drug abuse relates to methadone and heroin (diamorphine), cocaine, ecstasy (MDMA) and alcohol. It is also probable that you will be asked to comment on your emergency management. As with overdoses of therapeutic drugs, the examiners will be less interested in a generic approach than in your ability to apply appropriate pharmacological knowledge.

Opiates

Methadone and heroin are the main opiates of abuse.

- **Mechanisms:** for details see page 213.
- **Features of overdose:** the features of opiate overdose are well known. The life-threatening complication of opiate overdose is profound central respiratory depression. Patients may be sedated, comatose and bradypnoeic. Hypotension is common, and this may be associated with both tachycardia and bradycardia. The other numerous effects of opiates are of less relative importance. Methadone has a similar spectrum of action to diamorphine, although it is less euphoriant and less sedative. It has a much longer elimination half-life (>24 hours).
- **Management:** the specific opiate antagonist naloxone is the initial drug of choice. The intravenous dose is higher than is used for typical postoperative respiratory depression, being 0.8–2.0 mg, repeated after 2–3 minutes to a maximum of 10 mg. If there has been no response by this stage then the diagnosis should be reviewed.

Cocaine

- **Mechanisms:** cocaine is an indirect sympathomimetic which blocks the presynaptic re-uptake of noradrenaline. It also exerts central dopaminergic and serotonergic effects.
- **Features of overdose:** these include agitation and disorientation, together with other features of sympathetic hyperstimulation. Hypertension, hyperpyrexia, convulsions and coma may all be evident. The drug increases myocardial oxygen demand and causes coronary vasospasm. Ventricular fibrillation may supervene.
- **Management:** it would be logical to treat the sympathetic overactivity with α- and β-adrenoceptor blockers, although some authorities dispute the place of β-blockers because of their unopposed α-effects on the circulation. These can be offset by using, for example, phentolamine (5 mg intravenously, repeated as necessary). Otherwise, the management of cocaine poisoning is supportive.

MDMA (ecstasy)

This is a popular recreational drug, which has caused well publicized deaths among a small number of young people. These deaths are not necessarily related to overdose, although, because the drug is illegal, information about quantity, quality and formulation is almost impossible to obtain. The clinical features may, therefore, be caused by an idiosyncratic reaction.

- **Mechanisms:** 3,4-methylenedioxy methamphetamine (MDMA) is related structurally both to methamphetamine and to mescaline, which is a potent hallucinogen. Amphetamines are centrally-acting sympathomimetics which appear to stimulate central aminergic pathways, particularly those mediated by dopamine and noradrenaline. They inhibit re-uptake of neurotransmitter, stimulate its presynaptic release, and act as direct agonists at postsynaptic receptors. These effects occur peripherally as well as centrally. MDMA also acts as an agonist at 5-HT$_2$ receptors to produce psychotomimetic effects. This may also be partly responsible for the hyperthermia that may be evident.
- **Features of overdose:** ecstasy use is associated with the club scene and so patients may present having been dancing violently in a hot environment without taking adequate isotonic fluid. They may be delirious or unconscious, with grand mal convulsions. They are frequently diaphoretic and febrile. This hypermetabolic state is associated with a metabolic acidosis, and also with rhabdomyolysis. Disseminated intravascular coagulation may supervene, followed by multi-organ failure.
- **Management:** patients may require full intensive care management, including renal support if indicated. Dantrolene (1 mg kg^{-1} initially) has been used to control hyperpyrexia, although support for its use is not universal.

Alcohol
This may be taken alone in overdose, or as part of a cocktail of substances (page 253).

Cannabis
Overdose is not a common problem, given that most users in the UK smoke the drug, rather than ingesting it. Nor is acute excess directly life-threatening. A brief account is included for completeness in the event that the examiners may raise the topic.

- **Mechanisms:** central cannabinoid receptors (CB$_1$ subtype) exert an inhibitory effect on nociceptive afferents and on transmission via the dorsal horn. Like opiates they are typical G protein-linked receptors, which inhibit adenyl cyclase, hyperpolarize cell membranes by facilitating the opening of potassium channels, and decrease neurotransmitter release via calcium channel inhibition. Tetrahydrocannabinol (THC) is analgesic, sedating, anti-emetic, antispasmodic, euphoriant, anxiolytic and bronchodilatory. (These features would actually make the drug an ideal premedicant.)
- **Features of acute excess:** the main features are sedation and confusion, although the drug can also cause vasodilatation and tachycardia. Paranoid delusions of the kind that may be seen with hallucinogenic drugs can occur with stronger preparations.
- **Management:** unless patients have complicated cannabis use by concurrent ingestion of other substances they will require only modest supportive therapy.

Direction the viva may take
You may be asked about the anaesthetic implications of drug abuse. There are three main considerations: the patient may be under the residual influence of the drug; they

may suffer an acute withdrawal syndrome; and they may have continued physiological dependence. (Drug-associated co-morbidity such as infection with HIV and hepatitis B should also be considered.) It may be very difficult to obtain an accurate history.

- **Opiates:** recent ingestion in a habituated patient will do little more than act as opiate premedication. Withdrawal is characterized by autonomic hyperactivity with clinical features of both sympathetic and parasympathetic stimulation. These include agitation, tachycardia, diaphoresis, vomiting and abdominal cramps. It is important not to precipitate a withdrawal syndrome in the perioperative period by giving inadequate doses of opioid. Postoperative pain requirements should be added to their estimated daily 'maintenance' requirement. PCA doses may need to be increased significantly and must be given via a device that is secure and tamperproof.
- **Cocaine and amphetamines:** residual sympathetic stimulation will complicate anaesthesia, but its manifestations are easily treated. Cocaine withdrawal is characterized mainly by psychological craving for the drug. This may be mediated by dopamine and/or 5-HT, but the use of antagonists is not widespread.
- **Cannabis:** this has many of the properties of a useful drug for premedication, and residual effects may even confer some benefit, as long as these are recognized and the sedation is not compounded by excessive anaesthetic and analgesic doses. A withdrawal syndrome has been described that manifests mainly as restlessness, irritability, insomnia and anorexia.

Drugs affecting mood

Commentary

These commonly prescribed drugs are of interest because some have specific implications for anaesthesia. You are unlikely to be asked about all the classes of drugs, and the viva may concentrate on one group with only supplementary reference to the others. Even if you are hazy on their precise details of action (these being drugs which anaesthetists almost never prescribe), at least make sure that you are aware of their clinical significance in the context of anaesthesia and surgery.

The viva

You will be asked to discuss the anaesthetic implications for one or more of the groups of drugs that are used to treat affective disorders.

Lithium

Lithium (Li^+) is an inorganic ion, which is used prophylactically to control the mood swings of bipolar manic depression. In the acute situation it may help to control mania, but not depression. The drug has a very narrow therapeutic index; it is effective at plasma levels of $0.5–1.0\,mmol\,L^{-1}$, produces side effects at $>1.5\,mmol\,l^{-1}$, and may be fatal at a plasma concentration of $3.0–5.0\,mmol\,l^{-1}$.

- **Mechanisms:** as an inorganic ion it can mimic the role of sodium in excitable tissue by entering cells via fast voltage-gated channels that generate action potentials. Unlike sodium, however, it is not pumped out of the excitable cell by Na^+/K^+-ATPase and so accumulates within the cytoplasm, partially replacing intracellular potassium. Its therapeutic effect is thought to be mediated by its interference with two second messenger systems: cAMP and inositol triphosphate. It may increase 5-HT synthesis in the CNS. Its actions are enhanced by diuretics, which reduce clearance, and by dehydration.

- **Adverse effects and implications for anaesthesia:** side effects include polydipsia and polyuria secondary to ADH inhibition, diarrhoea and vomiting, hypothyroidism, lassitude and renal impairment. Acute toxicity causes cardiac arrhythmias, ataxia, confusion, convulsions and, in extreme cases, coma and death. Plasma levels must be measured before anaesthesia. The drug enhances the effects of all muscle relaxants (both depolarizing and non-depolarizing) and potentiates anaesthetic agents. It has a long plasma half-life and so can be withheld for 2 days preceding surgery. Good hydration is important, as is sodium balance. Low serum sodium increases lithium toxicity, and electrolytes should be restored to normal levels before surgery. NSAIDs may reduce Li^+ clearance and increase plasma levels.

Monoamine oxidase inhibitors (MAOIs)

Potentially dangerous interactions led to a fall in the number of patients receiving MAOIs for refractory depressive illness. Recently, however, newer agents have been synthesized and this class of drugs has enjoyed resurgence. Monoamine oxidase (MAO) describes a non-specific group of enzymes, which is subdivided into two main classes.

- **MAO-A:** this is mainly intraneuronal and degrades dopamine, noradrenaline and 5-HT (serotonin). Inhibition of the enzyme increases levels of amine neurotransmitters, some of which are associated with mood and affect.
- **MAO-B:** this is predominantly extracellular and degrades other amines such as tyramine. MAOs have only a minor role in terminating the actions either of noradrenaline at sympathetic nerve terminals (re-uptake is the more important mechanism) or of exogenous direct-acting sympathomimetics.
- **Drugs:** these fall into one of three groups – non-selective and irreversible MAOIs, selective and reversible MAO-A inhibitors, and selective MAO-B inhibitors.
  - *Non-selective and irreversible MAOIs:* drugs such as phenelzine, tranylcypromine, iproniazid, isocarboxazid and pargyline potentiate effects of amines (especially tyramine) in foods. Patients are given strict dietary restrictions because the hazard of hypertensive crisis is real. Such drugs will potentiate the action of any indirectly acting sympathomimetics, although the use of directly acting sympathomimetics is less dangerous. The drugs may also interact with opiates, particularly with piperazine derivatives such as pethidine and fentanyl. Co-administration may result in hyperpyrexia, excitation, muscle rigidity and coma. The mechanism for this reaction is unclear.
  - *Selective and reversible MAO-A inhibitors:* drugs such as moclobemide cause less potentiation of amines and so fewer dietary restrictions are necessary.

Vasopressors which have an indirect action such as ephedrine and metaraminol should none the less be avoided.

— *Selective MAO-B inhibitors:* the main example is selegiline, whose primary use is in the treatment of Parkinson's disease. MAO-B predominates in dopamine-rich areas of the CNS.

- **Implications for anaesthesia:** patients should ideally discontinue these drugs (apart from selegiline, whose sudden withdrawal may exacerbate symptoms) at least 2 weeks before anaesthesia, because the range of interactions is wide and the response is unpredictable. There is an obvious danger in discontinuing treatment in severely depressed patients, and so expert opinion should be sought. If emergency surgery cannot be deferred, the anaesthetic management must take into account any likely interactions. This mandates caution with use of extradural or subarachnoid anaesthesia because of the possible need for vasopressors, and caution with the use of opiates. Pethidine should not be used, but morphine is considered to be safe.

TCAs, tetracyclics and SSRIs

All are antidepressants. Typical examples are amitriptyline and imipramine (TCAs), mianserin, which is a tetracyclic compound, and fluoxetine (Prozac) and paroxetine (Seroxat), which are SSRIs.

- **Mechanisms:** TCAs block the re-uptake of amines, primarily noradrenaline and 5-HT (page 251).
- **Implications for anaesthesia:** the effects of sympathomimetic drugs may be exaggerated, and anticholinergic drugs may precipitate confusion (by causing the central anticholinergic syndrome).

Benzodiazepines

These are anxiolytics and hypnotic (page 252).

- **Implications for anaesthesia:** benzodiazepines cause sedation and, when given in combination with other CNS depressants, may be associated with profound respiratory depression.

Drugs affecting coagulation

Commentary

Patients presenting for surgery or neuraxial anaesthesia who are receiving anticoagulants and antiplatelet drugs are of particular interest to anaesthetists. The examiners are not likely to ask you to write down the entire coagulation cascade, but you will need to be knowledgeable about those parts of it which are affected by the drugs that you are discussing. You must also be able to formulate a coherent management plan for patients who are receiving these agents.

The viva

You may be asked to outline your approach to a surgical patient who is taking anti-coagulants. This may either take the form of a discussion of general principles or you may be given a specific scenario. Hospital protocols vary so describe the management with which you are familiar. The approach depends both on the reasons why the patient may be anticoagulated and on the type of surgery that they face. Some examples follow below.

- **General management:** this will need to be adapted according to the specific clinical situation, but warfarin is usually stopped at least 48 hours preoperatively. If the international normalized ratio (INR) remains unacceptably high, then the patient should be given vitamin K (1.0 mg iv) and fresh frozen plasma (FFP; 15 ml kg^{-1}). After minor surgery the warfarin can be resumed on the first postoperative day. After major surgery, anticoagulation should be maintained by heparin infusion (typically at a rate of 1000–2000 units h^{-1}) or by subcutaneous low molecular weight heparin (LMWH). If necessary, the actions of heparin can be reversed by protamine (1 mg for every 100 units of heparin), whose positive charge neutralizes the negatively charged heparin.
- **Sample scenario (1):** a 70-year-old man requires inguinal hernia repair. He is on long-term warfarin for atrial fibrillation with an INR of 2.8. Plan: aim for an INR <2.0. Stop warfarin without substituting another anticoagulant and restart normal dose after surgery.
- **Sample scenario (2):** a 65-year-old man requires colonic resection. After mechanical mitral valve replacement, his INR has been kept between 3.0 and 4.0. Plan: stop warfarin early enough to allow the INR to fall below 2.0, and follow one of two main options. 1) Heparin: infuse iv heparin to maintain activated partial thromboplastin time (APTT) at 1.5–2.5, stop 2 hours prior to surgery and then restart 6 hours postoperatively. Restart warfarin as soon as oral intake is restored. 2) LMWH: e.g. tinzaparin 100 units kg^{-1} daily, increasing to 175 units kg^{-1} post-operatively. If surgery is urgent, then a high INR should be reduced by FFP and vitamin K. Restart warfarin as soon as oral intake is restored.
- **Surgery:** neurosurgery requires normal coagulation; cataract surgery may be performed safely with an INR of up to 2.5. Some surgeons will even undertake emergency procedures such as hemiarthroplasty in patients whose INR is even higher. They do so because clinical experience suggests that, contrary to expectation, blood loss under these circumstances is not excessive. Many surgeons would be prepared to perform routine surgery such as day case arthroscopy on a patient with an INR of 2.0.

Direction the viva may take

You will then be asked about the specific anticoagulants that are in use.

- **Haemostatic mechanisms:** understanding the actions of anticoagulant drugs requires an appreciation of normal haemostasis. The process of coagulation ends with a haemostatic plug that forms following platelet activation, and which is subsequently reinforced by fibrin. This final step involves the conversion of soluble fibrinogen to insoluble strands of fibrin, in a reaction catalysed by thrombin. Thrombin is one of several important serine proteases that are present in the coagulation cascade, and is formed from prothrombin (factor II) in the presence of activated factor X. Both coagulation pathways activate factor X which, as Xa (the suffix 'a' denotes 'active'), converts prothrombin to thrombin.

- **Coagulation pathways:** there are two pathways – the 'intrinsic', or contact, pathway, all of whose components are present within blood, and the 'extrinsic', or in vivo pathway, in which some components are found outside blood. The intrinsic system is triggered by contact with exposed collagen in endothelium, while the extrinsic system is activated by the release of tissue thromboplastin. The protein coagulation factors are present in blood as inactive precursors, which are then activated by proteolysis, particularly of serine moieties. The cascade is amplified, with each step producing greater quantities of activated clotting factors than the one preceding it. The process in health is held in check by antithrombin III, which neutralizes all the serine proteases involved in the cascade.

- **Vitamin K:** clotting factors II, VII, IX and X are glycoproteins which contain glutamic acid. The interaction of these factors with calcium, and with negatively charged phospholipid, requires the presence of a carboxyl moiety on their glutamate residues. Reduced vitamin K (named from the German word 'Koagulation') acts as an essential co-factor in this hepatic γ-carboxylation reaction, during which vitamin K is oxidized from the reduced active hydroquinone form to the inactive 2,3-epoxide. In the presence of vitamin K reductase, this process is then reversed.

- **Warfarin:** warfarin is a competitive inhibitor of vitamin K reductase, and so prevents the regeneration of the reduced active form and the addition of the essential carboxyl moiety to the four coagulation factors. It was first isolated from natural coumarins by American researchers after whom the compound was named (**W**isconsin **A**lumni **R**esearch **F**oundation). Its effect takes some days to develop because of the different rates at which the carboxylated coagulation factors degrade. The elimination half-life of factor VII is only 6 hours, whereas that of factor II is 60 hours (the $t_{1/2}$ of factors IX and X are 24 and 40 hours, respectively). The effect of warfarin on the prothrombin time (or INR) starts at 12–16 hours and lasts for 4–5 days. It is metabolized by the hepatic mixed function oxidase P450 system, and there are a number of drugs which can interfere with its metabolism. Its effects are potentiated by agents that inhibit hepatic drug metabolism, such as cimetidine, metronidazole and amiodarone. Its effects are attenuated by dietary vitamin K and by drugs such as barbiturates and carbamazepine which induce hepatic cytochrome P450. Some drugs, such as NSAIDs, displace warfarin from binding sites and increase plasma concentrations, but this is of only modest clinical significance.

- **Heparins:** heparin is not a single homogenous substance. Heparins are a family of sulphated glycosaminoglycans (extracted first from liver, hence the name) whose actions are assayed biologically against an agreed international standard. They are therefore prescribed in units of activity and not of mass. Heparin fragments, or LMWHs, are increasingly being used instead of unfractionated preparations. Heparin inhibits coagulation by potentiating the action of antithrombin III (ATIII). ATIII inactivates thrombin and other serine proteases by binding to the active serine site, and so inhibits factors II, IX, X, XI and XII. Heparin binds specifically to

ATIII. To inhibit thrombin, heparin needs to bind both to the protease enzyme as well as to ATIII, whereas to inhibit factor Xa it needs to bind only to ATIII. The larger molecules of unfractionated heparin bind both to the enzyme and to the inhibitor, but the smaller LMWHs increase the action of ATIII only on factor Xa. (The in vitro effect of unfractionated heparin is measured by the APTT, which is not prolonged by LMWHs.)

- **Antiplatelet drugs:** drugs with antiplatelet actions include non-steroidal anti-inflammatory drugs (NSAIDs), of which aspirin (acetyl salicylic acid) is a typical example. Aspirin inactivates the enzyme cyclo-oxygenase(COX) by irreversible binding to COX-1 via acetylation of a serine residue on the active site. Platelet synthesis of thromboxane (TXA_2), which promotes platelet aggregation, then falls. TXA_2 also reduces the synthesis of prostaglandin PGI_2 (also known as epoprostenol or prostacyclin) in vascular endothelium. This substance inhibits platelet aggregation. The persistent inhibition of platelet aggregation results from the fact that vascular endothelium is able to synthesize new PGI_2 whereas platelets are unable to produce new TXA_2.

- **Clopidogrel:** this drug irreversibly blocks the (P2Y12) ADP receptor that is found on platelet cell membranes, and which mediates platelet aggregation. Receptor blockade inhibits fibrin cross-linking by preventing activation of the glycoprotein IIb/IIIa pathway. This is a calcium-dependent process that is required for normal aggregation and endothelial adherence. The drug acts within 2 hours of oral administration and its effects last for the lifetime of the platelet (usually 7–10 days). (Other drugs: Abciximab is a monoclonal antibody and specific GPIIb/IIa receptor antagonist which inhibits all pathways of platelet activation.)

Further direction the viva may take

You might be asked how you would manage a patient with a high INR (usually >8.0) who is bleeding.

- FFP does not contain sufficient quantities of the vitamin K-dependent clotting factors for complete reversal of warfarin-induced bleeding, although it does reduce the INR. Prothrombin complex concentrate (PCC, Beriplex) contains factors II, VII, IX and X and, in a dose of 50 units kg^{-1}, will correct such acquired coagulation factor deficiencies within 1 hour. It costs around £0.35 per unit (£17.50 kg^{-1}) and theoretically may exacerbate the underlying hypercoagulable states that are associated with warfarin therapy.

Alternatively, you may be asked about your views on central neuraxial blockade in patients who are receiving anticoagulants.

- You can take a firm line, which is that anticoagulation of any type is an absolute contraindication to extradural or subarachnoid block. The reality of clinical practice, however, is that the hard line may not always be in the patient's best interest, and that some form of pragmatic risk-benefit analysis will be needed. Most anaesthetists would agree that full anticoagulation either with warfarin or heparin is an absolute contraindication to central neuraxial block. For patients on a typical twice-daily dose of 5000 units of subcutaneous unfractionated heparin, 3 hours should elapse before a block is established or an epidural catheter is removed. If a patient is receiving LMWH, these intervals extend to 12 hours.

- Some anaesthetists are nervous about siting an epidural catheter in vascular patients who may receive large doses of heparin intraoperatively. There is no prospective evidence which attests to the safety of this practice, but observational studies in large numbers of patients (3000) have not found any increased incidence of epidural haematoma formation.
- There is little agreement in the UK about the potential dangers to patients who are taking clopidogrel, aspirin or other NSAIDs.
- Best practice in these cases is regular postoperative testing of sensory and motor function and of deep tendon reflexes (which will be impaired by a compressive spinal haematoma).

Finally, you could be asked about venous thromboembolism.

- **Risk factors:** the long list includes age (exponential increase); pregnancy (which as a hypercoagulable state increases risk 5×); obesity (3× increase in risk if BMI exceeds 30); previous positive history; congenital thrombophilic states such as protein C deficiency, or factor V Leiden; thrombotic states such as malignancy (7× increase) and heart failure; immobility (hence the importance of thromboprophylaxis in critical care); and hormone therapy, including HRT, the oral contraceptive and oestrogen-receptor antagonists such as tamoxifen. Trauma surgery, and lower limb and pelvic surgery also increase risk.
- **Prevention:** these conditions should be tailored to likely risk to include early mobilization; hydration (to minimize haemoconcentration); graduated elastic compression stockings; intermittent pneumatic compression devices; and pharmacological intervention, usually in the form of low molecular weight or unfractionated heparins.

Cyclo-oxygenase (COX) enzymes

Commentary

The use of non-steroidal anti-inflammatory drugs (NSAIDs) in anaesthetic practice is widespread, but side effects are common and there is continued interest in selective COX-2 inhibitors. The viva is likely to be linked to a discussion of the cyclo-oxygenase enzyme system. It will help if you can show broad familiarity with the (simplified) information summarized below.

The viva

You may be asked a token introductory question about the clinical indications for NSAIDs before being asked about their effect on the COX enzyme system. The actions of the prostaglandins that are synthesized are too diverse to cover in any detail, except insofar as they are affected by NSAIDs.

- **Indications:** these include acute surgical pain (but note the withdrawal of piroxicam for this indication), treatment of chronic inflammatory conditions, acute gout, dysmenorrhoea and pyrexia.
- **COX enzymes:** it is now recognized that these exist in at least two isoforms: a 'constitutive' COX-1 enzyme that is present in all tissues, and an 'inducible' COX-2 enzyme which is produced in high concentrations within cells at inflammatory sites. (A COX-3 isoform has also been identified, which is thought to mediate pyrexia, but fuller details have not yet been elucidated.)
- **Mechanisms:** COX enzymes catalyse the production of prostanoids, which comprise a family of lipid mediators with numerous diverse biological roles. The preferential substrate for COX enzymes is arachidonic acid. This is a 20-carbon unsaturated chain which is cleaved from the phospholipid of membranes by phospholipase A_2 (PLA_2). (This exists in at least 10 isoforms. Glucocorticoids inhibit PLA_2 as well as decreasing the induction of COX.) The initial step in prostanoid biosynthesis is the conversion of arachidonic acid to prostaglandin PGG_2 and thence to PGH_2, which is the precursor to all the compounds in the series, including PGE_2, PGD_2, PGF_{2a}, PGI_2 (prostacyclin) and thromboxane (TXA_2). COX enzymes are involved in two different biosynthetic reactions; in addition to catalysing the production of prostaglandin PGG_2, a secondary peroxidase reaction then converts PGG_2 to PGH_2.

Direction the viva may take
You will be asked about the drugs which affect COXs.

- **NSAIDs:** these include non-selective drugs in common use, such as diclofenac, ketoprofen, ibuprofen, aspirin and paracetamol, as well as the newer selective COX-2 inhibitors (the '-coxib' class), e.g. parecoxib, celecoxib and rofecoxib. The beneficial effects of NSAIDs are mediated largely through COX-2 inhibition, whereas adverse effects are related to COX-1 inhibition.
- **Antipyretic action:** NSAIDs inhibit prostaglandin production in the hypothalamus. IL-1 release during an inflammatory response stimulates the hypothalamic production of prostaglandin PGEs, which effectively 'reset' the hypothalamic thermostat upwards. PGD_2 in the brain is also involved in temperature homeostasis. COX-2 is induced centrally by pyrogens, with an increase in PGE_2 production.
- **Analgesia:** NSAIDs decrease production of the prostaglandins PGE_2 and PGI_2 that sensitize nociceptors to inflammatory mediators such as serotonin and bradykinin. They probably also exert central effects at spinal cord level, with COX-2 mediating hyperalgaesia secondary to increased neuronal excitability.
- **Anti-inflammatory effects:** the inflammatory response is complex, involving a large number of mediators (page 398). NSAIDs influence mainly those components in which the products of COX-2 reactions are important. These include vasodilatation, oedema formation and pain. Some NSAIDs (such as sulindac) also act as oxygen free radical scavengers which may reduce tissue damage and inflammation.
- **Antithrombotic effects:** NSAIDs reduce platelet aggregation by inhibiting thromboxane TXA_2 synthesis. This is unaffected by COX-2 inhibitors, which have no antithrombotic effect.

- **Antineoplastic effects:** the regular use of aspirin (and, by extension, any of the NSAIDs) almost halves the risk of colonic cancer. Their potentially protective role relates to the suppression of COX-2, whose expression is markedly increased in adenocarcinomas as well as in other tumours of the oesophagus and pancreas.
- **Mechanisms:** NSAIDs affect only the main cyclo-oxygenation step and do not influence the peroxidase conversion stage of prostanoid synthesis. Non-selective drugs act mainly by competitive inhibition of the arachidonic acid binding site. This is reversible, except in the case of aspirin, which irreversibly acetylates hydroxyl groups on serine residues. The -coxib class are non-competitive, time-dependent COX-2 inhibitors, whereas the -oxicam class (meloxicam, tenoxicam) are competitive.

Further direction the viva may take

You are likely to be asked about adverse effects, and about the potential benefits of COX-2 inhibitors.

Adverse effects

These relate mainly to the inhibition of the COX-1 'housekeeping' enzyme.

- **Gastrointestinal tract effects:** gastrointestinal complications are common, with gastric damage present in around 20% of chronic users. Prostaglandins decrease gastric acid secretion, increase mucus production and improve the microcirculatory bloodflow.
- **Renal effects:** two prostaglandins are important in renal function. PGE_2 has a role in water reabsorption and also mediates compensatory vasodilatation to offset the action of noradrenaline or angiotensin II. PGI_2 also maintains renal dilatation and blood flow, but does so only under circumstances of physiological stress such as hypovolaemia. Concurrent administration of NSAIDs, therefore, can cause acute renal impairment. The situation is made more complex by the fact that COX-2 is constitutively expressed in the kidney. This explains why trials of high-dose COX-2 selective inhibitors have shown an association with hypertension and fluid retention. (The chronic use of NSAIDs may also lead to irreversible analgesic nephropathy.)
- **Respiratory effects:** bronchoconstriction can be triggered in about 10% of asthmatic subjects. This may be due partly to the inhibition of PGE_2-mediated bronchodilatation.
- **Cardiovascular effects:** endothelial COX-1 releases PGI_2 to mediate vasodilatation and inhibition of platelet aggregation. COX-2 can also be expressed in vascular smooth muscle with the release of PGI_2 and PGE_2. COX enzymes may therefore have a cardioprotective function. This may explain the findings of the large VIGOR trial (VIOXX Gastrointestinal Outcomes Research Study), which showed an unexplained increase in the incidence of myocardial infarction in the COX-2 (rofecoxib) group in comparison with the non-selective (naproxen) group.
- **COX-2 inhibitors:** these drugs have a safer side effect profile in respect of the gastrointestinal system, which is the commonest site of adverse effects. They should still be used with caution in patients with renal impairment and there remains concern about cardiovascular effects.

Magnesium sulphate

Commentary

When this topic was first asked in the Final FRCA it caused some consternation because most candidates were unaware of its physiological importance and wide range of clinical applications. These are now better recognized, and the question seems more reasonable.

The viva

You will be asked about the clinical uses of magnesium sulphate.

- **Pre-eclampsia and eclampsia:** magnesium sulphate decreases systemic vascular resistance and reduces CNS excitability. Following the MAGPIE Trial its use in the UK to pre-empt eclamptic convulsions is now well established.
- **Tocolysis:** it causes uterine relaxation.
- **Acute arrhythymias:** it is effective at abolishing tachyarrhythmias (particularly ventricular), those induced by adrenaline, digitalis and bupivacaine, and torsade de pointes associated with a long Q–T interval. The ECG of hypermagnesaemia shows widening QRS with a prolonged P–Q interval.
- **Hypomagnesaemia:** this may have endocrine and nutritional causes (normal intake is 12 mmol daily). It may be caused by malabsorption and is also associated with critical illness. Acute decreases may follow subarachnoid haemorrhage.
- **Tetanus:** this is rare in the UK, but magnesium sulphate by infusion is the primary treatment for the muscle spasm and autonomic instability caused by this condition.
- **Epilepsy:** it can be used to control status epilepticus.
- **Subarachnoid haemorrhage:** it has been used to prevent cerebral vasospasm following aneurysmal subarachnoid haemorrhage.
- **Asthma:** magnesium sulphate is a bronchodilator that can be effective in severe refractory asthma. (Initial dose is 25 mg kg^{-1} by infusion.)
- **Analgesia:** as a physiological NMDA receptor antagonist it has been used as an epidural adjunct to local anaesthetics for postoperative analgesia.
- **Constipation and dyspepsia:** magnesium is a laxative and an antacid.

You will then be asked to describe its basic pharmacology and physiology.

- **Mode of action:** many processes are dependent on magnesium (Mg^{2+}), including the production and functioning of ATP (to which it is chelated) and the biosynthesis of DNA and RNA. It has an essential role in the regulation of most cellular functions.
  - It acts as a natural calcium (Ca^{2+}) antagonist. High extracellular Mg^{2+} leads to an increase in intracellular Mg^{2+}, which in turn inhibits Ca^{2+} influx through Ca^{2+} channels. It is this non-competitive inhibition that appears to mediate many of its effects. It also competes with calcium for binding sites on sarcoplasmic reticulum, thereby inhibiting its release. It acts as a physiological NMDA receptor antagonist.
  - High concentrations inhibit both the presynaptic release of ACh as well as postjunctional potentials.

— Mg^{2+} has an antiadrenergic action; release at all synaptic junctions is decreased and it inhibits catecholamine release.
- **Physiology:** magnesium is the fourth most abundant cation in the body, as well as being the second most important intracellular cation. It activates at least 300 enzyme systems. It affects the activity of neurons, of myocardial and skeletal muscle fibres, and of the myocardial conduction system. It also influences vasomotor tone and hormone receptor binding.

Effects on systems

- **Central and peripheral nervous systems:** magnesium penetrates the blood–brain barrier poorly, but it nevertheless depresses the CNS and is sedating. It acts as a cerebral vasodilator, and it interferes with the release of neurotransmitters at all synaptic junctions. Deep tendon reflexes are lost at a blood concentration of $10\,\text{mmol}\,l^{-1}$. High Mg^{2+} levels do not, as once was thought, potentiate the action of depolarizing muscle relaxants. Predictably, however, they do decrease the onset time and reduce the dose requirements of non-depolarizing relaxants.
- **Cardiovascular:** magnesium mediates a reduction of vascular tone via direct vasodilatation. It also causes sympathetic block and the inhibition of catecholamine release. It decreases cardiac conduction and diminishes myocardial contractile force. This intrinsic slowing is opposed partly by vagolytic action.
- **Respiratory:** magnesium has no effect on respiratory drive, but it may weaken respiratory muscles. It reduces bronchomotor tone.
- **Uterus:** it is a powerful tocolytic, which has implications for mothers who are being treated with the drug to control hypertensive disease of pregnancy prior to delivery.
- **Renal:** magnesium acts as a vasodilator and diuretic.

Direction the viva may take

You may be asked about magnesium toxicity.

- Many of these are predictable from its known actions.
  - $0.7–1.0\,\text{mmol}\,l^{-1}$ – normal blood level.
  - $4.0–8.0\,\text{mmol}\,l^{-1}$ – therapeutic level.
  - $15.0\,\text{mmol}\,l^{-1}$ – respiratory paralysis.
  - $15.0\,\text{mmol}\,l^{-1}$ – at these levels SAN and AV block is complete.
  - $25.0\,\text{mmol}\,l^{-1}$ – cardiac arrest.
  - Magnesium crosses the placenta rapidly, and so may exert similar effects in the neonate, which may be hypotonic and apnoeic.

Tocolytics (drugs which relax the uterus)

Commentary

Tocolysis is indicated either to inhibit premature labour in an attempt to save a threatened fetus, or to attenuate uterine contractions which are compromising fetal oxygenation. Anaesthetists are involved frequently with mothers in these situations and so you should know about the principles of management. There are a number of drugs which exert a tocolytic effect; ensure that you are familiar with at least the one that you have seen used most often.

The viva

You may be asked about the clinical situations in which you (as an anaesthetist rather than as an obstetrician) might use tocolysis.

- There is no placental blood flow during a contraction, and in a case of fetal distress in which the decision has been made to proceed to operative delivery it is logical to try to relax the uterus. Inhibiting uterine contractions is also important in situations in which urgent caesarean section is indicated. An example of this is cord prolapse, in which although there may not necessarily be fetal distress the pressure of the presenting part on the umbilical cord can cut off the fetal blood supply. A rare but serious complication is acute uterine inversion, in which relaxation is usually necessary before the uterus can be replaced back through the cervix.

You will then be asked to describe the classes of drugs which relax the uterus.

β_2-adrenoceptor agonists

- **Drugs:** these include salbutamol and terbutaline. (Ritodrine is no longer recommended.)
- **Mechanisms:** the smooth muscle of the myometrium contains numerous β_2-receptors on the outer membrane of myometrial cells. β_2-agonists bind to these specific adrenergic receptors. This stimulation activates adenyl cyclase with the formation of cAMP, the second messenger which in smooth muscle mediates relaxation. (The process is complex, but there is always the risk that some examiners may ask for more detail. Smooth muscle contraction depends on the interaction of actin and myosin, an energy-dependent process that is reliant on the hydrolysis of ATP. The interaction of the myofilaments is dependent also on the phosphorylation of myosin by myosin light-chain kinase. This enzyme is activated by calmodulin, which requires intracellular calcium ions for its activation. Increased cAMP decreases intracellular calcium and thereby inhibits myosin light-chain kinase.)
- **Effects:** their selectivity is limited and all these drugs have some β_1- as well as β_2-activity. Hypotension, tachycardia and chest pain can complicate their use, as can tachyarrhythmias. Pulmonary oedema has been reported, to which associated high infusion rates may contribute. Patients may become agitated and tremulous. β_2-agonism stimulates glucagon release and hepatic glycogenolysis, which lead to hyperglycaemia. Increased insulin secretion occurs both in response to this rise in blood glucose and to direct β_2-stimulation. While this maintains glucose homeostasis, the net effect is to lower serum potassium, which moves into cells.

    β_2-agonists cross the placenta, increase fetal heart rate and can also cause hyperglycaemia and hyperinsulinaemia followed by hypoglycaemia.

Magnesium sulphate

- $MgSO_4$ is an effective tocolytic (page 265).

Calcium channel blockers

- **Drugs:** the only drug that is used as a tocolytic is nifedipine.
- **Mechanism:** nifedipine blocks voltage-dependent calcium channels and also antagonizes the release of calcium from sarcoplasmic reticulum.

Oxytocin antagonists

- **Drugs**; atosiban (Tractocile) is the only available drug of this type.
- **Mechanism:** it is a specific oxytocin antagonist, which has an effect on the pregnant uterus that is similar to ritodrine but with a better side effect profile. Atosiban inhibits the second messenger release of free intracellular calcium which mediates uterine contraction. It can be used in conjunction with other tocolytics.

Nitrates

- **Drugs:** glyceryl trinitrate (GTN) is the only nitrate used for tocolysis.
- **Mechanism:** effects are mediated via nitric oxide (page 184), which relaxes smooth muscle. It is synthesized in the uterus and helps to maintain uteroplacental blood flow. Exogenous GTN is effective transdermally, sublingually or by intravenous infusion. The drug may cause hypotension as well as pulmonary oedema owing to an increase in vascular permeability. It may be less effective after 34 weeks' gestation.

Miscellaneous

- Other tocolytics include ethanol (ethyl alcohol), which is effective but which may cause maternal intoxication, hypotension and hyperglycaemia. Significant side effects also limit the use of diazoxide, which otherwise is another effective agent. Volatile anaesthetic agents cause a dose-dependent relaxation of uterine smooth muscle.

Drugs which stimulate the uterus

Commentary

Successive reports of the Confidential Enquiry into Maternal Mortality have confirmed that uterine atony is the most important cause of fatal postpartum haemorrhage. A knowledge of the range of drugs that is available is therefore of obvious importance. The list is not very long, and so the viva will also include consideration of postpartum haemorrhage.

The viva

You will be asked about the causes of postpartum haemorrhage and its predisposing factors. (See page 382 for a more detailed discussion.)

- **Uterine causes:** atony is the most important cause, and in the UK accounts for one-third of all deaths associated with maternal haemorrhage. Other causes include uterine disruption or inversion, complications of operative or instrumental delivery and retained products of conception. Abnormal placentation (placenta accreta, increta and percreta) occurs in 1 in 3000 deliveries.

- **Non-uterine causes:** the main causes are genital tract trauma and coagulopathies.
- **Risk factors:** uterine atony is associated with augmentation of labour, with multiple births, with polyhydramnios and with large infants (>4 kg). It is also associated with prolonged labour, with tocolytics and with maternal hypotension. (Ischaemia due to hypoperfusion impairs effective uterine contraction.)

Direction the viva may take

You will then be asked to describe the drugs which stimulate the uterus.

You could begin by outlining the normal contractile mechanisms of the gravid uterus.

- **Uterine activity:** uterine smooth muscle demonstrates considerable spontaneous electrical and contractile activity. Gap junctions between myometrial cells enhance the spread of electrical activity, and these junctions increase during pregnancy to provide a low resistance pathway. Depolarization takes place in response to the influx of sodium ions, while the availability of calcium ions enhances the response of uterine smooth muscle. These cross the cell membrane to stimulate further release of calcium from the sarcoplasmic reticulum. The uterus contains α_1-adrenergic (excitatory), β_2-adrenergic (inhibitory) and serotoninergic receptors, as well as specific excitatory receptors for oxytocin. These increase in number in late pregnancy.

Oxytocins

- **Syntocinon:** this is an oxytocin analogue which is largely free from the arginine vasopressin effects of the endogenous compound.
- **Mechanism of action and effects:** it acts via specific excitatory receptors, as above. In the presence of oestrogen, oxytocin stimulates both the force and frequency of uterine contraction. It also has vasodilator properties which decrease systolic and diastolic pressures, and which provoke a reflex tachycardia. It also appears to have amnesic properties. Its elimination $t_{1/2}$ is between 5 and 12 minutes. Problems associated with its use include hypotension and pulmonary oedema.

Ergot alkaloids

- **Ergometrine:** This is one of the powerful ergot alkaloids derived from the fungus *Claviceps purpurea*.
- **Mechanism of action and effects:** it acts via α_1-adrenergic and also serotoninergic myometrial receptors, but the precise mechanism whereby it mediates its oxytocic effect is not fully understood. It causes uterine contraction. On the already contracted uterus it has little effect, but it is a potent oxytocic if the postpartum uterus is relaxed. Ergometrine also increases blood pressure via arterial and venous constriction. It can cause coronary vasospasm and may even precipitate angina pectoris. It is emetic, probably through a direct dopaminergic effect on the chemoreceptor trigger zone.

Compound preparations

- **Drugs:** the main compound preparation is syntometrine, which is a mixture of syntocinon (5 units) and ergometrine (500 µg).
- **Mechanism of action and effects:** the drugs act in combination as above to cause uterine contraction. The opposing cardiovascular effects of the two drugs in combination minimize the separate cardiovascular effects of each. The preparation is less emetic than ergometrine alone.

Prostaglandins

- **Drugs:** the main prostaglandin used to counteract uterine atony is 15-methyl $PGF_{2\alpha}$ (carboprost – Hemabate). PGE_2 (dinoprostone, 'Prostin') is used for induction and augmentation of labour.
- **Mechanism of action and effects:** endogenous prostaglandins are usually synthesized and inactivated locally in the tissue in which they are active. PGE_2 and $PGF_{2\alpha}$ mediate strong uterine contractions. The uterus becomes more sensitive to their effects as pregnancy progresses. Exogenous prostaglandins stimulate smooth muscle and can cause diarrhoea and vomiting. $PGF_{2\alpha}$ is also a potent constrictor of bronchiolar smooth muscle. In addition, this synthetic preparation has hypothalamic effects which may lead to pyrexia. Flushing and hypotension are common. (It is no longer recommended that carboprost be injected myometrially because of the risk of inadvertent intravenous injection into venous sinuses.)

Target-controlled infusion (TCI)

Commentary

Target-controlled infusion (TCI) for sedation or for total intravenous anaesthesia (TIVA) is now a common technique, but only a proportion of this viva will dwell on the reasons for its clinical popularity. The remainder of the questioning will relate to the pharmacokinetics of these systems. You will not be asked about pharmacokinetic mathematical modelling, but you need to be able to define some of the main terms and describe the basic concepts with sufficient confidence to persuade the examiners that you do understand the principles which underlie their effective use. The subject may be linked to the topic of conscious sedation (page 273).

The viva

You will be asked to describe the pharmacokinetic principles that are relevant for a target-controlled infusion system, almost certainly using propofol as the example.

- **Introduction:** a TCI system incorporates a computer-controlled infusion pump (with safety features to prevent the risk of overdose), which is programmed with a pharmacokinetic model specific to the drug that is being infused. A microprocessor computes the infusion rate that is required to maintain a predicted blood concentration and an adequate concentration of drug at the effector site throughout the duration of the procedure. Examples of such drugs include propofol, alfentanil and remifentanil. The uptake kinetics of intravenous agents mean that the infusion rate needs to be changed exponentially to maintain a steady plasma concentration as peripheral compartments fill up and metabolism and elimination begin. When a lower blood concentration is selected, the pump stops infusing and then resumes at a slower rate.

- **Propofol:** propofol is a highly lipophilic hypnotic that distributes rapidly from blood to the effector site. It then undergoes further rapid redistribution to muscle and fat before being metabolized mainly in the liver, undergoing conjugation to glucuronide and sulphate prior to renal excretion.
- **Remifentanil:** this is an ultra-short-acting opioid agonist which is metabolized in the blood by non-specific esterases, and whose pharmacokinetics are unimpaired by renal or hepatic dysfunction. Its duration of action is between 5 and 10 minutes, it has a very short context-sensitive half-life and has minimal accumulation even after prolonged infusion.
- **Pharmacokinetic model:** the decay in blood concentrations following a bolus dose or a continuous infusion of propofol is best identified by a three-compartment model, which describes its distribution, redistribution and clearance. (Such a model is used in the Diprifusor, which is pre-programmed with pharmacokinetic data.) At the starting target concentration a bolus dose fills the central compartment. This is then followed by an intial high infusion rate which compensates for rapid distribution. Thereafter, the rate slows to maintain the steady state. The microprocessor employs continuous calculations of the concentrations in the different compartments by employing pharmacokinetic information about the elimination and distribution of the drug. (Arguably, there should be an additional compartment to represent the effector site, the brain.) The maintenance infusion rate has to compensate for clearance, and for redistribution to the peripheral compartments which is governed by different rate constants: K_{10}, which is the elimination rate constant from the central compartment; and K_{12}, K_{21}, K_{13} and K_{31}, which are the rate constants governing movement of drug between the peripheral compartments (1, 2 and 3). In the early phase of drug administration, distribution to other compartments is much the most important of the factors which decrease drug effects. With propofol the initial distribution half-life, a, is short (2–3 minutes) while intermediate distribution, β_1, takes 30–60 minutes. The terminal phase decline, β_2, is less steep, and takes 3–8 hours. The immediate volume of distribution is $228 \, ml \, kg^{-1}$, but the steady state volume of distribution in healthy young adults is around 800 litres.
- **Context-sensitive half-time (CSHT):** this is the time taken for the plasma concentration to halve after an infusion designed to maintain constant blood levels is stopped. This is different not only for dissimilar drugs but also for the same drug depending on the duration of infusion. The CSHT for remifentanil is about 4.5 minutes after 2 hours of infusion, and 9.0 minutes after 8 hours. Fentanyl, in contrast, has a CSHT after 2 hours of infusion of 48 minutes, which extends after 8 hours to 282 minutes. The figures for alfentanil are 50 and 64 minutes, and for

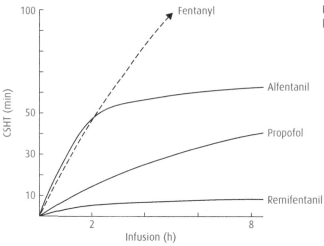

Fig. 4.5 Context-sensitive half-time (CSHT).

propofol 16 and 41 minutes. This makes it clear why remifentanil is such a suitable drug for administration in this way (Figure 4.5).

- **Volume of distribution (V_d):** the concept of the apparent V_d assumes that a drug is distributed evenly throughout a single compartment. (If, for example, 100 mg of a drug given intravenously yields a plasma concentration of 1 mg l^{-1}, then the V_d is $100/1 = 100$ litres. V_d equals the dose/initial concentration.) Were a drug to remain entirely within the circulation its V_d would approximate the plasma volume (0.05 l kg^{-1}). Were it to distribute through the extracellular compartment its V_d would be about 14 litres (0.2 l kg^{-1}). Were it to distribute throughout all fluid compartments its V_d would approximate to total body water (0.6 l kg^{-1}). If, however, it is sequestrated by ion-trapping, cellular uptake or specific tissue binding, then its V_d will be much larger. The volumes of distribution of drugs used in TCI are useful in explaining their clinical behaviour, being 800 litres for propofol and 30 litres for both alfentanil and remifentanil. V_d is, however, affected by such factors as pregnancy, age and volaemic status.
- **Clearance:** one of several definitions of clearance is the rate of drug elimination per unit time per unit concentration. An alternative (and neat) model-independent method of determining clearance is to divide the dose of drug by the area under its concentration–time curve. The whole body clearance of propofol is 2500 ml min^{-1}.

Direction the viva may take
You may be asked about some clinical aspects of TCI and TIVA.

- **Target concentration:** this clearly will vary according to the procedure. For 'conscious sedation' a target plasma concentration below 1.0 μg ml^{-1} might prove sufficient, whereas surgical anaesthesia might require upwards of 8.0 or 10.0 μg ml^{-1}. In practice, the range is from around 2.0–8.0 μg ml^{-1}. It is much lower if propofol is used in conjunction with remifentanil. This reflects the considerable pharmacokinetic and pharmacodynamic inter-patient variability. Influences include age, body weight, genetic factors, concurrent disease and administration of other drugs. Alfentanil, for example, reduces the distribution and clearance of propofol.

- **Repeated infusion:** if a patient has to return to theatre soon after TCI has been discontinued, the microprocessor will no longer be storing the pharmacokinetic information. When the TCI is restarted, therefore, the system will deliver another bolus and rapid initial infusion as if there were no residual propofol in the body. The shorter the interval between cessation and resumption, the greater the risk of overdose.

Conscious sedation

Commentary

Sedation techniques have usually been an afterthought in anaesthetic practice, but reports from various central bodies have brought them into more recent focus. One such was a review of general anaesthesia and sedation in non-hospital dental care that was produced by the chief medical and dental officers in 2000. Entitled 'A Conscious Decision', it ensured that the concept of conscious sedation became more familiar to anaesthetists. It remains of less immediate interest to most, however, because, as we have the experience and skills to manage the situation safely, we tend to be unconcerned should sedation in our hands deepen. That perhaps means that we are not as good at providing it as we think; hence its appearance in the exam.

The viva

You will be asked what you understand by the term 'conscious sedation' and under what circumstances you might use it.

- **Conscious sedation:** this is a level of sedation in which the patient remains conscious, retains protective reflexes, and can still respond to commands. (The full definition is more cumbersome: ' . . . it is a technique in which the use of a drug or drugs produces a state of depression of the central nervous system, which enables treatment to be carried out, but during which verbal contact with the patient can be maintained throughout. The drugs used should have a margin of safety wide enough to render loss of consciousness unlikely. The level of sedation must be such that the patient remains conscious, retains protective reflexes, and is able to respond to verbal commands.') Note that polypharmacy is not proscribed.
- **Indications:** the technique provides anxiolysis and relaxation in patients unable otherwise to tolerate a surgical or medical procedure. It is used commonly for dental treatment, and for surgery performed under local, regional or neuraxial anaesthesia, interventional radiology and endoscopy.

You will then be asked how you achieve it.

- **Local anaesthesia:** satisfactory conscious sedation for patients is crucially dependent on effective local anaesthesia. The only way that an inadequate block can be overcome is by edging towards deeper sedation and general anaesthesia.
- **Intravenous sedation**
  - *Propofol:* this is usually delivered by TCI (page 270), although it is possible for patients to administer their own sedation using a system analogous to PCA. Propofol (page 195) is particularly suitable for TCI because of its short onset of effect, its rapid redistribution and a short CSHT (16 minutes after 2 hours of infusion), which means that accumulation is modest. For conscious sedation a target plasma concentration below 1.0 $\mu g \, ml^{-1}$ can prove sufficient, but there is considerable inter-individual variability in response.
  - *Midazolam:* this is the commonest used benzodiazepine. It is anxiolytic and hypnotic and potentiates the inhibitory effects of GABA on $GABA_A$ receptors throughout the CNS. It is water-soluble at pH levels below 4, but at body pH the imidazole ring closes and the molecule becomes highly lipophilic. The doses required to achieve conscious sedation are usually small (0.5–1.0 mg increments to a total of about 5 mg). In most patients, higher doses are associated either with sedation that is not 'conscious' or, less commonly, with paradoxical disinhibition. (This is particularly true of benzodiazepine use in children.) Midazolam can also be given orally, nasally and bucally. Bolus dosing by the oral route is unpredictable, but the high bioavailability of intranasal and buccal midazolam (both ∼75%) makes it more feasible to use these routes. Overdose is readily treated with flumazenil (Anexate), the specific antagonist which displaces the drug from its binding sites. The normal dose is up to 500 µg titrated against response. Its effective duration of action is 1–2 hours.
- **Inhalation sedation:** also known as 'relative analgesia', this is a technique that produces a maintained level of conscious sedation by the administration of a varying concentration of nitrous oxide in oxygen up to a maximum of 50%. It is used primarily in dental practice. There are some sceptics, but proponents for its use claim that uniquely among single agents it provides analgesia, anxiolysis and mild amnesia while preserving laryngeal reflexes and the maintenance of verbal contact. The sceptics might be wrong. It is possible that at low concentrations of nitrous oxide patients are in Guedel's first stage of anaesthesia (analgesia), and there is some historical evidence to suggest that within a very narrow (but unpredictable) range of concentrations this analgesia can be profound.
- **Ketamine:** subhypnotic doses of ketamine ($<0.5 \, mg \, kg^{-1}$) are used by some anaesthetists as part of a conscious sedation technique (usually in combination with another drug). Ketamine has complex neuropharmacology (page 197) and there are enough anecdotal reports to suggest that in some hands this technique is ill advised.
- **Complications:** if the sedation remains 'conscious' as defined, then problems such as respiratory depression with hypoxia or hypotension should not occur. Complications usually arise when increased levels of sedation risk the loss of protective reflexes with an unsecured airway. This is more likely to happen when combinations of drugs are used. (In addition, there are the generic complications such as allergic reactions.)

Drugs used to treat diabetes mellitus

Commentary

Diabetes is a common multisystem disorder that gives the anaesthetist the challenge of managing potential co-morbidity while maintaining effective perioperative glucose homeostasis. This question will also focus on an understanding of intermediary metabolism. The range of drugs is expanding, but you will not be asked in any detail about newer agents such as the meglitinides and glitazones. You will, on the other hand, be expected to know about insulin and something about the well established biguanides and sulphonylureas.

The viva

You may be asked to outline the problems associated with anaesthetizing patients with diabetes mellitus, some 50% of whom will present for surgery. (You can preface your answer with a brief definition of the two types of diabetes mellitus.)

- Type 1, or insulin-dependent diabetes mellitus, is caused by an absolute deficiency of insulin. Type 2, or non-insulin-dependent diabetes, is caused by a relative deficiency. This comprises either insulin resistance (as in obesity), reduced insulin secretion from the ß-cells in the pancreatic islets of Langerhans, or both.
- **Diabetic morbidity:** potential problems include ischaemic heart disease, hypertension, peripheral vascular disease, cerebrovascular disease and renal impairment secondary to microangiopathy. Peripheral and autonomic neuropathy can occur, with attendant problems such as diabetic gastroparesis and postural hypotension. Affected patients may also lose the normal sympathetic response to hypoglycaemia, of which they may remain unaware. Stiff joint syndrome can make tracheal intubation more difficult. Some 20% of diabetics harbour occult infection which may evolve into overt sepsis under the stress of surgery.
- **Perioperative glucose control:** there are numerous different protocols and you are unlikely to be asked about these in great detail. The main principle should be to restore the patient's normal regimen as soon as possible while maintaining adequate glycaemic control in the meantime (blood glucose $6-10 \text{ mmol l}^{-1}$). Major surgery will require postoperative insulin infusion, either in the form of a GKI regimen (glucose $10\% \times 500 \text{ ml}$ + KCl 10 mmol + Actrapid insulin 15 units) infused at 100 ml h^{-1}, or as a separate infusion (typically using the patient's total daily insulin dose/24 as the starting rate). Once the examiner is satisfied that your approach is sensible and safe, the viva will move on to the basic pharmacology.

Direction the viva will take

You will be asked about the range of drugs that is available.

Insulin

- This is a major anabolic hormone, which controls intermediary and not solely carbohydrate metabolism.

— *Carbohydrate:* it stimulates glycogen synthesis and inhibits glycogenolysis in the liver while also increasing glucose uptake and utilization in muscle.
— *Fat:* it increases lipid synthesis (fatty acids and triglycerides) and inhibits lipolysis.
— *Protein:* it enhances protein synthesis (hence its abuse amongst bodybuilders) by enhancing amino acid uptake by muscle. It decreases protein catabolism.

- **Mechanisms:** the hormone binds to a specific insulin receptor on the cell membrane. This is a large transmembrane glycoprotein complex, comprising two α-extracellular-binding sites and two β-intracellular and transmembrane proteins.
- **Insulin preparations:** there are numerous formulations whose purpose is to help diabetics stabilize blood glucose levels. Soluble insulin (such as human Actrapid) works rapidly but its action is evanescent. Longer-acting preparations are made by precipitating insulin with substances such as zinc and protamine to form an insoluble depot compound from which insulin is more slowly absorbed. Insulin glargine is a modified insulin analogue which, because of slow absorption, provides a basal insulin supply to mirror the normal physiological state. Other forms of insulin can then be given according to the patient's particular requirements.

Oral hypoglycaemic agents
Biguanides
The only biguanide in routine clinical use is metformin.

- **Mechanisms:** biguanides increase glucose uptake and utilization in skeletal muscle while decreasing hepatic gluconeogenesis. They also reduce the plasma concentrations of low density and very low density lipoproteins (LDL and VLDL). Rarely, they may cause a severe lactic acidosis, particularly in patients with impaired renal function. Their precise mode of action is not fully known, but they act only in the presence of residual endogenous insulin.
- **Pharmacokinetics:** metformin has an elimination $t_{1/2}$ of 3 hours. It is excreted renally and will accumulate if renal function is compromised (common in diabetics).

Sulphonylureas
These include chlorpropamide (now largely obsolete), tolbutamide, and the second generation sulphonylureas, glibenclamide and glipazide.

- **Mechanisms:** sulphonylureas promote insulin secretion from β-cells after binding to high affinity receptors on the cell membrane. They block an ATP-sensitive potassium channel, thereby allowing membrane depolarization, calcium influx and insulin release. They can cause prolonged and severe hypoglycaemia, particularly in the presence of other drugs such as NSAIDs. These can compete for metabolizing enzymes and alter plasma protein binding.
- **Pharmacokinetics:** tolbutamide has a shorter $t_{1/2}$ (6–12 h) and duration of action (4 h) than glibenclamide ($t_{1/2}$ 18–24 h and duration 10 h) or glipazide ($t_{1/2}$ 16–24 h and duration 7 h). Some (e.g. glibenclamide) have active metabolites, and these, like the parent compound, are excreted by the kidney. Renal impairment mandates caution with their use.

α-glucosidase inhibitors

The only drug of this class that is available is acarbose.

- **Mechanisms:** acarbose inhibits intestinal α-glucosidase, which delays the breakdown and absorption of carbohydrates (sugars and starch). Its inhibitory action is maximal against sucrase.
- **Pharmacokinetics:** most of the drug remains within the gut, with only about 1–2% being absorbed systemically. Duration of action varies greatly according to intestinal transit times.

Glitazones

The agents available are pioglitazone and rosiglitazone.

- **Mechanisms:** the drugs reduce peripheral insulin resistance, enhance glucose uptake by muscle and decrease hepatic gluconeogenesis. Their mechanism of action is complex, but they are agonists at the nuclear PPAR γ-receptor which mediates lipogenesis and uptake both of glucose and of free fatty acids. They also lower LDL concentrations. The glitazones increase plasma volume and some weight gain is common. Their onset of action develops over weeks and they should not be used as single component therapy.
- **Pharmacokinetics:** time to peak action is 2 hours and the $t_{1/2}$ for each is around 7 hours. Both drugs have active metabolites: weakly active in the case of rosiglitazone, but with a long $t_{1/2}$ of 150 h more active in the case of pioglitazone, but with a shorter $t_{1/2}$ of 24 h.

Meglitinides

These are analogous in action to the sulphonylureas. The two that have been developed are nateglinide (licensed only for use in combination with metformin) and repaglinide.

- **Mechanisms:** these also promote insulin secretion from ß-cells by blocking the ATP-sensitive potassium channel in the cell membrane. The drugs are less potent than the sulphonylureas.
- **Pharmacokinetics:** the time to peak effect is short, at about 55 minutes, and they also have a rapid $t_{1/2}$ of around 3 h. Inadvertent hypoglycaemia is therefore less likely with their use.

Bioavailability

Commentary

Bioavailability is a straightforward concept whose value is disputed by some authorities. It is a subject, however, that can fit readily into the time frame of the viva. Make sure that you are able to define it, and that you can draw simple curves of concentration plotted against time of a drug that is given intravenously and one that is given by some other route. The questioning is likely to revert thereafter to a general discussion of the factors that may affect drug absorption.

The viva

You will be asked to define the term 'bioavailability' and to describe how it could be measured.

- Bioavailability is that fraction of the dose of an administered drug that gains access to the systemic circulation, and is therefore available to act at its receptor sites. It is assumed that the bioavailability of an intravenous dose is 100% (or 1.0). Alternatively, bioavailability can be defined simply as the ratio of the effective dose to the administered dose. It has been used most commonly as a measure following oral administration, but it applies equally to drugs given by other routes, of which there are many. These include rectal, vaginal, nasal, ocular, pulmonary, sublingual, extradural, intrathecal and transdermal routes.
- Critics who doubt the usefulness of the term cite the cumbersome American Food and Drug Administration (FDA) definition of bioavailability as 'The rate and extent to which the therapeutic moiety is absorbed and becomes available to the site of drug action.' 'Rate' and 'extent' are separate entities and the expression being 'available to the site of action' is imprecise. Most such definitions are of limited use because they relate bioavailability only to the total proportion of drug that reaches the systemic circulation while ignoring the rate. Clearly, if absorption is complete by 30 minutes then the clinical effect is likely to be more marked than if that process takes 6 hours. The bioavailability of a particular oral drug is affected both by its formulation and by the physiology of its recipient (as discussed below), and so, strictly speaking, it cannot accurately be quantified, except in a particular individual on a given occasion.
- It is, none the less, important to be aware of the concept, particularly in relation to drugs such as digoxin, which have a narrow therapeutic index. Different formulations of digoxin, which contain the same mass of drug, can give rise to plasma levels that vary over sevenfold. It is also useful to be aware of the bioavailability of drugs that can be given by multiple different routes. That of ketamine, for example, is 20% (orally), 25% (rectally), 50% (nasally), 77% (epidurally) and 90% (intramuscularly).

Direction the viva may take

You may be asked how you would measure bioavailability.

- **Measurement:** bioavailability is measured by first giving a drug intravenously and then plotting the plasma concentration against time. When the drug has been completely removed from the system, the same agent is administered by a different route and a second elimination curve is plotted. Both curves are continued until they reach the x-axis and the plasma concentration is zero. Bioavailability is given by the ratio of the areas under the curves, $AUC_{non-iv}:AUC_{iv}$ (Figure 4.6).
- **Analysis of low bioavailability:** if bioavailability is low, then urinary or plasma metabolites may indicate broadly the reasons why. High concentrations of metabolites suggest that a drug has undergone extensive first pass metabolism in

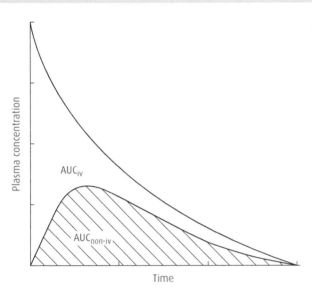

Fig. 4.6 Bioavailability.

the liver. Low concentrations suggest either that there is poor gastrointestinal absorption or that significant biotransformation has taken place in the gut.

Further direction the viva could take

You may be asked about the factors that can influence bioavailability.

- **Physicochemical characteristics:** bioavailability is affected by the physicochemical characteristics of a drug and its formulation. Salts which are highly soluble have a much greater dissolution rate than drugs that are presented as strong acids or bases. Drugs of low lipid solubility, of which acidic and basic salts are an example, are in general absorbed poorly from the gut. Acidic drugs are absorbed better from the stomach, however, because low gastric pH reduces the proportion of drug that is ionized. In the more alkaline environment of the small gut, it is basic drugs whose ionization is reduced and which are therefore absorbed more effectively. There may also be significant interactions within the gut; the absorption of tetracyclines, for example, is prevented if they bind to dietary calcium. Particle size is important, in that smaller particles have a greater surface area : mass ratio and therefore dissolve more rapidly. Formulation in a crystalline form also aids dissolution, as does crystal hydration, anhydrous salts of drugs being more water-soluble. Excipients also affect the rate of absorption, with water repellents such as magnesium stearate decreasing the rate of dissolution. These properties are utilized in slow release and enteric-coated drugs.
- **Physiological factors:** orally (and rectally) administered drugs are absorbed into the portal circulation where they undergo first pass metabolism by hepatic enzymes. Extensive first pass metabolism clearly reduces bioavailability. Absorption of oral drugs is related to intestinal motility and integrity, as well as the extent to which they are subject to the action of enzymes in the gut wall. Glyceryl trinitrate is an

example of a drug that undergoes hydrolysis by enzymes residing in the intestinal epithelium.

- Most of the above is relevant for drugs that are given orally. There is probably less extra chemistry and science to discuss in respect of other routes of administration, and there is unlikely to be sufficient time to deal with them in any detail. A logical approach using first principles should be sufficient. Skin, for example, is an effective physical barrier, but lipid-soluble drugs in adequate concentration can be delivered via patches. (Fentanyl, hyoscine, nicotine and sex hormones are examples of drugs that can be given in this way.) Mucous membranes, in contrast, offer less impediment to absorption, because the physical barrier is thinner.

Design of a clinical trial for a new analgesic drug

Commentary

Drugs are at the core of the specialty of anaesthesia, and so you should not find it unreasonable to be asked about the broad principles that underpin randomized controlled clinical trials (RCTs). The subject is not too difficult, and you should be able to work out the important aspects of this kind of research even if you do not have the information readily to hand. It is inevitable that statistics will form part of the discussion. You will always do well to start simply when the subject of statistics arises, because a demonstration that you understand the basic concepts will usually be sufficient to get you through.

The viva

You will be asked to describe how you would design a clinical trial for a new drug, typically an anaesthetic or analgesic agent.

- A clinical trial for a new agent is carried out during phase II or phase III of the drug's development. (Preclinical development involves animal studies into aspects such as safety, efficacy and mutagenicity. Phase I involves small group studies of fewer than 100 healthy volunteers, looking at pharmacokinetics, pharmacodynamics and adverse effects. Phase II recruits larger numbers of patients, typically 200–300, in which the findings of the phase I studies are refined. Phase III involves still larger numbers of patients, usually in the thousands, who are entered into definitive RCTs. Phase IV occurs after the drug has been licensed for use, and involves post-marketing surveillance of its effects in much greater numbers of individuals.)
- **Ethics committee approval:** no clinical trial can proceed without the approval of an appropriately constituted ethics committee, which will include lay people amongst its members. These committees are increasingly rigorous, and in essence they seek to preserve the full protection of the rights of every potential participant. Individuals must receive full information about every aspect of the trial before they

consent, and must be free to withdraw at any stage without compromising their future care. Committees will scrutinize intensely any trial in which financial inducements are involved.

- **Trial design:** the best-designed clinical trials seek to answer a single simple question: in this case, whether the new analgesic is superior to established treatments. It is essential to have a control in the study, which in this instance would be an analgesic in clinical use that was of proven benefit. Trial design must therefore involve defining endpoints for efficacy, and must also ensure that data relating to adverse effects are collected. The use of placebos in trials of analgesics is considered to be unethical, and so the drugs in all limbs of the trial will be pharmacologically active.

- **Subject selection:** it is important that the groups are matched as far as possible. Such matching should include age, gender, American Society of Anesthesiologists (ASA) status and racial characteristics. Exclusion criteria must also be established. If the drug is to be used for treatment of chronic pain, then the trial can be a double blind crossover trial (see below) in which the patient can act as their own control. Sufficient time must elapse between administrations of the two drugs to ensure that the first one that the patient has received is no longer exerting any effect.

- **Sample size:** the conclusions of any trial can be erroneous. The study can determine either that there is a difference between treatments when none exists, or it can determine that there is no difference between treatments when a difference does in fact exist. The first (false positive) conclusion is known as a type I error. The second (false negative) conclusion is a type II error. The probability of avoiding a type II error and missing a significant difference between treatments is known as the power of the trial. In other words, the power of a study is its ability to reveal a difference of a particular size. The power calculation allows the investigator to determine the sample size necessary to demonstrate this difference. It is calculated from $1-\beta$, where β is the type II error. Trials are usually designed with a power of 80% ($\beta = 0.2$) or better, 90% ($\beta = 0.1$). The investigators must also decide the magnitude of the difference that is sought.

- **Randomization:** randomization of patients to one or other limbs of the trial is intended to remove bias. The bias may be unconscious or hidden. Patients may not have been allocated randomly to an operating list, for example, and so assigning alternate patients to trial groups might be unreliable. Simple methods such as tossing a coin are valid, although it is more common to use computer-generated randomization.

- **Blinding:** it is ideal for the trial to be double blind, so that neither the patient nor the investigator knows to which group they have been assigned. This is of particular importance when the outcome data are subjective, as in a comparison of analgesic drugs or techniques.

- **Data collection:** obvious considerations apply to the scrupulous collection of data. Inherent variation can be avoided by minimizing the number of investigators involved in the process.

- **Statistical evaluation:** the appropriate statistical tests must be chosen for the question that is being asked. In this case the null hypothesis is that there is no difference between new analgesic A and established analgesic B. The tests of statistical significance aim to define whether the null hypothesis has been disproved; in other words, that there is a difference between drugs A and B, and at what level of probability. The investigators must also decide whether the data are continuous and normally distributed, in which case a parametric test is appropriate. If the data do not follow a normal distribution, then a non-parametric test should be used. The evaluation of an analgesic would almost certainly involve the use of visual analogue scales, about which statisticians may disagree. Some argue that response to pain is a biological variable with a normal distribution; others contend that the data are not normally distributed and that non-parametric tests should be applied.

- **Clinical and statistical significance:** trial data will be cited according to the strength of its statistical significance, although clinical significance is more important. The bigger the sample size, the more likely it is that a small effect will be statistically significant, even though clinically its impact may be negligible.

Physics, clinical measurement, equipment and statistics

Depth of anaesthesia

Commentary

The discovery of anaesthesia transformed the human condition, and unplanned awareness returns a patient to the nightmare that was surgery before anaesthesia and analgesia. Significant advances in the pharmacology and technology of anaesthesia have still not brought us much closer to a reliable means of monitoring its depth, although because awareness is such a serious complication considerable research effort has been dedicated to the search for methods of detection. Many remain research tools or are not yet in widespread use, but you should have some idea about which may in due course find their way into clinical practice.

The viva

You may be asked about the types of awareness under general anaesthesia, the commonest causes, patients particularly at risk, and possible sequelae.

- **Definitions:** awareness can be 'explicit' or 'implicit'. Explicit awareness is defined by spontaneous or prompted recall of intraoperative events, which may or may not include pain. Its accurate incidence is hard to determine, but commonly quoted figures are up to 0.2% in non-obstetric and non-cardiac anaesthesia, up to 0.4% in emergency caesarean section under general anaesthesia, and up to 1.5% in cardiac surgery. (The Royal College of Anaesthetists patient information leaflet quotes an incidence of 0.1–0.2%.)
- **Causes:** its causes lie in equipment and its (mis)use, in pharmacology and its application, and, very rarely, in the physiology of patients.
- **Equipment and apparatus:** awareness may result from a failure of the apparatus to deliver adequate concentrations of anaesthetic agent. The anaesthetic machine must

deliver an accurate fresh gas flow via an appropriate breathing system using a vaporizer. For total intravenous anaesthesia (TIVA), an accurate syringe driver is required, together with a reliable system of infusion tubing. Awareness may result if there are failures in any part of these systems. Such failures include leaks, faulty or empty vaporizers, a misconnected or disconnected breathing system, inaccurate pumps, misplaced venous cannulae and occluded infusion tubing.

- **Use of equipment and apparatus:** awareness may result from a failure of the anaesthetist to use the equipment properly. Circle systems can present a particular difficulty.

- **Monitoring:** failure to monitor the concentrations of inspired and expired volatile agents may result in inadequate anaesthetic agent being delivered. TIVA is more difficult to monitor in this respect.

- **Pharmacology:** awareness, by definition, results from inadequate anaesthesia. The dose of induction agent may have been inadequate, as may be the alveolar concentration (it is important to remember that the MAC value that is quoted is only the MAC^{50}) or the computed blood concentration in target-controlled infusion (TCI). Awareness is not prevented by hyperventilation, by the use of nitrous oxide and oxygen alone, nor by the use of opiates. Muscle relaxant drugs are not anaesthetics, and anaesthesia must not be discontinued until their effects have been reversed.

- **Physiology:** very rarely, a patient may be 'resistant' to anaesthetic agents. Alcohol and other drugs of abuse are convenient scapegoats but the evidence is unconvincing. Similarly, high anxiety is frequently cited as the reason that some patients may need larger than normal induction doses. In any of these situations the anaesthetist should be alert to the clinical signs indicative of inadequate anaesthesia. On occasion, a patient may be so moribund (or so inadequately resuscitated) that adequate anaesthesia may be incompatible with maintaining cardiac function.

- **Airway problems and bronchoscopy:** during a difficult intubation, the effects of the induction agent may wear off before those of the muscle relaxant. Awareness is also a potential problem during some anaesthetic techniques for rigid bronchoscopy (such as those using insufflation or injectors).

- **Sequelae:** it is very unusual to cause physical morbidity as a result of cardiovascular stresses provoked by being aware, although it is a theoretical possibility. Much more common are manifestations of a post-traumatic stress syndrome, whose typical features may include nightmares, insomnia, panic attacks and agoraphobia.

Direction the viva may take

You will be asked about methods of determining depth of anaesthesia.

The list of techniques that have been described is a long one, and so a systematic approach may help you to recall them. It does not matter how you do this, but in the description below the methods are ranked broadly according to their usefulness and practicality. Clinical signs are therefore discussed first, not because they are the most reliable, but because every anaesthetist will use them. Some of these sections below contain more detail than you could be expected reasonably to know, but they are none the less considerable oversimplifications of a scientifically complex subject. You will, however, need to deliver some of this detail because it will look otherwise as though you are simply reciting a list.

- **Clinical signs:** in the spontaneously breathing patient who is not paralysed, awareness may be manifest by purposeful movement. Movement is a reliable indicator of light anaesthesia although a patient may have no recall.
- **Sympathetic stimulation:** the main clinical signs are tachycardia, hypertension, diaphoresis and lachrymation. Attempts have been made to quantify these objectively by using the PRST scoring system (blood **p**ressure, heart **r**ate, **s**weating, **t**ear formation), but without any real evidence of its benefit. In the absence of other causes, sympathetic signs may be reliable if present, but the main problem is that their absence does not exclude awareness.

Effective methods

- **Evoked potentials (EPs):** visual, somatosensory and auditory EPs have been investigated as indicators of the depth of anaesthesia. The few microvolts that are generated by each potential have to be separated from the overall electrical noise that is produced by the brain as a whole. Auditory EPs appear to be the most effective because they are the last to disappear and are the best indicators of anaesthetic depth. The patient's auditory system is stimulated by repetitive clicks at around 6–10 Hz. The EEG is recorded immediately after each stimulus and is amplified, before the auditory EPs are extracted by taking the average of a large number of responses. This is covered in greater detail on page 287.
- **Compressed spectral array:** this is a method of simplifying the EEG in which the signals are subjected to Fourier analysis. Fourier transformation is the mathematical technique whereby complex waveforms are analysed into their simpler sine wave components. Spectral analysis calculates the total power contained within the different frequencies of cerebral activity over a period of time (known as an epoch). The graph of power against frequency forms a spectral array. As an anaesthetic continues or deepens, each linear plot obtained during successive epochs can be superimposed to give the typical peak and trough or 'hill and valley' display. This compressed display is what constitutes 'compressed spectral array'. In an anaesthetized patient, power shifts to the lower frequencies.
- **Spectral edge:** this is the frequency above which there is only 5% of the total EEG power. A decrease in the spectral edge frequency accompanies increasing concentrations of anaesthetic agents. The relationship between the two does not appear to be linear, and in the transition between light and deeper anaesthesia there is a poor correlation between spectral edge frequency and drug concentration.
- **Median frequency:** this is another number determined from compressed spectral array, and is the frequency above and below which lies 50% of the total power of the EEG. It may correlate better with drug concentrations, but the spectral array shows a pattern that is not consistent between different anaesthetic agents.

- **Bispectral analysis and bispectral index:** this is another modification of the EEG, in which there is analysis of the phase and power relationships between the numerous frequencies. The term 'bispectral' describes the phase and power relationships between any two frequencies in the EEG. The bispectral index is a number generated from these phased and power frequencies that are the components of the EEG, and in essence compares frequency harmonics in the frontal EEG. The dimensionless scale of 0 (cortical electrical silence) to 100 (normal cortical electrical activity) has been derived from EEG recordings in volunteers and patients undergoing transitions between consciousness and unconsciousness. A bispectral index score of between 40 and 60 suggests surgical anaesthesia. This device has a rapid response time. It appears to be accurate in respect of hypnotic drugs, both inhalational and intravenous, but reflects less well the synergistic sedative effects of opiates when used as part of 'balanced anaesthesia'. It has no predictive value for any particular individual's threshold for loss of consciousness.
- **Respiratory sinus arrhythmia and R–R interval variation:** this method does have promise, although it is only useful in the presence of an intact autonomic nervous system and healthy myocardial conducting system. Its value is greatly restricted in patients, for example, who are being treated with β-adrenoceptor blockers, who have autonomic neuropathy or dysfunction (common in the elderly), sepsis, or who have cardiac conduction abnormalities. It provides a measure of brainstem function, which decreases with increasing depth of anaesthesia.

Methods of limited value

- **Isolated forearm technique:** this is not strictly a monitor of the depth of anaesthesia, but it is included as a method of detecting awareness that is simple and ingenious. It was described originally by Tunstall, who was interested in preventing awareness during obstetric general anaesthesia. An arterial tourniquet isolates the arm from drugs which enter the systemic circulation and, prior to the procedure, the anaesthetist agrees with the patient the hand signals that they will use to convey awareness. The method is effective, but its practical use is limited both by the considerable degree of cooperation that is necessary and by the fact that after about 20 minutes of tourniquet inflation, ischaemic paralysis supervenes and prevents any further arm movement.
- **EEG:** the formal EEG is a highly complex monitor, which produces too much data to be of any practical use in theatre. The raw EEG demonstrates differing patterns in response to different anaesthetic agents and changes in response to events such as hypoxia and hypercarbia. It also processes a lot of information from the cerebral cortex which may not be the area most appropriate for examining depth of anaesthesia.
- **Cerebral function monitor (CFM):** this is a processed and simplified EEG which displays only part of the frequency range. It has been used in neurointensive care units as an indirect monitor of cerebral oxygenation. It is of limited value in measuring depth of anaesthesia.
- **Cerebral function analysing monitor (CFAM):** this is a refinement of the CFM, which separates out the main frequencies of cerebral activity. It is technically

easier to use but has a slow response time and may also obtain a disproportionate amount of information from the temporal lobe.

- **Oesophageal contractility:** the amplitude and frequency of contractions of lower oesophageal smooth muscle reduce with increasing depth of anaesthesia. The technique is of limited value because of the high rate of false positive and false negative results.
- **Frontalis (scalp) electromyogram (EMG):** this technique measures the amplitude of the EMG, which decreases with increasing depth of anaesthesia. It is of very restricted benefit if for no other reason than it cannot be used in paralysed patients.

Evoked potentials

Commentary

EPs are one means of monitoring the depth of anaesthesia, and they are also used to assess spinal cord function during surgery. The first usage remains confined mainly to research centres and the second to specialist centres, yet the topic is of some general anaesthetic interest. The underlying neurophysiology and the signal processing are too complex to explore in a short viva, and a broad knowledge of the principles will suffice.

The viva

You may be asked about the clinical applications of EPs.

- **Anaesthetic depth:** EPs have been investigated as indicators of the depth of anaesthesia. Visual and somatosensory EPs show less promise than auditory evoked responses (below).
- **Spinal surgery:** EPs are used to monitor spinal cord function, which can be compromised by distraction during scoliosis surgery. Historically, patients were subjected to the intraoperative wake-up test, during which anaesthesia was lightened (with appropriate analgesia) to the point at which the subject could respond to a request to move both arms and legs. This technique actually worked better than it may sound to those who have never seen it done, but it is none the less crude in comparison to somatosensory EPs. The potentials are of very low amplitude, and the signal is averaged. The latency and amplitude are measured, as above, usually by electrodes which monitor the cerebral cortex. This technique is based on the assumption that if sensory pathways are intact then motor pathways will not have been damaged. This is not always true, but evoked motor potentials are depressed by general anaesthetic agents. An alternative is to test cord function by means of epidural motor EPs which are relatively unaffected by anaesthetic agents. Somatosensory potentials are also depressed by high-concentration volatile agents and by high-dose opiates (such as fentanyl in doses greater than $50\,\mu g\,kg^{-1}$), but the normal clinical use of these drugs does not compromise the technique. Hypoxaemia and hypoperfusion of the cord are confounding factors which may influence the response. They decrease the amplitude of the response but do not have any effect on its waveform.

- **Neurology:** EPs are used to aid the diagnosis of a number of neurological conditions. These include multiple sclerosis and other demyelinating diseases, tumours in the posterior fossa, in which auditory EPs are useful, and global head injury.

Direction the viva may take

You may then be asked to explain in more detail what is meant by an 'evoked potential'.

- An EP, also known as an evoked response (ER) or event-related potential (ERP), is an aspect of EEG monitoring. The signal in the EEG is produced when an individual receives a visual, auditory or somatosensory stimulus, and the EPs are detected by an electrode which is positioned over the primary receiving area for that sensory modality.
- The potentials are only a few microvolts in amplitude and so are swamped by the noise of the global EEG. Each can measure from as low as $0.1\ \mu V$ up to around $2\ \mu V$, compared with the EEG background amplitude of $10–300\ \mu V$. These low potentials are extracted from the EEG by a process of computer averaging. The patient is subjected to a large number of repeated stimuli, and the EEG is recorded during a fixed period after each one. It is then amplified before the EPs are extracted by taking the average of this large number of responses.
- **Auditory ERs:** the processed signals comprise a series of peaks and troughs, which represent the response time or 'latency'. This has been mapped most thoroughly in respect of auditory ERs, which produce a series of waves as the repetitive 6–10 Hz stimulus activates pathways from the cochlea to the cortex. (The separate waves relate to their anatomical origin.) Neither the brain stem response (0–10 ms latency) nor the late cortical response (50–500 ms latency) correlates with depth of anaesthesia. It is examination of the waveform of the middle latency section (10–50 ms latency) which provides this information. (It originates in the auditory cortex.) This mid-latency region contains two troughs separated by a peak. The amplitude and latency of the peak (Pa) and second trough, or nadir (Nb), are analysed. Signals beyond around 100–1000 ms represent the late cortical response which arises from the frontal cortex and association areas.
- **Visual EPs:** these are produced in response to a pulsed flash of light and elicit mainly a cortical response. They are more variable than auditory EPs and so give more qualitative than quantitative information.
- **Somatosensory potentials:** as outlined above.

Pulse oximetry

Commentary

Pulse oximetry has been widely available in the UK only since the late 1980s, but rapidly became established as, arguably, the single most important form of monitoring in anaesthetic practice. You might even be asked to discuss this proposition in the viva. In any event, most anaesthetists believe that continuous measurement of oxygen saturation during anaesthesia is essential. You will be expected to have a broad understanding of how the technique works, with particular reference to its limitations and potential sources of error.

The viva

The clinical relevance of oximetry is so obvious that you might well start with the science rather than the application.

- Oxygenated haemoglobin (HbO_2) and deoxygenated haemoglobin (Hb) have differential absorption spectra.
- At a wavelength of 660 nm (red light), HbO_2 absorbs less than Hb, hence its red colour.
- At a wavelength of 940 nm (infrared light), this is reversed and Hb absorbs more than HbO_2. At 800 nm – the isobestic point – the absorption coefficients are identical.
- The pulse oximeter uses two light-emitting diodes which emit pulses of red (660nm) and infrared (980nm) light every 5–10 μs from one side of the probe. The light is transmitted through the tissue to be sensed by a photocell on the other side.
- The output is submitted to electronic processing, during which the absorption of the blood at the two different wavelengths is converted to a ratio, which is compared to an algorithm produced from experimental data.
- Oximetry aims to measure the saturation in arterial blood, and so the instrument detects the points of maximum and minimum absorption (during cardiac systole and diastole). It measures the pulsatile component and subtracts the non-arterial constant component before displaying a pulse waveform and the percentage oxygen saturation. Hence, strictly defined, it is measuring the Sp (*p*lethysmographic) O_2 rather than the Sa (*a*rterial) O_2.

Direction the viva may take

You may be asked about potential sources of error, limitations of the technique, and problems in interpreting the results.

- Pulse oximetry is calibrated against volunteers and so calibration against dangerously hypoxic values is impossible. The instruments are less accurate at SpO_2 values below 70%. (You can use this fact to reassure colleagues who are less composed than you in the face of a patient's saturation that otherwise seems alarmingly low.)
- Interference by ambient light. This can occur if light is bright and direct, but the pulsed nature of the emissions is intended to allow detection of, and compensation for, any ambient light.
- Loss of the pulsatile component. This occurs in conditions of hypoperfusion, hypothermia and peripheral vasoconstriction, when there is a narrow pulse pressure, arrhythmias which distort the points of maximum and minimum absorption, or venous congestion. These are all common reasons for a poor signal.
- Movement artefact or electrical interference (neither are major problems).
- Infrared absorption by other substances, such as nail varnish or nicotine staining.

- More significant errors are associated with absorption by abnormal haemoglobins and other compounds:
  - *Carboxyhaemoglobinaemia:* this is seen in heavy smokers or in CO poisoning. COHb has a similar absorption coefficient to HbO_2 and will give an abnormally high SpO_2 reading of about 96%.
  - *Jaundice:* bilirubin has a similar absorption coefficient to deoxygenated Hb and will give abnormally low saturation readings.
  - *Methaemoglobinaemia:* metHb has absorption similar at both wavelengths and gives a saturation reading of around 84%.
  - Dyes in the circulation such as methylene blue or disulphine blue give falsely low readings.

Problems in interpretation

- Pulse oximetry does not detect respiratory failure. A high FiO_2 may mask ventilatory failure by ensuring high SpO_2% readings despite a rising CO_2.
- The slope of the oxygen–haemoglobin dissociation curve means that there is a lag of 20 seconds or more between any drop in arterial oxygen tension and the resultant fall in oxygen saturation.
- In very anaemic patients SpO_2% readings may show high saturations, although oxygen delivery to the tissues may be impaired.
- The amplitude of the pulse waveform is not a reliable indicator of the pulse volume. Many instruments automatically augment the trace to fill the display.

Further direction the viva could take

If you have done well on the above, the examiner may have time to explore, for example, the proposition that pulse oximetry is the single most important monitor. There are no correct examination answers to this, but it can make briefly for an interesting discussion. If you do have views, then argue your case. Points to consider might include the fact that, in contrast to end-tidal CO_2 measurement, pulse oximetry gives information some of which can be obtained by clinical observation. The examiner might ask what single, theoretical monitoring device you would use, were you to be allowed only one. An answer might be a device that measured reliably the state of cerebral oxygenation. If you do find yourself in such an interchange then you should be able to relax. The examiner will be satisfied that you know the facts, but just wishes to discover whether you have thought further about the subject and are prepared to advance an independent argument.

Measurement of CO_2

Commentary

The capnograph is an essential monitor which is used in all but the briefest of anaesthetics. There is not a vast amount to ask about the principles of the commonest

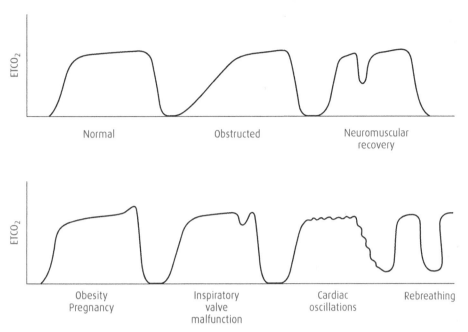

Fig. 5.1 Capnography waveforms (capnograms). ETCO$_2$, End-tidal CO$_2$.

method of CO$_2$ measurement (infrared absorption), and unless you are unfortunate enough to encounter an examiner who has a passion for Raman scattering, the viva will concentrate equally on clinical uses. Make sure that you are able to interpret the range of capnograph traces that you may commonly encounter. It may help if you can draw them.

The viva

You may be asked what information can be obtained from a capnograph trace (Figure 5.1).

- **Cardiovascular information:** CO$_2$ production can occur only if the patient has a cardiac output. A falling CO$_2$ may indicate a decreasing cardiac output, a sudden fall may be a sign of pulmonary embolus, and a flat trace will be seen if there is complete circulatory arrest. Normal end-tidal CO$_2$ usually reassures the anaesthetist that ventilation is adequate.
- **Respiratory information:** there are many possible variations of a capnograph trace, some of which may be quite subtle, such as the waveform you may see with intermittent malfunction of an inspiratory valve, or the small rise at the end of the rising plateau phase that may be seen in obese and pregnant patients. (This is attributed to fast- and slow-emptying alveoli with different time constants.) You will be asked about the traces which convey more commonly important information.
  — *No CO$_2$ trace:* this may indicate oesophageal intubation, tracheal tube displacement, or disconnection of the breathing system.
  — *Low or falling end-tidal CO$_2$:* this may be due to overventilation if IPPV is being used, or to hyperventilation in a patient breathing spontaneously.

— *High or rising end-tidal CO_2:* this may be caused by inadequate ventilation, respiratory depression, rebreathing, or exhaustion of the soda lime. It may rarely be a sign of a hypermetabolic state, of which the most extreme example is malignant hyperpyrexia, in which there is a massive increase in CO_2 production.

— *Abnormal capnography waveforms:* a slow upstroke and slowly rising plateau indicates chronic or acute airway obstruction. The obstruction can be anywhere in the system; either in the upper or lower airway, or in the breathing circuit. A trace that shows inspiratory dips in the waveform may be indicating partial recovery from neuromuscular blockade. A raised baseline indicates rebreathing.

Direction the viva may take
You will be asked about methods of measuring CO_2.

- **Infrared absorption:** this is the main method of measuring CO_2 in theatre.
- Its principle is that a molecule will absorb infrared radiation (wavelength 1–40 μm) as long as it contains at least two different atoms. This applies to CO_2, as well as to N_2O and to all other inhalational agents.
- The system comprises an infrared source, a filter to ensure that only radiation of the desired wavelength is transmitted, a crystal window (glass absorbs infrared), a sample chamber and a photodetector.
- The fraction of radiation absorbed is compared with a reference gas (so regular calibration against zero and known CO_2 concentrations is essential) before the value is displayed.
- The infrared wavelength absorbed varies with the gas, thereby allowing its identification. For CO_2, this absorption is maximal at 4.28 μm. There is some overlap between CO_2 and N_2O for which modern instruments can compensate; collision broadening would otherwise falsely elevate the CO_2 readings.

Further direction the viva may take
You will be asked what other methods can be used.

- **Colorimetric:** carbonic acid forms from CO_2 and water, and will change a pH-sensitive colour indicator. This principle is used in portable devices intended to confirm correct tracheal tube placement in emergency situations in which formal capnography is not available.
- **Mass spectrometry:** this technique is extremely accurate, has a very rapid response time and allows the simultaneous measurement of different compounds. The instruments, however, are very large and expensive and are not used for routine gas monitoring in the UK. The gas sample is introduced into an ionization chamber in which some of its component molecules pass through an electron beam and become charged. The ionized particles are then accelerated out of the chamber into a strong magnetic field, which deflects the particles according to their mass.
- **Raman effect:** the interaction of electromagnetic radiation with a molecule may result in a partial, as opposed to a complete, transfer of energy. Intermolecular bonds

absorb the energy and some is then re-emitted at different wavelengths. There is usually a decrease in wavelength which is characteristic of the individual molecule.

The fuel cell (oxygen measurement)

Commentary

It is a little hard to know why this question continues to appear, given that fuel cell oxygen analysers are no longer widely in use. The subject may broaden to include other methods of measuring oxygen concentrations, although there is no obvious clinical angle to leaven the science. A few examiners may be excited by the topic; most will be rather less enthusiastic and so do not worry if the viva seems a bit flat at this stage. It is likely to be because of the line of questioning that the examiners are constrained to follow rather than the fact that they are depressed by your answers.

The viva

You will be asked about the mode of action of a galvanic fuel cell.

- A reliable method of analysing oxygen in the common gas outlet of the anaesthetic machine is fundamental to patient safety.
- The fuel cell is similar in principle to a polarographic (Clark) oxygen electrode. It comprises a lead anode and a gold mesh cathode, bathed in an electrolyte solution. At the anode, lead reacts with hydroxyl ions to produce electrons. At the cathode, oxygen reacts with the electrons and water, and generates hydroxyl ions.
- The current flow is proportional to the partial pressure of oxygen. The response time is around 30 seconds.
- The fuel cell produces its own voltage and needs no other electrical source. Protecting it from oxygen (air) during the periods when it is not in use will prolong its life. Its function is not affected by water vapour.
- Fuel cells are bulky, heavy and are not robust. They may also be affected by the accumulation of nitrogen that occurs if nitrous oxide is passed though the cell.

Direction the viva may take

You may be asked what other methods you know of measuring oxygen.

- **The Clark electrode:** this comprises a silver/silver chloride anode and platinum cathode bathed in an electrolyte solution. A small potential is applied across the electrodes and the current measured. The electrode works in an analogous way to the fuel cell, in that current flow is proportional to the oxygen tension at the cathode. The Clark electrode measures oxygen in a blood sample from which it is separated by a plastic membrane.
- **Paramagnetic analyser:** oxygen is paramagnetic, with unpaired electrons in the outer shell, which means that it is drawn into a magnetic field. (Most other gases

are diamagnetic.) The traditional paramagnetic analyser comprises a chamber containing a nitrogen-filled glass dumbbell, which is suspended on a wire and allowed to rotate within a non-uniform magnetic field. When oxygen enters the chamber, it is attracted by the magnetic field and displaces the dumbbell. The degree of rotation is proportional to the amount of oxygen present. Modern analysers comprise two chambers separated by a pressure transducer. One is a reference chamber containing 20.93% oxygen (air); the other contains the sample to be measured. Both chambers are then subjected to a changing magnetic field, which increases the activity of the oxygen molecules. This agitation changes the pressure in each chamber; the oxygen partial pressure difference is proportional to the pressure difference across the transducer. These analysers are very accurate and have a rapid response time which allows breath-by-breath measurement.

- **Mass spectrometry:** this technique is accurate, has a very rapid response time and allows the simultaneous measurement of different compounds, including oxygen (page 292).

Supply of medical gases

Commentary

Conceptually this is not a difficult question and it requires of you no judgement and little science. It requires simply facts, and facts which are mostly of modest clinical relevance, albeit of some general interest. The question is not a very good discriminator, so you might as well learn the basic information, repeat it gratefully to the examiner, and hope that the next subject about which you are asked is rather more enticing.

The viva

You will be asked how medical gases (namely oxygen, nitrous oxide, entonox and medical air) are supplied to a typical hospital.

- **Gas cylinders:**
  - The cylinders on an anaesthetic machine are usually size 'E', which contain 680 litres of oxygen and 1800 litres of nitrous oxide. Designed to withstand very high pressures (they are tested to 250 bar), they are made of molybdenum, chromium steel, manganese and high carbon manganese steel. (Cylinders for domiciliary oxygen can be made of lightweight aluminium alloy.)
  - Their features include colour coding (which is not international; oxygen cylinders in the UK are black with white shoulders, whereas in the USA they are green), a pin index system to ensure attachment only to the correct yoke, and information about the contents of the cylinder. The coloured plastic collar indicates the date of the last cylinder test (the interval is between 5 and 10 years). The bodok seal is a neoprene washer enclosed within an aluminium surround which provides a gas-tight seal between the cylinder head and the yoke.

- **Cylinder contents**
  - Oxygen is stored as a gas at a pressure of 13 700 kPa (137 bar).
  - Nitrous oxide is in a mixed liquid and vapour phase whose pressure is 4400 kPa.
  - Entonox is a 50:50 gas mixture of oxygen and nitrous oxide at a pressure of 13 700 kPa.
- **Central gas supply**
  - Piped gas (oxygen, nitrous oxide, entonox and medical air) is supplied through high quality copper pipelines. The outlets have a non-interchangeable coupling in the form of a Schrader-type valve. The hoses from the gas outlet to the anaesthetic machine are colour-coded. Gas is supplied at a pressure of 4 bar, apart from the medical gas that is used to drive surgical instruments which is supplied at 7 bar.
  - The gases may come from a manifold of large cylinders. They may be arranged in banks of cylinders, each of which should contain enough gas to supply a hospital for at least 2 days.
  - Oxygen is usually supplied from a liquid oxygen source. Liquid oxygen is stored below its critical temperature (−118°C) at around −160°C and at a pressure of 7 bar, which is the vapour pressure of oxygen at that temperature. The low temperature is maintained both by a vacuum insulated shell, and by the fact that as the oxygen evaporates its temperature will fall. The contents of the storage device can be determined either by weight or by pressure gauges, which measure the pressure difference between the top and bottom of the liquid oxygen.
- **Oxygen concentrators**
  - These provide an alternative method of providing oxygen, although their low flow rates (4 lmin^{-1}) and pressures (70 kPa) mean that they are more commonly used to provide domiciliary supplies for individual patients.
  - They comprise zeolite-containing columns. Zeolites are hydrated aluminium silicates which are ion-exchangers and molecular sieves. The flow of air into the cylinders is directed so that nitrogen and water vapour are absorbed from one cylinder, while absorbed gas from the other is extracted by a vacuum pump. Every 30 seconds a solenoid valve switches the flow to ensure a constant flow of 95% oxygen to the reservoir. The remaining 5% is argon, which appears to have no adverse effects.
- **Medical air:** this can be supplied from a central compressor or from cylinders. It must be dry, free from particulate matter, including the mineral oils used to lubricate the compressor, and free from bacteria. The air is, therefore, desiccated and filtered.

Direction the viva may take

You may be asked some miscellaneous definitions before questions about safety, safe storage and supply failure.

- **Filling ratio:** this is the mass of gas used to fill a cylinder divided by the mass of water needed to fill the cylinder completely. It applies to gases that are stored in the liquid phase, and for nitrous oxide, it is 0.75. If the cylinder is to be used in hotter climates this is reduced to 0.67. An overfilled cylinder that is exposed to high ambient temperatures will generate dangerously high pressures.

- **Safe storage:** this is largely common sense. Cylinders should be kept in a secure and dry environment, free from extremes of temperature. Full and empty cylinders should ideally be kept in separate areas to avoid the risk of substitution. Large cylinders are usually stored upright; smaller ones may be laid horizontally.
- **Entonox:** this is a 50:50 mixture of nitrous oxide and oxygen at a pressure of 13 700 kPa. Cylinders should be stored flat to prevent delivery of 100% nitrous oxide when the cylinder is first used.
- **Nitrous oxide:** you may be asked what happens when a nitrous oxide cylinder empties. In theory, the pressure, which is the vapour pressure, should remain constant until the liquid phase is exhausted, after which the pressure would fall to zero as the cylinder emptied. In practice, because the temperature of the liquid nitrous oxide falls as it vaporizes, the cylinder pressure also drops. The pressure returns to 4400 kPa only if the gas flow ceases and the cylinder is allowed to return to room temperature.
- **Gas supply or oxygen failure:** failure of the liquid oxygen source triggers supply from a reserve manifold of large oxygen cylinders, which are also remote from the site of delivery to the patient. There should also be reserve cylinders available in theatre. Should there be a complete failure of oxygen delivery, the anaesthetic machine should discontinue the flow of nitrous oxide, and entrain air.

The anaesthetic machine

Commentary

This topic may be asked in various ways. The viva may deal with overall safety features, or it may concentrate on prevention of barotrauma or hypoxia. A structured approach should allow you to answer the question adequately, from whichever direction it is approached. It is a core subject, but not one which is difficult. The safety features of the anaesthetic machine are numerous and you will have little time to do more than list them.

The viva

- The modern anaesthetic machine delivers accurate mixtures of anaesthetic gases and inhalational agents at variable, controlled flow rates and at low pressure. It accomplishes this via a number of features that are best described by tracing the gas flow through the system from the cylinder or pipeline to the fresh gas outlet.
- **Gas pipelines:** these are colour-coded for the UK, but there is no international consistency. A Schrader coupling system ensures that the pipeline connections are non-interchangeable. Reducing valves reduce the pressures to 4 bar. The pipeline hose connection to the rear of the anaesthetic machine is permanent. The threads

are gas-specific (NIST – non-interchangeable screw thread) and a one-way valve ensures unidirectional flow.

- **Gas cylinders:** these too are colour-coded for the UK, but there is no international standard. They are made from molybdenum steel. They are robust and undergo rigorous regular hydraulic testing (as does the cylinder outlet valve). A pin-index system, which is unique to each gas, prevents connection to the wrong yoke, and side guards on each yoke ensure that the cylinders are vertical. Bodok (**bo**nded **dis**k) seals ensure a gas-tight fit. A Bourdon pressure gauge indicates cylinder pressure.

- **Pressure regulators:** primary pressure regulators/reducing valves decrease the high cylinder pressures to 4 bar, and a relief valve is located downstream in case of regulator failure. Adjustable pressure-limiting (APL) valves are part of the breathing system rather than the anaesthetic machine itself, but are designed to minimize the risk of barotrauma by venting gas when a pre-set pressure is exceeded. When fully closed, the APL will open at a pressure of 60 cmH$_2$O.

- **Flow restrictors:** these are placed upstream of the flowmeter block and protect the low pressure part of the system from damaging surges in gas pressure from the piped supply. They may sometimes be used downstream of the vaporizer back bar to minimize back pressure associated with IPPV.

- **Flow control valves:** these govern the transition from the high pressure to the low pressure system, and reduce the pressure from 4 bar to just above atmospheric as gas enters the flowmeter block.

- **Oxygen failure and interlock devices:** systems vary, but a British Standard specifies that the failure alarm should be powered by the O$_2$ supply pressure in the machine pipeline and activated by a pressure reduction to below 2 bar. In most systems the gas mixture is then vented, and an audible warning tone is activated. The same valve opens an air-entrainment valve so that the patient cannot be exposed to a hypoxic mixture resulting from failure of O$_2$ delivery. An interlock system between the O$_2$ and N$_2$O control valves prevents the administration of a hypoxic mixture. The machine cannot deliver a nitrous oxide concentration greater than 75%.

- **Emergency oxygen flush:** O$_2$ is supplied direct from the high pressure circuit upstream of the vaporizer block and provides 35–75 l min^{-1} (if the O$_2$ flowmeter needle valve is opened fully, it delivers about 40 l min^{-1}). Both methods may cause barotrauma in vulnerable patients.

- **Flowmeters:** these are constant pressure variable orifice flowmeters (Rotameter is a trade name) which are calibrated for a specific gas. Accuracy is to within 2.5%. The tubes have an antistatic coating to prevent sticking, and there are vanes etched into the bobbin to ensure rotation. In the UK the oxygen knob is always on the left, is larger, is hexagonal in profile and is more prominent than the others. This is said to be because Boyle, who designed one of the original anaesthetic machines, was left-handed. This position does, however, put the patient at risk of breathing a hypoxic mixture if there is damage to a downstream flowmeter tube. Thus, modern O$_2$ flowmeters feed distal to other gases should there be a proximal leak. CO$_2$ has disappeared from most machines; where it is still delivered it is usually governed to prevent a flow of greater than 500 ml min^{-1}. Not all machines use flowmeters: some control gas flow by microprocessors and produce an electronic display.

- **Vaporizers and back bar:** the most common vaporizers are temperature-compensated variable bypass devices which allow accurate and safe delivery of the dialled concentrations. A locking mechanism on the back bar prevents more than one vaporizer being used at the same time. A spring-loaded non-return valve on the back bar prevents retrograde flow caused by the pumping effect of IPPV. A pressure relief valve on the downstream end of the back bar protects against increases in the pressure within the circuit.
- **Common gas outlet:** this receives gases from the back bar and from the emergency O_2 flush. It has a swivel outlet with a standard 15-mm female connection.

Direction the viva may take

The features listed above will take most of the viva to describe, and if you can add some extra detail in one or two key areas, there will be little opportunity for the examiners to take it much further.

If the viva concentrates on protection from barotrauma, then key features from the list above include:

- Pressure-reducing valves, both pipeline and cylinders.
- Flow restrictors.
- Flow control valves.
- Pressure relief valves downstream of the vaporizer back bar.

If the viva concentrates on protection from hypoxia, then key features from the list above include:

- Gas pipelines colour coding and NIST connections.
- Gas cylinders colour coding and pin indexing.
- Oxygen failure devices.
- Interlock system.
- Emergency oxygen flush.

Flowmeters

Commentary

There are few anaesthetics given which do not involve the use of at least one flowmeter, although microprocessor-controlled gas flow is becoming more widespread as older anaesthetic machines are replaced. It is important, none the less, to be aware of how traditional flowmeters function as well as of the potential sources of inaccuracy. This is a predictable and straightforward question, but it is fairly thin, and so you will be expected to know the basic physics.

The viva

You will be asked about the physical principles which underlie the function of flowmeters.

- A flowmeter is a variable orifice, fixed pressure difference device, which gives a continuous indication of the rate of gas flow. (Rotameter is a trade name which continual use has given generic status.)

Physical principles

- A bobbin floats within a vertical conical glass tube, supported by the gas flow which is controlled by a needle valve.
- At low flows the orifice around the bobbin is an annular tube, and the gas flow is laminar. Flow rate through a tube is related to the viscosity of the gas and the fourth power of the radius.
- At higher flows and further up the tube the area of the annular orifice is larger in relation to the bobbin and the flow is turbulent. Flow rate through an orifice is related to the density of the gas and the square of the radius.
- These factors mean, therefore, that flowmeters have to be calibrated for the specific gases that they are measuring. They are not interchangeable for different gases. They are accurate to ±2.5%.
- The pressure across the bobbin at any flow rate remains constant, because the force to which it gives rise is balanced exactly by the force of gravity acting on the bobbin.

Other features of flowmeters

- The bobbin is designed with small slots or fins in its upper part so that it will rotate centrally within the gas stream without touching the flowmeter tube. This is to prevent its sticking to the sides because of dirt or static electricity.
- To prevent the accumulation of static charge, tubes have either a conductive coating or a conductive strip at the back.
- The flowmeter blocks are designed to ensure that the bobbin remains visible at the top of the tubes, even when the gas flow is at its maximum.

Direction the viva may take

You may be asked about potential sources of inaccuracy.

- Accumulation of dirt or static electricity (despite the design features above).
- A flowmeter block may not be vertical; the bobbin must not impinge on the sides of the tube.
- Back pressure on the gas flow may still be a problem on some anaesthetic machines, although this is normally prevented by a spring-loaded non-return valve.
- Cracked seals or tubes may provide a source of error. Oxygen is often the last gas to be added to the mixture that is delivered to the back bar, although some modern flowmeter blocks are designed to deliver oxygen downstream of the other gases should there be a proximal leak.

Further direction the viva could take

At some stage the viva may divert into the subject of laminar and turbulent flow. This is covered in more detail below.

Laminar and turbulent flow

Commentary

Precise physical principles underlie the concepts of laminar and turbulent flow, and the viva is likely to concentrate more on these than on their practical implications. Factors which influence flow are important in relation to intravenous fluid therapy and to the administration of inhaled gases, but their relevance is obvious, and the potential for discussion is relatively limited. Examiners tend to view this as a straightforward and predictable question. They do not expect candidates to have much difficulty with it, and so you should know the topic well.

The viva

You may be asked first about the practical relevance of laminar and turbulent flow.

- **Gas flow:** turbulent flow increases resistance and so it is important to minimize angles and constrictions in breathing systems. Increased velocity may increase turbulence, which can be of significance, for example, in a hyperventilating asthmatic patient. In an infant with bronchiolitis, a small decrease in the calibre of the airways due to inflammation and oedema may critically impair the capacity of the exhausted baby to maintain effective ventilation. (These are some of several possible examples.)
- **Fluid flow:** the Poiseuille–Hagen equation is well known to anaesthetists because of its clinical relevance. The flow of fluid via an intravenous infusion will double if the driving pressure is doubled, or if the length of the cannula is halved. Fluid resuscitation through long central venous catheters may, therefore, may not be effective. Flow, however, in theory will increase by 16 times if the internal diameter of the cannula is doubled. (In practice, the increase may not be quite as impressive; a typical 14G cannula of 2.20 mm (external) diameter has a flow rate of 315 ml min^{-1}, in contrast to an 18G cannula with a diameter of 1.30 mm through which distilled water flows at 100 ml min^{-1}.) The difference remains significant enough, however, to mandate the use of short, wide-bore cannulae for rapid restoration of circulating volume.

You will then be asked to define more precisely laminar and turbulent flow.

- **Flow:** flow is the amount of a fluid (gas or liquid) passing a point in unit time.
- **Laminar flow:**
  — This describes the situation in which a molecule of the given substance maintains a constant spatial relationship to all the others that are flowing in

the same layer, or lamina, down the tube. The flow is greatest in the centre of the tube, being approximately twice the mean flow, whereas at the walls of the tube the flow reduces almost to zero.

— A number of factors influence flow: these include the pressure differential between the ends of the tube ($P_1 - P_2$), the radius of the tube (r), the length of the tube (l), and the viscosity of the fluid (η).

— These factors have been combined (together with a proportionality constant π / 128) to derive the Poiseuille–Hagen equation:

$$\text{Flow rate} = (P_1 - P_2) \times r^4 \times \pi / 128 \times l \times \eta.$$

— This applies only to an ideal or Newtonian fluid, which is defined as any fluid that demonstrates a linear relation between the applied shear stress and the rate of deformation. A flowing liquid can be visualized as a series of parallel laminae. If the flow is to double, therefore, it must overcome a resistive force that is twice as great. Water is a Newtonian fluid, but blood is not.

— Fluids resist flow because of the phenomenon of viscosity. Viscosity describes the frictional forces which act between the layers of the fluid as it moves down the tube. (Its units are Pascal seconds.)

• **Turbulent flow:** this describes fluid flow in which the orderly arrangement of the molecules is lost and the fluid swirls and eddies, thereby increasing the resistance. In contrast to laminar flow, in which flow is directly proportional to the pressure differential (ΔP), when the flow is turbulent then fluid flow is proportional to the square root of the differential ($\sqrt{\Delta P}$).

• **The transition from laminar to turbulent flow**
  — This is given by the Reynolds number, which is an index derived from a combination of linear velocity (v), the density of the fluid (ρ), the diameter of the tube (d) and the viscosity of the fluid (η). Reynolds number = $v\rho d/\eta$.
  — When the Reynolds number exceeds 2000, turbulent flow supervenes. (This information has been obtained empirically from in vitro experiments.)
  — Critical flow and critical velocity refer to the situation in which the Reynolds number is 2000, and the flow is liable to become turbulent.
  — Any local increase in velocity such as occurs in the angles or constrictions of a breathing system, is likely to change gas flow from laminar to turbulent, with a resultant increase in resistance and the work of breathing.

Vaporizers

Commentary

Vaporizers, volatile agents and circle systems are of obvious clinical relevance, but this being the science viva it is the basic principles which will dominate the questions. The oral should follow a relatively predictable course, including the 'trick' question about the use of vaporizers at altitude.

The viva

You may be asked about the physical principles of vaporization and the problems that these cause for vaporizer design.

- **Saturated vapour pressure (SVP):** vaporizers have to overcome the fact that the SVP of volatile agents at 20°C is many times greater than that required to produce anaesthesia. (The SVP of sevoflurane is 22.7 kPa and so its maximum achievable concentration is 22.4% (22.7/101.325). For desflurane, with an SVP of 89.2, the figure is 88%). Vaporizers have to be designed to allow the addition of a controlled amount of volatile anaesthetic agent to the fresh gas flow, having changed the liquid to a vapour. This is done by streaming the fresh gas flow (FGF).
- **Splitting ratio:** as the FGF enters the vaporizer it is split into two streams; approximately 20% passes into the vaporization chamber while the rest enters a bypass chamber. The gas leaving the vaporizing chamber should be fully saturated with vapour. This is achieved by increasing the available surface area by the use of wicks or a series of baffles.
- **Latent heat of vaporization:** as a liquid vaporizes so its temperature falls, and compensation for this change is essential. If there is no such compensation then the SVP of the agent and its delivered concentration will also fall. Vaporizers are made of material with high thermal conductivity, which supplies energy for the heat of vaporization by allowing heat to flow from the vaporizer into the anaesthetic in its liquid phase. The splitting ratio must also be altered as the temperature changes, hence the design of the bimetallic strip, which allows more gas into the vaporizing chamber as the temperature drops.
- **Calibration:** vaporizers are calibrated for individual agents, and should one inadvertently be filled with a different volatile anaesthetic then it will deliver either excessive or inadequate vapour concentrations depending on the respective vapour pressures. If a volatile with a high SVP (such as desflurane, 89.2 kPa) is used in a sevoflurane vaporizer (SVP 22.7 kPa), then vapour output will be high. If the situation is reversed, then vapour output will be low. Even if the SVP differences are small, the effect is still significant; isoflurane (SVP 32.5 kPa) in a halothane vaporizer (SVP 32.1 kPa) will deliver a concentration that is 25–50% higher than is dialled up.

Potential problems

- **Flow rate dependence:** modern vaporizers function independently of flow rates between 0.5 and 15 l min^{-1}. Outside these limits they will deliver less than the dialled concentration.
- **Overfilling:** volatile agent may get directly into the bypass chamber if the vaporizer is overfilled, leading to the delivery of dangerously high concentrations.
- **'Pumping' effect:** if a ventilator produces cyclical changes in the pressure in the back bar, this may force gas back into the vaporizing chamber and saturated gas in the vaporizing chamber back into the bypass channel. The forward flow as the ventilator cycles then increases the concentration of delivered vapour. This occurred with minute volume divider ventilators which are now used much less commonly.

- **'Pressurizing' effect:** this occurs if the overall pressure in the vaporizer is raised (as happens in large vaporizer chambers at high flows). When the gas reaches the common outlet it expands to atmospheric pressure, with a lowering of the effective concentration.
- **Monitoring:** monitoring volatile agent concentrations minimizes these theoretical risks.

Direction the viva may take

You may be asked a number of miscellaneous, but usually predictable, questions which may include the use of vaporizers at altitude or under hyperbaric conditions, the characteristics of the desflurane vaporizer and the use of vaporizers inside and outside circle systems.

- **Effects of altitude:** at altitude the atmospheric pressure is reduced, but the SVP remains unchanged. The actual output of vapour in volumes percent increases, but the partial pressure remains unchanged. As it is the partial pressure of the agent that is responsible for anaesthesia, the vaporizer can be used in the same way at 5000 m as at sea level. The same applies to vaporizers used under hyperbaric conditions.
- **Desflurane:** the physical properties of desflurane require a more complex vaporizer; one that is designed like no other in current use. At 23.5°C, the boiling point of desflurane is close to room temperature. Small changes in operating theatre temperature could therefore cause large changes in the SVP of desflurane, with an increase in vapour output. To control this accurately, the vaporizer is heated to 39°C. This produces a gas under pressure (200 kPa) which is then injected into the FGF. This vaporizer design obviates the need for any temperature compensation devices. (It is technically easier to heat a vaporizer than to cool it, which would be the alternative technique.)
- **Position in the circuit**
  - *VOC (vaporizer outside circle):* plenum vaporizers (in which positive upstream pressure drives the gas) have high internal resistance, are unsuitable for use within circle breathing systems, and deliver volatile agent from the back bar of the anaesthetic machine. At low flows, large changes in the dialled concentration are reflected only very slowly within the circle system. A change in FGF rather than vapour concentration may be necessary to effect a more rapid change in the depth of anaesthesia.
  - **VIC (vaporizer inside circle):** drawover vaporizers (in which a subatmospheric pressure generated distal to the vaporizer either mechanically or by the patient's spontaneous respiration, draws the gas through the system) have minimal resistance to flow and can be used within a circle. At low flows the vapour concentration rises, because rather than being diluted it is being added to each inspiration. If the minute volume is large then the risk of delivering very high concentrations of volatile agent is increased.

Further direction the viva could take

If there is time you may be asked about some of the characteristics of the volatile agents. There is unlikely to be time to explore these in any depth, but you should try to demonstrate in your answers that you are confident clinically and practically in their use.

Anaesthetic breathing systems

Commentary

This is a standard topic, which will inevitably involve a discussion either of the circle system or of the Mapleson classification. Alternatively, you might be asked to talk about both, which means that you will not have to go into the subject in any depth. You will probably be invited to draw some of the different arrangements, and a useful way of dealing with this request is to give a running commentary as you draw the components. If you do this you will not find yourself sitting at the table drawing in silence while the examiners watch, and it will allow you to demonstrate that you understand how these breathing systems behave. Analysis of the behaviour of the systems can be complex, and so you are more likely to be asked about those (such as the Magill attachment and the circle system) that can be explained within the time available.

The viva

You may be asked to draw (and describe) the typical components of a circle system.

- **Circle system:** the fresh gas flow (FGF), together with volatile anaesthetic (if used), enters the inspiratory limb and travels through a one-way non-return valve to the patient. Expired air enters the expiratory limb and passes through a second non-return valve. Excess gas (mixed expired air) is vented through the pressure relief valve on the reservoir bag with the remainder passing through the CO_2-absorbing soda lime and back into the inspiratory limb (Figure 5.2).

You may then be asked in more detail why the components are arranged in this way, and what would be the effects of altering their positions in the system. There are numerous potential combinations, but you should be able to answer most variations of this question if you have understood the basic principles of the circuit. (For example, were the pressure relief valve and reservoir bag to be sited between the patient and the inspiratory one-way valve, then rebreathing would occur.)

Direction the viva may take

You may be asked to describe the advantages and disadvantages of the circle system before going on to outline the principles that underlie its use. Detailed discussion of anaesthetic uptake and gas exchange risks entering complex (and time-consuming) territory and so it is more likely that you will have to show only that you can use a circle system logically and safely.

- **Advantages:** the circle is very efficient in terms of conservation of gases, heat and moisture. It is therefore more economical and less polluting than semi-closed systems.

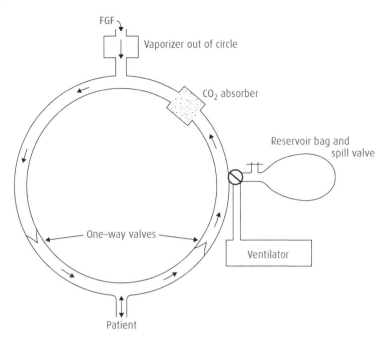

Fig. 5.2 Schematic arrangement of a circle system.

- **Disadvantages:** the circle is simple in outline theory but much more complex in detailed execution. The uptake and excretion of the different components within the system can vary greatly, and it is essential to monitor the FiO_2, CO_2 and agent concentration within the circle. The system is slow to react to changes in the inspired volatile concentration. If nitrous oxide is used in a closed system, then hypoxia is a potential risk (see below). Should soda lime be allowed to dry it may react with the CHF_2 group of desflurane, isoflurane and enflurane to produce carbon monoxide.

- **Principles of use**
  - *Closed:* the circle system can be used as a genuine closed circuit in which expired gases and volatile agents recirculate. No more oxygen is added than is required for the patient's metabolic demand and CO_2 is removed by passage of the gases through soda lime. Volatile anaesthetic agents enter the system via vaporizers that can be sited either outside (VOC) the circuit or, much less commonly, within the circuit (VIC) as a drawover vaporizer. In a truly closed system delivering only basal flows, it is important to realize that prolonged anaesthesia with nitrous oxide can cause hypoxia. Consider a situation in which $1\,l\,min^{-1}$ is being delivered, 0.25 l of which is oxygen. At the end of one tidal volume breath this basal oxygen will be absorbed, leaving the alveoli filled with 100% N_2O which will dilute the next breath. Equilibrium takes a long time to achieve, however, and N_2O uptake is still $100\,ml\,h^{-1}$ after 2 hours. It is prudent, nevertheless, to flush out the system periodically. (At

the beginning of anaesthesia there is the opposite problem. The rapid N_2O uptake of $450 \, ml \, min^{-1}$ reduces the partial pressure in the system with the risk of inadequate anaesthesia.)

— *Semi-open:* in this arrangement the circle is used with a higher than basal FGF with the excess gas being vented through the pressure relief spill valve. Under these circumstances the concentrations of gases and volatile agent in the fresh gas supply are closer to those in the circle and can be changed more quickly. This represents a compromise between economy and ease of use.

- **Practical considerations:** the total volume of the system, including the breathing hoses, the air in the absorber, reservoir bag and the patient's FRC, is around 5 l. Immediate delivery of low flows at $1 \, l \, min^{-1}$ would clearly result in inadequate anaesthesia. An additional factor which reduces anaesthetic partial pressures in the breathing system is the very rapid uptake of N_2O (if used) and volatile agent during the early part of the anaesthetic. This means that high flows must be used for the first 5–10 minutes. A VOC will always show a higher concentration than is being inspired (unless equilibrium has been reached), and rapid changes can only be initiated by a reversion to high flow. If a fully closed system is used, then monitors which measure inspiratory gas and volatile concentrations as close to the patient as possible must be used, and the system should be flushed at regular intervals to minimize the risk of dilutional hypoxia.

You may then be asked to compare the behaviour of the circle with one or more of the systems described by Mapleson.

The Mapleson classification

There are more logical ways of analysing breathing systems, but this system has become hallowed by tradition and familiarity, and shows little sign of being superseded. (Mapleson was Professor of Medical Physics in Cardiff who, in 1953, published his analysis of the behaviour of the various combinations of the valve, tubing, reservoir bag and FGF that were used in breathing systems.) Strictly speaking, these should be described as breathing *systems* rather than *circuits*, but common usage makes the term permissible, although technically incorrect.

- **Classification:** the systems were classified as A to F, and they all potentially allow rebreathing. They are 'semi-closed' ('semi-open' in the USA) and supply more gas than the patient needs, with the excess being vented to the atmosphere. If rebreathing of CO_2 does occur, a healthy patient who is breathing spontaneously will respond by increasing alveolar ventilation which will rise, by up to 20 times if necessary, to keep the $PaCO_2$ normal. These systems are defined, therefore, in terms of the FGF that is needed to maintain an unchanged $PaCO_2$ in the face of unchanged ventilation.
- **Mapleson A:** this is most commonly used in the form of the Magill attachment and comprises a reservoir bag into which the FGF is directed, a length of corrugated tubing (which is resistant to kinking) and, at the patient end, an adjustable pressure-limiting (APL) valve (Figure 5.3).
  - *Spontaneous respiration:* the system is very efficient. At the end of inspiration the valve is closed and the reservoir bag is emptying. During expiration, the

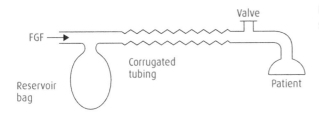

Fig. 5.3 Mapleson A breathing system. FGF, Fresh gas flow.

FGF is filling the reservoir bag, while expired air (dead space gas and then alveolar gas) is passing into the tube. Hence the pressure in both the reservoir bag and the breathing system increase to the point at which the valve opens and vents expired air. The FGF continues to flow down the tube. At an FGF equal to the alveolar ventilation, it is alveolar gas and not dead space gas that is expelled preferentially. This analysis is based on the assumption that there is no longitudinal mixing of dead space and alveolar gases, and Mapleson recommended that the FGF should equal the minute ventilation. (Subsequent investigation suggested that 70% of minute ventilation, i.e. the alveolar ventilation, would be adequate.)

— *Controlled ventilation:* if controlled ventilation is used, the circuit loses all its economy; fresh gas is vented during inspiration, while during expiration the valve tends to close, and all expired air passes back into the system which selectively retains expired air. To prevent rebreathing the FGF should be at least twice the minute ventilation.

— *Co-axial versions:* co-axial versions, of which the commonest is the Lack system, function in the same way. Early narrow co-axial systems effectively reduced the capacity of the outer expiratory limb to store gas, and hence expired gas could reach the reservoir bag. Increasing the dimensions solved this problem, but at the cost of increasing the bulk of the system.

- **Mapleson B and C:** the Mapleson C comprises an APL at the patient end with the FGF entering just proximally. A short length of tubing connects this to the reservoir bag which, in the classic 'Waters' circuit, includes a CO_2-absorbing canister. The Mapleson B includes a length of corrugated tubing between the FGF and the reservoir bag. The Mapleson C circuit is used in resuscitation and in areas such as theatre recovery. Both systems allow mixing of expired air with the FGF, which must approximate three times minute ventilation to flush the system and prevent rebreathing. A Mapleson B circuit, nevertheless, is still more efficient than the Mapleson A during controlled ventilation (Figure 5.4).

- **Mapleson D, E and F:** these systems all function as T-pieces, being inefficient for spontaneous respiration but not for controlled ventilation. Analysis of their behaviour is much more complex than that of the Mapleson A system, although, as a simplification, they require up to three times the minute ventilation to prevent rebreathing during spontaneous respiration ($150–200\,\mathrm{ml\,kg^{-1}}$) but only $70\,\mathrm{ml\,kg^{-1}}$ to achieve normocapnia during IPPV. Analysis is complicated by, amongst other factors, the influence of the respiratory pattern. The respiratory cycle is a sinusoidal waveform, and, in order to prevent rebreathing, the FGF must

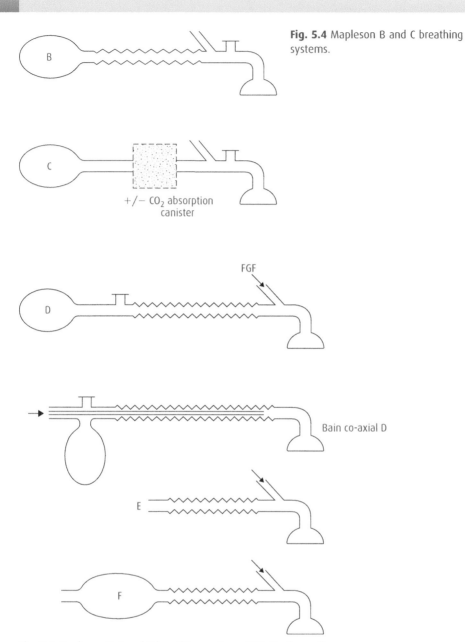

Fig. 5.4 Mapleson B and C breathing systems.

+/− CO_2 absorption canister

FGF

Bain co-axial D

Fig. 5.5 Mapleson D, E and F breathing systems. FGF, Fresh gas flow.

equal or exceed the peak inspiratory flow rate (PIFR). At end-expiration, alveolar gas has moved into the expiratory limb where it mixes with the FGF, and, to prevent rebreathing, the FGF should approach three times the minute ventilation. If, however, there is an expiratory pause, some alveolar gas will be expelled by the FGF and theoretically the flow rate can be decreased (Figure 5.5).

— *Mapleson D:* the Bain circuit is the co-axial version of the Mapleson D circuit.
— *Mapleson E:* this is the original Ayre's T-piece. It can allow both rebreathing of CO_2-containing gas as well as entrainment of ambient air. There is no reservoir bag and expiratory resistance is negligible.
— **Mapleson F:** this differs from the E only in that it has a reservoir bag, added by Jackson–Rees to allow controlled ventilation. The system has no valves and so there is minimal expiratory resistance, hence its traditional use in paediatric anaesthesia. Effective scavenging is difficult from both the E and F systems.
- **Humphrey ADE system:** the Humphrey block is located at the common gas outlet and exists in both parallel and co-axial versions (of equal efficiency). It comprises an APL valve, a pressure relief valve, a reservoir bag, a ventilator port and a lever for selection of spontaneous ventilation (in the A mode) or controlled ventilation (in D/E mode).
- **Monitoring:** it is worth commenting that, although it is important to understand the functional behaviour of these breathing systems, the modern ability to measure the concentrations of gases and volatile agents has removed many of the potential hazards posed by imprecision of the analyses and by inter-patient variability.

Soda lime

Commentary
This question appears in the Final FRCA, although it is a topic that you may already have encountered in the Primary. The potential clinical problems with the use of soda lime are almost entirely theoretical, but there will be insufficient time for a discussion of low-flow anaesthesia, which, logically, is where the viva should lead. The subject is conceptually not difficult and so this is another one of those questions about which you will just have to know some of the facts.

The viva
You will be asked about the composition of soda lime and its mode of action.

- Soda lime is used to absorb CO_2. The discovery is not recent; it has been known for over two centuries that CO_2 is absorbed by strong alkali (caustic soda).
- Its main use is to allow the rebreathing of exhaled gases within breathing systems. This is most commonly the circle system, although it was also used in the original Waters circuit. To-and-fro breathing was allowed by the insertion into the system of a small soda lime canister.
- Its chemical constituents are calcium hydroxide ($Ca(OH)_2$) 80%, sodium hydroxide (NaOH) 4%, potassium hydroxide (KOH) 1% (this accelerates the reaction), and water (H_2O) 15%.
- Also added are silicates in trace amounts which harden the granules which otherwise would disintegrate into powder. An indicator dye is present which changes the colour of the soda lime as it is progressively exhausted. This is either

phenolphthalein (the colour changes from red to white) or, less commonly, ethyl violet (the colour changes from white to purple). As these colour changes are in opposite directions it is clearly important to know which dye is being used.
- Soda lime is formed either into granules whose size is 4–8 mesh (mesh describes the number of openings per inch in a uniform metal strainer) or into spheres. The more uniform the shape, the greater the likelihood of uniform flow through the canister. The size of the granules or spheres is a compromise between providing the largest surface area for absorption without providing excessive resistance to flow.
- Under ideal conditions, 1 kg can absorb 250 of CO_2.
- In the presence of water and with NaOH and KOH as activators, the chemical reaction can be summarized as follows:

$$CO_2 + Ca(OH)_2 \longrightarrow CaCO_3 + H_2O$$

- Partially exhausted soda lime may regenerate on standing, with the migration of unused hydroxide ions from the core to outer areas. Its absorptive capacity in this state is minimal.

Direction the viva may take

You may be asked what other compounds can be used to absorb CO_2.

- **Barium lime (Baralyme):** this comprises calcium hydroxide ($Ca(OH)_2$) 80% and barium hydroxide ($Ba(OH)_2$) 20%. Water is incorporated into the structure of $Ba(OH)_2$. The chemical reaction is similar to that of soda lime, although it is less efficient.
- **Amsorb:** this compound (developed in Belfast) contains $Ca(OH)_2$, calcium chloride and two setting agents. Its absorption capacity is comparable to other agents but its use is associated neither with carbon monoxide (CO) nor compound A formation.

Further direction the viva could take

You may be asked about potentially dangerous reactions between CO_2 absorbents and anaesthetic agents.

- **CO:** modern anaesthetic machines continue to deliver a FGF of 200 ml min^{-1} of oxygen even when the flowmeters are turned off. If the machine goes unused for some time, then this constant flow may dry out a canister of soda or barium lime. Under these circumstances, the reaction of the desiccated absorbent with the CHF_2 group of isoflurane, enflurane or desflurane can produce high levels of CO.
- **Compound A:** sevoflurane reacts with strong monovalent hydroxide bases, such as those which are used in soda lime and barium lime CO_2-absorbers, to produce a number of substances, including compound A. (The reaction with barium lime is about five times more rapid than with soda lime.) Of the degradation products (compounds A, B, D, E and G), only compound A, a vinyl halide, has been shown to have any toxicity. However, the dose-dependent renal damage noted in rats has never been seen in humans. Amsorb appears to be safer in this respect. Compound A production is substantially reduced if the absorbent is cooled.

- **Trilene (trichloroethylene):** of historical interest, and included just in case you should be asked, is the reaction between trilene and soda lime. This produced dichloroacetylene, which is a potent neurotoxin that affected particularly the trigeminal and facial nerves.

Scavenging

Commentary

This topic is rather dry, but it is hard to argue with the importance of minimizing pollution within the theatre environment, and so scavenging is something that you will have to know about, even though the direct clinical implications are only modest.

The viva

You may be asked first why there is a need to scavenge anaesthetic gases.

- **Purpose of scavenging:** the safe removal of waste theatre gases is a health and safety issue and, since 1989, with the government introduction of 'Control of Substances Hazardous to Health' (COSHH), has been a legal requirement. It is only the local environment that is protected, because the gases are pollutants that are vented to atmosphere.
- **Staff health issues:** some studies have identified increased risks of spontaneous abortion in women exposed to trace concentrations of anaesthetic gases, and also that male anaesthetists were more likely to father daughters than sons. There was, in addition, the suggestion of an increase in haematological malignancies. The association is not strong, because other studies have not replicated these data. Moreover, sufficiently large numbers of anaesthetics are administered annually in the developed world, to suggest that were there to be an emphatic problem of this kind, then its provenance would be a lot more obvious.

You will then be asked about the basic components of the scavenging systems that are in use.

- **Scavenging system:** the basic arrangement comprises collection, transfer, receiving and disposal systems.
  - *Collection system:* this is usually a shroud that is connected to the APL or expiratory valves of the ventilator via a 30-mm connector (which prevents confusion with components of the breathing system).
  - *Transfer system:* this comprises wide-bore tubing to remove the gases.
  - *Receiving system:* this is a reservoir system, which is protected against excessive pressures by valves. The positive pressure relief valve is set at 1000 Pa (1 kPa); the negative pressure relief valve is set at −50 Pa (0.05 kPa).
  - *Disposal system:* this simply vents the exhaust to atmosphere and makes the pollution someone else's problem. Ejector systems include fans, vacuum and venturi devices.

- There are two main types of system: **passive** and **active**.
  - *Passive systems:* the components of the system are as described above, and the gases are vented to atmosphere either by the patient's spontaneous respiratory efforts or by the mechanical ventilator.
    The 'Cardiff Aldasorber' is another passive device which comprises a canister containing charcoal particles that absorb halogenated volatile anaesthetic agents. Absorption does not render the agents inert; if the canister is disposed of by incineration, the inhalational agents are released to atmosphere. This device does not absorb nitrous oxide.
  - *Active systems:* the basic components of the system are again as described above, but the vacuum created by a fan or a pump in the disposal system draws the anaesthetic gases through the system. It is important that the negative pressures so generated cannot be transmitted to the patient.

Direction the viva may take
You may then be asked how else you might minimize theatre pollution.

- Theatre air changes (at least 15 times per hour).
- Substitution of total intravenous anaesthesia (TIVA) and regional anaesthesia for inhalational anaesthesia.
- Use of low- and ultra-low-flow breathing systems.

Further direction the viva could take
You may finally be asked about the maximum permitted exposures, which are expressed as an 8-hour time-weighted average. The practical relevance of knowing these numbers is elusive, and it also seems suspicious both that there is such a big variation in levels between the UK and the USA, and that in the UK the permitted maxima are all multiples of 10. The science underlying these data may not therefore be robust.

- Permitted maxima:
  - *Nitrous oxide:*　　100 parts per million (ppm)　(25 ppm in the USA).
  - *Isoflurane and enflurane:*　　50 ppm.
  - *Sevoflurane and desflurane:*　　50 ppm. As yet there are no maximum limits; COSHH states that their similarity to enflurane means that 50 ppm would be appropriate.
  - *Halothane:*　　10 ppm.
  - In the USA, all halogenated volatiles:　　2 ppm.

The gas laws

Commentary
This is the kind of question that you thought you had left behind when you passed the Primary FRCA exam, but it does reappear in the Final. It will not be asked of you in any

greater detail, and the examiner is expecting you to list each gas law and indicate their relevance to anaesthetic practice. If you enunciate each of them slowly and carefully, perhaps writing them down as you go, and even volunteering a little biographical information, then maybe there will be little time for the examiner to ask you in detail about anything else.

The viva

You will be asked to describe the gas laws.

- **Boyle's law**
  - This is the first perfect gas law. It states that at a constant temperature, the volume of a given (fixed) mass of gas varies inversely with the absolute pressure. It can be expressed the other way round, namely that at a constant temperature, the pressure of a given mass of gas is inversely proportional to the volume. Pressure $(P) \times$ volume (V), therefore, is a constant.
  - This law was described in 1662 by Robert Boyle (1627–1691), born in Ireland as the youngest of 14 children, but who lived and studied in England and who was one of the founders of the scientific method.
- **Charles's law**
  - This is the second perfect gas law. It states that at a constant pressure, the volume of a given mass of gas varies directly with the absolute temperature (T). The relationship is linear, which means that at absolute zero that fixed mass of gas would have no volume.
  - This law was described in 1787 by Jacques Charles (1746–1823), a French physicist who constructed the first gas balloon and who later made an ascent to an altitude of over 10 000 feet.
- **Universal gas law**
  - Boyle's Law and Charles's Law can be combined to give the universal gas law, in which $P \times V = T \times nR$, where R is the universal gas constant (8.1 J K^{-1} mol^{-1}) and n is the number of moles of a gas.
- **Gay-Lussac's law**
  - From the equation $PV = nRT$ it is evident that, for a fixed mass of gas at constant volume, the pressure varies directly with temperature.
  - The enunciation of this relationship is attributed to another physicist (and balloonist), Joseph Gay-Lussac (1778–1850). In some texts this is described as the *third perfect gas law.*
- **Dalton's law of partial pressures**
  - This states that the pressure that is exerted by each gas in a mixture of gases is the same as it would exert if it alone occupied the container.
  - This law was described in 1801 by John Dalton (1766–1844), an English chemist from Manchester. He also did early work on colour blindness, which for a while became known as Daltonism.
- **Henry's law**
  - This states that the amount of gas that is dissolved in a liquid at a given temperature is proportional to the partial pressure in the gas in equilibrium with the solution.

— This law was described in 1801 by William Henry (1774–1836), an English chemist and physician. He also identified as methane the gas known as 'firedamp' that was responsible for the death of miners.

- **Avogadro's law**
  - This states that equal volumes of gases at the same temperature and pressure contain the same number of molecules. This also means that 1 g molecular weight of any gas occupies the same volume (22.4 litres at standard temperature and pressure, STP, which is 273.15 K (0° C) and 101.325 kPa).
  - The law was described in 1811 by Amadeus Avogadro (1776–1856), an Italian professor of mathematical physics who lived and worked in Turin. This theory went unremarked for over 50 years, partly due to the scepticism and opposition of scientists such as Dalton.
- **Combined gas laws:** the gas laws can be combined so that

$$P_1 \times V_1 / T_1 = P_2 \times V_2 / T_2.$$

Direction the viva may take

It would be more logical were you to be asked to give examples of the anaesthetic relevance of the gas laws as you describe them. In practice, however, this discussion tends to be deferred until the second part of the viva. The reason for this is probably that if a candidate spends a lot of time struggling to identify the clinical application of the first one or two gas laws, then they may not have a chance to give the examiner the rest of the list that is expected.

Some practical applications include the following.

- **Boyle's law:** (At constant T, PV is a constant; so $P_1 \times V_1 = P_2 \times V_2$.)
  - This can be used to calculate the volume of gas remaining in a cylinder. A size E oxygen cylinder has an internal volume of 10 litres, and so contains 10 litres (V_1) at 13 800 kPa (P_1). (Remember that this is absolute pressure, so 100 kPa of atmospheric pressure must be included.) At atmospheric pressure (P_2) there will therefore be 1380 litres of oxygen (V_2) available from the cylinder.
- **Dalton's law of partial pressures:** (The pressure exerted by each gas in a mixture is the same as if it were alone.)
  - This is relevant for the partial pressure of gases in any mixture, whether it be in a cylinder or within the alveoli.
- **Henry's law:** (The amount of gas that is dissolved in a liquid at a given temperature is proportional to the partial pressure in the gas in equilibrium with the solution.)
  - This has relevance for hyperbaric therapy. At atmospheric pressure and breathing air, the O_2 solubility coefficient (0.003 ml dl^{-1} mmHg^{-1}) means that the dissolved oxygen content is about 0.26 ml dl^{-1}. In a patient breathing 100% oxygen, this increases to 1.7 ml dl^{-1} and at three atmospheres in a hyperbaric chamber it reaches 5.6 ml dl^{-1}. At this level of pressure, therefore, dissolved oxygen can make a significant contribution to delivery. If nitrogen is

present in the gas mixture then it will pass into the tissues, only to come out of solution in the form of bubbles if the pressure decreases too abruptly. This is the cause of decompression sickness.

- **Avogadro's law:** (Equal volumes of gases at the same temperature and pressure contain the same number of molecules.)
  — This can be used, for example, to calibrate a vaporizer. The molecular weight of sevoflurane is 200, 1 mole is 200 g and will occupy 22.4 litres at STP. Imagine, therefore, a vaporizer containing 40 ml of sevoflurane, which is 0.2 mol occupying 4.48 litres at STP. If this is vaporized fully into oxygen of volume 224 litres then the resulting concentration will be 4.48/224 or 2%.

Gases and vapours

Commentary

This is another area that could be seen more properly as being the province of the Primary exam, but subjects related to gases, vapours and pressures will be viewed inevitably as appropriate for discussion. Vivas on these subjects can be haphazard, and you may be asked for a number of definitions before moving on to one or more disparate topics, amongst which may be partial pressure, saturated vapour pressure (SVP), vaporizers, water vapour and humidification.

The viva

There is no obvious clinical entry point for this topic and so you may be asked first for some definitions.

- **Gas:** a gas is a substance above its critical temperature.
- **Vapour:** a vapour is a substance below its critical temperature.
- **Critical temperature:** this is defined as the temperature above which a gas cannot be liquefied, no matter how great is the pressure that is applied.
- **Critical pressure:** this is defined as the vapour pressure of the substance at its critical temperature. It is the pressure needed to liquefy the gas at its critical temperature.
- **SVP:** a saturated vapour is one that is in equilibrium with its own liquid, so the number of molecules entering the liquid phase equals those entering the vapour phase. If the temperature rises, more molecules enter the vapour phase and the vapour pressure rises. The SVP is the maximum partial pressure that can be achieved at a given temperature. The relationship of SVP and temperature is non-linear. You could be asked the maximum concentration of one or other of the volatile agents that can be obtained at 20°C. The SVP of sevoflurane at this temperature is 22.7 kPa; its maximum concentration is therefore 22.7/101 or approximately 22.5%.

- **Boiling point:** when the SVP is the same as the ambient pressure, the liquid boils and the vapour concentration at the surface of the liquid is 100%. Hence the boiling point is the temperature at which the vapour pressure of a liquid equals the ambient temperature above it. The boiling point will therefore decrease as the ambient pressure falls, for example, during ascent to altitude.
- **Latent heat:** when any substance changes from a liquid to a vapour or from a solid to a liquid, heat must be supplied despite the fact that this change of state takes place at a constant temperature. This is the latent heat of vaporization (if the change is from a liquid to a vapour) or the latent heat of fusion (if the change is from a solid to a liquid). In any particular homogenous fluid the molecules do not possess identical kinetic energy. Those with a higher velocity escape the surface of the liquid and are vaporized, thus the mean kinetic energy of the remainder diminishes and the liquid cools. The latent heat of vaporization is defined as the additional heat that is required to convert a given mass of liquid into vapour at the same temperature. Conversely, heat is generated as vapour condenses back to a liquid.
- **Pseudocritical temperature:** in a mixture of gases there is a specific critical temperature, the pseudocritical temperature, at which the gas mixture may separate into its different constituents. The only stored gas mixture in common use in anaesthesia is Entonox (50% O_2: 50% N_2O). The critical temperature of N_2O is 36.5°C, but the interaction with oxygen lowers this to −5.5°C (its pseudocritical temperature). Thus, below −6°C, liquefaction of nitrous oxide takes place. This is potentially dangerous because, although at this point the N_2O has about 20% oxygen dissolved in it, as the oxygen-rich supernatant is drawn off, the oxygen in the liquid comes out of solution, leading eventually to the delivery of a hypoxic mixture.

Direction the viva may take

You may be asked about the relevance of these concepts for clinical practice.

- **N_2O cylinders:** the critical temperature of N_2O is 36.5°C, and so under normal circumstances in temperate climates it is stored in a liquid phase with its vapour above it. In the UK the filling ratio (the mass of gas in the cylinder divided by the mass of water that would completely fill the cylinder) is 0.75, to allow for expansion and to limit increases in pressure. As the liquid expands it compresses its vapour, some of which then condenses back to a liquid and restricts the pressure rise. In hotter climates the filling ratio is 0.67. If a N_2O cylinder is used continuously, it will cool as it vaporizes and the saturated vapour and gauge pressures will drop. If the gas is turned off, then both will be restored to normal as the cylinder rewarms. The belief that the gauge pressure will remain unchanged until the moment just before the cylinder empties is a misconception.
- **Oxygen supplies:** liquid oxygen must be kept at a temperature lower than its critical temperature of 118°C (page 295).
- **Vaporization of volatile anaesthetic agents:** see page 302.
- **Water vapour and humidification:** see page 332.

Pressure

Commentary

Pressures and their measurement are so much part of anaesthesia that it is not surprising to find them appearing as examination topics. The viva may start with any one of the disparate clinical implications before moving on to the underlying principles of definition and measurement. Alternatively, some of the basic science outlined below may form part of an oral on one of many potential subjects.

The viva

You may be asked about one of the situations in which physiological pressures may be important in anaesthetic practice.

- **Non-invasive blood pressure:** automatic machines utilize the oscillometric principle. The movement of the arterial wall is transmitted to the cuff and the pressure changes are sensed by a transducer. Above systolic pressure and below diastolic pressure, the oscillations are minimal. As the cuff deflates automatically to systolic pressure, oscillations begin and increase in amplitude until mean blood pressure is reached, after which the amplitude decreases until the diastolic pressure point is reached. The fluctuations are analysed by a microprocessor prior to being displayed digitally.
- **Invasive blood pressure:** see page 319.
- **Central venous pressure:** see page 104.
- **Intravascular pressures – Laplace's law:** in a tube, such as the aorta, the transmural pressure gradient is given by the wall tension divided by the radius ($P = T/r$). For a sphere the relationship is $P = 2T/r$. This pressure relationship explains why an expanding aortic aneurysm is increasingly likely to rupture as the aorta dilates, and why a reservoir bag on a breathing circuit does not cause barotrauma to normal lungs if it is allowed to distend by tightening the valve.
- **The Venturi principle:** flowing gas contains potential energy (from its pressure) and kinetic energy (associated with its flow). At a constriction the flow, and hence the kinetic energy of the gas, increases. The total amount of energy must remain constant and so the potential energy, and hence the pressure, decreases, allowing the entrainment of gas or fluid.
- **Intracranial pressure:** see page 143.
- **Intrapleural pressures:** see page 102.
- **Intraocular pressure:** see page 151. The normal value is 10–22 mmHg and its prime determinants are choroidal bloodflow and volume (influenced by $PaCO_2$, venous drainage, hypoxia), the formation and drainage of aqueous humour, and external pressure on the globe by contraction of extraocular muscles and of the orbicularis oculi muscle (or by orbital local anaesthetic or retrobulbar haemorrhage). Coughing, straining or vomiting will transiently increase the pressure by 40 mmHg or more.

Direction the viva may take

The discussion may then move on to definitions and methods of measurement.

- **Definitions:** pressure is defined as force per unit area, force being that which changes or tends to change the state of rest or motion of an object. The unit of force is the newton (N), 1 N being that force which will accelerate a (frictionless) mass of 1 kg at $1 \, m \, s^{-2}$ (in a vacuum). The SI unit of pressure is the pascal (Pa), 1 pascal being a force of 1 N acting over an area of $1 \, m^2$. Gravity gives any mass an acceleration of $9.81 \, m \, s^{-2}$, so the force acting on 1 kg is 9.81 N. 1 N is therefore equivalent to 102 g. This is a small pressure, hence the use of the kilopascal (kPa) as the main unit of physiological pressure. Higher pressures are still quoted in bar (1 bar = 100 kPa = 1 atmosphere).
- (The relationship between force and pressure explains why a small syringe can generate far higher pressures than a larger one. The pressure developed is force divided by area. The smaller the area represented by the plunger in the syringe, then the greater is the pressure generated for a given applied force; hence a 2 ml syringe is much more effective than a 10 ml syringe in flushing a blocked intravenous catheter.)
- **Absolute pressure and gauge pressure:** an empty gas cylinder has a gauge pressure of zero, but the ambient pressure inside the cylinder is 1 atmosphere. Absolute pressure, therefore, is given by the gauge pressure plus atmospheric pressure.
- **Measurement**
  - *Liquid manometry:* the pressure in the column is equal to the product of the height of the column, the density of the liquid and the force of gravity. The width and shape of the column have no effect on the pressure reading. Surface tension provides a potential source of error in columns less than 10 mm in diameter, but in the clinical context of central venous pressure measurement, in which trends are commonly more important than absolute numbers, this is not significant.
  - *Aneroid gauges:* examples include the Bourdon gauge for high pressures, which comprises a flattened coiled tube which unwinds as pressures increase.
  - *Diaphragm gauges:* these are used for many physiological pressures. Pressure changes cause movement in a flexible diaphragm, and these are either read directly or transduced. Electromechanical devices are probably the commonest, employing wire strain gauges whose resistance changes in response to pressure. The sensing diaphragm can also be incorporated as one plate of a capacitor, the other being fixed. The charge that is carried varies with the separation of the plates.

Direction the viva will take

The discussion may include non-physiological pressures, of which the most obvious are those in gas pipelines and cylinders (pages 294–296).

Intra-arterial blood pressure measurement

Commentary

Invasive arterial blood pressure monitoring is a routine part of modern anaesthetic and intensive care practice and so the viva will include clinical aspects such as indications and complications. The rest of the oral will concentrate on the physics that underlies the behaviour of a measurement system. You will not, however, be asked to discuss Fourier analysis of complex waveforms; time constraints will not allow it and it would take the questioning too far away from applied clinical science. Make sure, none the less, that you can draw the main arterial waveforms because these are relevant to clinical practice.

The viva

You may be asked for some indications for invasive arterial blood pressure monitoring.

- **Indications:** these are not difficult to define. Intra-arterial monitoring gives beat-to-beat information which is particularly useful in patients with actual or potential cardiovascular instability. It is used routinely in the critically ill, both to measure pressures and to allow arterial blood gas analysis. It is helpful in high-risk patients undergoing surgery, and in patients facing high-risk surgery. Many anaesthetists would also regard its use as mandatory whenever intravenous vasoactive drugs are used to manipulate the blood pressure. It may also be indicated in very obese patients whose size makes other methods of blood pressure monitoring inaccurate.

This may move on to the additional information that such monitoring may provide.

- **Information:** this is not confined purely to numbers (Figure 5.6). The slope of the systolic upstroke gives some indication of the contractile state of the myocardium,

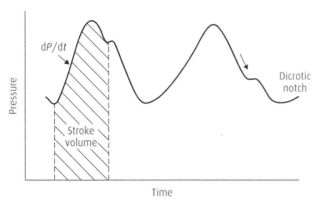

Fig. 5.6 The arterial pressure waveform.

and the maximum rate of rise of left ventricular pressure (dP/dt max) can be calculated. The area under the curve up to the position of the dicrotic notch gives an indication of stroke volume, and the position of the dicrotic notch on the downstroke of the waveform reflects systemic vascular resistance. In the presence of peripheral vasoconstriction, the dicrotic notch is high; if there is vasodilatation, then it moves lower down the curve. Pressure changes during IPPV can also be significant; a systolic pressure variation between the maximum and minimum recorded during the respiratory cycle of more than 10 mmHg suggests at least a 10% reduction in circulating volume.

Direction the viva may take

You may then be invited to describe the components of a system for direct blood pressure measurement, before being asked to explain how the arterial waveform is generated.

- The basic system for invasive blood pressure measurement comprises a parallel-walled intra-arterial cannula, a column of saline which is in continuity with blood, and a transducer (a device that converts the mechanical energy into an electrical signal that is processed and displayed on a monitor). The column of saline is pressurized to 300 mmHg and incorporates a manual flushing device.
- The fluid-filled catheter is in direct contact with the diaphragm of the transducer. Movement of this diaphragm is associated with alteration in the length of a strain gauge, which in some transducers is in the form of a wire resistor in a Wheatstone bridge circuit. (This contains four resistances, one of which is a strain gauge, another of which is variable. The variable resistance can be altered so that when $R_1/R_2 = R_3/R_4$ there is no current flow.) Most transducers include four strain gauges, comprising the four resistances of the bridge. The resistances of two gauges at opposite sides of the bridge are designed to increase as the pressure increases, while the resistances of the other two decrease. This gives rise to a larger potential change, with a deflection in the galvanometer that is amplified and displayed as a pressure.
- This whole system oscillates at the frequency of the arterial pulse, which is the fundamental frequency (the first harmonic). The arterial pressure waveform, however, comprises a series of sine waves of different frequencies and amplitude. For the system to reproduce the amplitude and phase difference of each harmonic to produce an accurate waveform, it requires a frequency response that is around 10 times the fundamental frequency (the heart rate). If the heart rate is 150 beats per minute the frequency response would need to be $(150 \times 10)/60 = 25$ Hz. The more rapid the rate of pressure change, the greater the number of harmonics. In practice, this means that the system requires a flat frequency response between 0.5 and 30 Hz.
- To reproduce the arterial waveform accurately, any recording system must also reproduce the amplitude and phase difference of each harmonic in the waveform. The system, therefore, needs a high resonant (or natural) frequency, which can then be optimally damped.
- This natural frequency is the frequency at which any system will resonate, and at which amplification of the signal will occur. If this frequency lies within the range

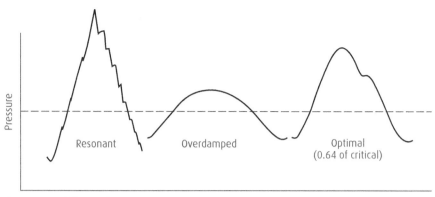

Fig. 5.7 Arterial waveforms.

of frequencies that comprise the pressure waveform, then that signal may be distorted by the superimposed sine wave that will be generated.

- The resonant frequency of the pressure-measuring system can be manipulated by altering the characteristics of its components. It is directly proportional to the diameter of the catheter, and is inversely proportional to the square root of the compliance or elasticity of the system, to the square root of the length of tubing, and to the square root of the density of the fluid within the system. This has clinical relevance, because stiffening the diaphragm of the transducer, shortening the length of the intra-arterial cannula or increasing its diameter, will lift the resonant frequency out of the frequency response range.
- If there is no damping, the system oscillates at its natural frequency. If the system is overdamped, the recorded signal falls slowly to the baseline. This can occur when there ceases to be free communication between the column of blood and the diaphragm of the transducer. A large air bubble, for example, will absorb pressure due to its compressibility, while clot or debris will restrict the pressure transmission even more effectively. The whole waveform trace is flattened as a result. If the damping is adjusted so that the output signal falls more rapidly to the baseline, but without any overshoot, then the system is described as being critically damped. In this situation, the amplitude is registered accurately but the speed of response is too slow. The best compromise between speed and accuracy is when the system is optimally damped, which is at 0.64 of critical. An underdamped waveform will increase systolic and decrease diastolic pressures, while an overdamped signal will decrease both (Figure 5.7). The mean arterial pressure in both instances will (largely) be unchanged.

Further direction the viva could take

If you have covered the main information you may be asked briefly about complications.

- **Complications:** vascular damage distal to the cannula may follow because of direct occlusion, of later occlusion due to thrombosis, or as a result of inadvertent intra-arterial injection (page 80). Disconnection is a potential hazard; fatal exsanguination can occur should it go unrecognized. Long-term cannulation, as is common in intensive care patients, may also be complicated by infection.

Measurement of organ blood flow

Commentary

This question may no longer stand alone, but details of these methods of determining flow may form part of questions on other topics. Examiners are likely to concentrate more on those methods that are useful clinically, such as Doppler ultrasonography and techniques based on the Fick principle.

The viva

You may be asked to describe how you can determine blood flow.

- **Direct cannulation and measurement:** this is possible, but impractical in any clinical context.
- **Doppler ultrasonography:** the Doppler effect describes the change in the frequency of sound (including ultrasound) if either the emitter or the receiver is moving. If a noise source, for example a siren, moves towards a listener, the wavelength of the sound decreases, its frequency increases, and so its pitch rises. This principle is utilized in Doppler ultrasonography, in which ultrasound is directed at a diagonal from one crystal and is sensed by a second crystal as it reflects off red blood cells. The frequency of these reflected waves increases by an amount that is proportional to the velocity of flow towards the receiving crystal. It is difficult to calibrate a Doppler ultrasound probe to provide accurate quantitative measurements because determinations of vessel calibre may be inaccurate, and the shape of the flow profile may not be uniform. None the less, the technique can provide some assessment of the adequacy of flow, particularly after vascular surgery to the carotid arteries or to vessels of the lower limb. It can also be used to give a non-invasive determination of cardiac output by measuring velocity in the arch of the aorta and relating it to aortic diameter. Transcranial Doppler ultrasonography can be used to give a measure of flow through large cerebral arteries.
- **The Fick principle:** this is the basis of several methods which are used to measure both cardiac output and regional blood flow. It underlies thermal and chemical indicator dilution tests, renal clearance estimations and measurement of cerebral blood flow. It has been described as an application of the law of conservation of matter, in that the uptake or excretion of a substance by an organ or tissue must be equal to the difference between the amount entering the organ (arterial flow×concentration) and the amount leaving the organ (venous flow×venous concentration). Rearrangement of this relationship gives the familiar formula, namely that: blood flow to an organ = rate of uptake or rate of excretion of a substance/arteriovenous concentration. If oxygen is used as the substance, for example, then cardiac output is given by: O_2 consumption (ml min^{-1}) / AV DO_2 (ml l^{-1}). (The Fick principle applies only to situations in which the arterial supply presents the only source of the substance that is taken up.)

- **Indicator dilution methods:** the commonest method in clinical use is the thermodilution technique for measuring cardiac output. Injection and sampling are both carried out via a catheter in the right side of the heart. Cold fluid (such as glucose 5% at 0°C) is injected into the right atrium, and the temperature change is detected by a thermistor at the distal end of the flotation catheter in the pulmonary artery. The recorded temperatures generate a concentration against time dilution curve analogous to that which would be seen had a chemical indicator been used. The equation that is used is: Flow (cardiac output) = 'heat dose' × 60/average concentration (AUC) × time (s). The injectate–blood temperature difference multiplied by the density, specific heat and volume of the injectate gives the numerator (the heat dose). The area under the curve (AUC) multiplied by the density and specific heat of blood gives the denominator. The potential complexity of these calculations means that the cardiac output determinations are computer-generated.
- **Electromagnetic flowmeters:** if a conductor (such as blood) flows at right angles to a magnetic field, then an electromotive force is induced which is perpendicular to the magnetic field and to the direction of fluid flow. The induced voltage is proportional to the strength of the field and to the velocity of blood flow. A determination of the diameter of the vessel allows calculation of flow.
- **Para-amino hippuric acid (PAH) clearance:** the clearance of PAH is used to determine renal blood flow, also using the Fick principle. PAH is not utilized or excreted by any other organ apart from the kidney, and so the peripheral venous PAH concentration will equal the arterial. Renal PAH uptake is given by the product of the urinary PAH concentration [U] and urinary volume (V). The final simplified equation is the same as that for PAH clearance: Renal blood flow = $[U] \times V/[P]$ Where $[P]$ is plasma PAH concentration. This actually measures plasma flow, because blood is not filtered at the glomerulus and the volume from which PAH is removed is plasma. Blood flow can thereafter be calculated if the haematocrit is known.
- **The Kety–Schmidt method:** this is an adaptation of the Fick principle which is used to make a global determination of cerebral blood flow (page 149).
- **PET and SPECT scanning:** positron emission tomography (PET) is a technique which monitors the uptake by different areas of the brain of 2-deoxyglucose labelled with a positron emitter. Scintillography and SPECT scanning use radioactive xenon to trace regional blood flow, with or without enhancement by CT or MR imaging.

Measurement of cardiac output

Commentary

Devices that determine cardiac output (CO) are popular; whether this popularity is deserved remains contentious. Certainly there are experienced anaesthetists and intensivists who believe that the ability to measure CO neither improves nor affects outcome. This debate is unlikely to occupy much of the viva, although the PACMAN study may warrant brief discussion. As there are now several different methods available, you are more likely to be asked to give a brief description rather than a detailed analysis. Moreover, many of the equations that are applied are quite complex; for example, determination of blood flow velocity using Doppler ultrasound is given by (v) velocity $= 2 \times$ ultrasound frequency (Fo)/ constant $\times$ Doppler shift (Fd) $\times \mathrm{Cos}\theta$, yet this is only part of the calculation. There is unlikely to be the time to explore this science in any detail.

The viva

You may be asked the rationale for measuring CO.

- CO delivers oxygen to tissues. Its prime determinants are heart rate and stroke volume (SV), in turn influenced by venous filling (preload), systemic vascular resistance (afterload), and myocardial contractility. Low CO states predict adverse outcomes both in the critically ill and in patients undergoing major surgery.

You will then be asked about some of the different methods of measuring CO.

- **Pulmonary artery flotation catheter (PAC):** although the use of the PAC has all but disappeared from most critical care units, it is still regarded as the most accurate method of determining CO, and is the one against which other techniques are judged. The principles of measurement are described on page 323.
- **Oesophageal Doppler monitor (ODM):** this non-invasive ultrasonic device measures the velocity of blood flow in the descending thoracic aorta. The shift in frequency is proportional to the velocity of ejected blood. The device generates a velocity/time waveform to which is applied a calibration factor derived from the patient's height, weight and age. The SV is then derived from the flow velocity, ejection time and aortic area. (A second transducer measures the cross-sectional area of the aorta.) The useful indices that the ODM produces are the CO, the SV and the corrected systolic flow time (FT_c). The FT_c is normally between 330 and 360 ms and is an indicator of volaemic status; a low (short) FT_c is associated with inadequate filling. Softer and smaller probes introduced nasally allow this technique to be used in the awake patient. Flow through the descending aorta is only around 70% of the total CO (the remainder is distributed through the subclavian arteries to the head, neck and upper limbs), but the device corrects for this proportion.
- **Transoesophageal echocardiography (TOE):** (see page 339). This technique also uses Doppler ultrasound. The TOE probe allows 180° views of the heart, and not only measures CO but also gives a range of information about ventricular function, wall motion abnormalities and valvular anatomy. It is very operator-dependent.
- **Pulse contour analysis:** it has long been recognized that arterial pressure changes during respiration may be an indicator of volaemic status and that a systolic pressure variation between the maximum and minimum recorded during one cycle of IPPV of more than 10 mmHg suggests at least a 10% reduction in circulating volume. Pulse contour analysis examines the arterial waveform, quantifies the SV and calculates the stroke volume variation (SVV). It is used both in LiDCO and PiCCO (see below).

- **Lithium dilution (LiDCO):** this is a bolus indicator dilution method of measuring CO. After intravenous injection of a small dose of lithium (0.15 mmol), the plasma concentration is measured by an ion-selective electrode attached to the arterial line. The resulting concentration/time curve allows the calculation of CO (given by: dose × 60/mean concentration (AUC) × time (s)). LiDCO can be used in combination with pulse contour analysis to provide continuous readings of CO, SV and SVV. (The technique cannot be used in patients who are receiving therapeutic lithium, nor in the first trimester of pregnancy.)
- **Pulse contour CO (PiCCO):** this technique uses a thermodilution technique in conjunction with pulse contour waveform analysis. Cold saline is injected through into a central vein and temperature is measured by a thermistor in an arterial cannula sited in a large artery (such as the brachial or femoral). This thermodilution CO measurement calibrates the system, after which the arterial waveform is analysed to produce beat-to-beat determinations of SV, SVV and a continuous measure of CO. (It is also claimed that PiCCO can provide information about other volumetric parameters: global end-diastolic volume (GEDV), intrathoracic blood volume (ITBV), and extravascular lung water (EVLW). You will not be asked how it does so.)
- **Thoracic electrical bioimpedance:** as the name suggests, this technique involves measuring the resistance to current flow through the thorax. This resistance changes both with the respiratory cycle and with pulsatile blood flow. High-frequency low-amplitude alternating current is emitted and sensed via electrodes on the neck and lower chest wall. Changes in impedance are detected as blood distends and then leaves the aorta. These changes allow continuous determinations of CO, SV, contractile state and SVR. The technique tends to over-estimate CO.

Direction the viva may take

You may be asked whether there is any evidence to support the use of these devices.

- The short answer is that there is none. The closest attempt to provide some evidence came in the form of the multicentre 'Pulmonary Artery Catheters in Patient Management (PACMAN)' study which investigated whether the use of PA catheters reduced hospital mortality in the critically ill (it was published in 2005). Over 1000 critically ill patients were randomized either to receive a PAC or to a control group in which management did not involve a PAC but could include the use of other devices to measure CO. There was no overall evidence of benefit or harm. (The 10% complication rate related largely to central venous access rather than the PAC itself.) The study was not flawless; there were, for example, no objective inclusion criteria, only the opinion of a clinician that a PAC was indicated. The fact that 80% of the patients in the no-PAC group had CO measured by a different means was potentially confounding, and sceptics were quick to point out that the outcomes in the other 20% of patients who had no CO measurement at all were very similar to those in patients who had PACs. Definitive evidence, therefore, will come only from one or more randomized controlled trials which compare CO measurement against none.

Jugular venous bulb oxygen saturation (SjVO$_2$)

Commentary

Jugular venous bulb oxygen saturation (SjVO$_2$) provides a measure of global cerebral oxygenation and finds uses in neurosurgery, in neurotrauma and in cerebral monitoring during cardiac surgery. This is an area of specialist practice which you may well not have encountered. If you are able to base your answer on first principles, it is likely that the examiners will make some allowances for lack of subspecialty knowledge.

The viva

The topic may be introduced via a question about the clinical value of this investigation, before you are asked how it can be measured.

- SjVO$_2$ is an indirect indicator of cerebral oxygen utilization.
- SjVO$_2$ is usually measured via an intravascular catheter which is threaded retrogradely up the internal jugular vein as far as the superior jugular bulb. (The jugular bulb is a dilatation at the origin of the vein, and lies just below the posterior part of the floor of the tympanic cavity.) The normal value is 55–75%.
- A fibreoptic catheter uses reflectance oximetry (as in pulmonary arterial catheter monitoring of mixed venous saturation) to provide continuous SjVO$_2$ monitoring. As with pulse oximetry, the apparatus uses the light absorption spectra of haemoglobin and deoxyhaemoglobin.
- Catheter placement can be facilitated by locating the vessel using ultrasound, and is verified by lateral skull X-ray, which should confirm the tip lying at the level of, and medial to, the mastoid process.
- Alternatively, a sample may be taken directly from the jugular bulb and the oxygen saturation measured by co-oximetry.

Direction the viva may take

You are likely to be asked to discuss in more detail the clinical value of SjVO$_2$ measurements.

- SjVO$_2$ is an indirect indicator of cerebral oxygen utilization: when O$_2$ demand exceeds supply, then O$_2$ extraction increases and SjVO$_2$ falls (desaturated at <50%). Conversely, when supply exceeds demand the SjVO$_2$ rises (luxuriant at >75%). Bulb O$_2$ saturation can be used as a specific measure of global cerebral oxygenation but it cannot provide information about smaller focal areas of ischaemia.
- The difference in oxygen content between arterial and jugular venous blood (AjvDO$_2$) is given by CMRO$_2$/CBF (cerebral metabolic rate for O$_2$/cerebral blood flow). The normal value is 4–8 ml O$_2$/100 ml of blood.
- If AjvDO$_2$ is <4, supply is luxuriant; if >8 it suggests ischaemia.
- **Factors decreasing SjVO$_2$:** an increased oxygen demand or a decrease in supply (leading to a fall in SjVO$_2$ and rise in AjvDO$_2$) results from raised intracranial pressure (ICP), severe systemic hypotension, hypocapnia (<3.75 kPa), arterial

hypoxia, seizure activity and cerebral vasospasm. During rewarming after profound hypothermia, the $SjVO_2$ may be below 40%, reflecting maximal O_2 extraction. It will also fall if the patient is pyrexial and in response to increased metabolic demand. A decrease in $SjVO_2$ always indicates potential cerebral dysfunction.

- **Factors increasing $SjVO_2$:** a decreased O_2 demand or increase in supply (leading to a rise in $SjVO_2$ and fall in $AjvDO_2$) results from decreased metabolic demand (such as occurs with hypothermia or sedation), brain death (in which there is minimal demand), an increased blood supply, hypercapnia and arterial hyperoxia. An increase in $SjVO_2$ may also presage cerebral damage.

Temperature and its measurement

Commentary

The maintenance and control of body temperature are of evident importance in clinical anaesthetic practice. It is more difficult to see how an intimate knowledge of thermistors and thermocouples is especially helpful, but this will form the bulk of the science component of the question.

The viva

You may be asked first about the clinical consequences of hypothermia. This is covered in more detail on page 330 and so the following is an outline summary.

- **Cardiorespiratory effects:** oxygen consumption increases and cardiac output decreases. Arrhythmias and myocardial ischaemia are more likely. The oxygen–haemoglobin dissociation curve shifts to the left and reduces oxygen delivery. Blood viscosity increases.
- **Coagulation:** platelet function is impaired, intraoperative blood loss increases, and transfusion requirements rise.
- **Metabolic effects and effects on drugs:** within a few degrees of normal core temperature, metabolic rate decreases by 6–7% for each 1°C fall. Enzymatic reactions and intermediary metabolism are slower at core temperatures below 34°C. Drug actions are prolonged, especially those of muscle relaxants. Glucose utilization decreases and hyperglycaemia can result. Metabolic acidosis may supervene.
- **Surgical outcome:** hypothermia compromises immune function and increases postoperative infection rates. Wound healing is adversely affected and hospital stay may be extended.

Direction the viva will take

You will then be asked about methods of measuring temperature.

- Heat is an energy form related to the activity, or kinetic energy in the molecules of the particular substance. Temperature is a way of quantifying the thermal state of a substance.

- **Units of measurement:** the SI unit is the Kelvin (K), which equals Celsius (°C) plus 273.15. As 1° is the same as 1 K, the unit is used universally in medicine.
- Most of the body heat content (66%) lies within the central core compartment comprising the brain and the organs of the trunk, whose temperature is maintained between 36.5 and 37.5°C. The remaining 33% is accounted for by the periphery, the temperature of which can undergo much wider fluctuation. It is essential, therefore, to measure core temperature.
- There are three main types of device for measuring temperature: electrical, non-electrical and infrared.
- **Electrical**
  - *Thermistor:* a small bead of a semiconductor material, usually a metal oxide, is incorporated into a Wheatstone bridge circuit. The resistance of the bead decreases exponentially as the temperature rises. These beads are both robust and very small, and are used in the tips of pulmonary artery flotation catheters and in arterial lines for thermodilution measurements.
  - *Thermocouple:* if two dissimilar metals are joined, a small potential difference develops which is proportional to the temperature of the junction. (This is known as the Seebeck effect.) Another junction between the metals is necessary to complete an electrical circuit, although another temperature-dependent voltage will develop at this junction. The metals that are used are commonly copper and a copper/nickel alloy. When the thermocouple is used as a thermometer, one of the junctions forms the temperature probe, while the other is kept at a constant temperature and acts as a reference. Thermocouples are stable and accurate to ±0.1°C.
  - *Resistance thermometer:* these are based on the principle that electrical resistance in metals shows a linear increase with temperature. These systems are not used clinically.
- **Non-electrical**
  - *Mercury and alcohol thermometers:* volume increases with temperature. Like all thermometers, these are calibrated against fixed points, such as the triple point (at which water, water vapour and ice are in equilibrium) and boiling point of water.
  - *Dial thermometers:* these may use a coil comprising two metals with differential coefficients of expansion. As the temperature changes, the coil tightens and relaxes, and an attached lever moves across a calibrated dial.
- **Infrared**
  - *Tympanic membrane thermometers:* the living body emits infrared radiation, whose intensity and wavelength varies with temperature. This property is utilized in tympanic membrane thermometers. These use pyroelectric sensors, which comprise an electrically polarized substance whose polarization alters with temperature. This change can be used to generate an electrical output, which is proportional to the temperature. Their response time is very rapid compared with other types of clinical thermometer. The tympanic membrane is the favoured site for temperature measurement in anaesthesia because it offers the most accurate indication of cerebral temperature.

Further direction the viva could take

You may be asked finally about mechanisms by which patients lose heat. This is also covered in more detail below.

Mechanisms of heat loss

- **Radiation (50%):** the body is an efficient radiator, transferring heat from a hot to cooler objects.
- **Convection (30%):** air in the layer close to the body is warmed by conduction, rises as its temperature increases and is carried away by convection currents.
- **Evaporation (20–25%):** moisture on the body's surface evaporates, loses latent heat of vaporization and the body cools.
- **Conduction (3–5%):** this occurs only if the patient is lying unprotected on an efficient heat conductor.
- **Respiration (10%):** heat loss is via evaporation and the need to heat inspired air.
- **Anaesthesia:** this causes vasodilatation and also affects central thermoregulation.

Heat loss

Commentary

This topic incorporates some basic science and is also of clinical importance, given evidence of the morbidity that is associated with perioperative heat loss.

The viva

You may be asked about the clinical consequences of hypothermia. (This question is directed at mild falls in perioperative temperature rather than profound hypothermia, although if you have covered the basic ground then the questioning may extend to the latter.)

- Mild perioperative hypothermia, as defined by a fall in core temperature of 1–3°C, is common during anaesthesia. General anaesthesia not only causes vasodilatation and a diversion of core blood to the periphery, but it also decreases the threshold at which thermoregulatory vasoconstriction is activated. This leads to the rapid fall in temperature of 1–1.5°C that is seen in many patients undergoing even short procedures. As surgery continues, patients lose heat more slowly via the mechanisms described below. Typically this is of the order of 1°C over 2–3 hours. Usually the temperature reaches a plateau at this point which is where the lowered vasoconstriction threshold is activated, and where heat loss is compensated by metabolic heat production.
- Severe hypothermia occurs either as a result of environmental exposure or when a patient's body temperature is deliberately lowered to allow specialized forms of

surgery. In deep hypothermic circulatory arrest, the core temperature may be reduced as low as 15°C for aortic arch replacement or cerebral aneurysm repair.

- **Cardiorespiratory effects:** oxygen consumption increases during mild hypothermia, although it may increase by 500% during shivering as a patient rewarms. Cardiac output is decreased and hypothermia increases the incidence of arrhythmias. The oxygen–haemoglobin dissociation curve shifts to the left, increasing oxygen affinity and reducing oxygen delivery. Blood viscosity increases and, with it, the risk of intravascular sludging. Studies have suggested that a drop in core temperature to around 35°C is associated with a 6% incidence of myocardial ischaemia or arrhythmia (1% in control groups).
- **Coagulation:** hypothermia impairs platelet function such that intraoperative blood loss increases and with it the need for blood transfusion (demonstrated in patients undergoing total hip replacement).
- **Metabolic effects and effects on drugs:** metabolic rate decreases initially by around 6–7% for each 1°C fall in core temperature from normal. (This fall is exponential. At 15°C, for example, a further 1°C drop results in a decrease in $CMRO_2$ of only 1%.) Enzymatic reactions are slowed and all the reactions of intermediate metabolism are affected at core temperatures lower than 34°C. The effects of most drugs, therefore, are prolonged, particularly neuromuscular blocking agents whose duration of action at 35°C is extended by around 50%. Hypothermia leads to a progressive acidosis. Renal and hepatic function are depressed, but diuresis can result from the failure of active reabsorption of sodium and water. Hyperglycaemia may occur as glucose utilization falls.
- **CNS effects:** there is a progressive deterioration in mental function to the point at which the EEG will record no cerebral activity. This occurs at a core temperature of around 18°C. (The brain is still metabolically active and will exhaust energy substrate after around 25 minutes.)
- **Surgical outcome:** wound healing is adversely affected both because of the reduction in subcutaneous wound tissue oxygenation and because of direct impairment of neutrophil function. Thus, hypothermia compromises immune function and increases postoperative infection rates, with the result that hospital stay may be prolonged.
- **Prevention:** heat losses owing to the mechanisms above can be minimized by the use, for example, of insulated operating table warmers, heat and moisture exchangers in the breathing system, warm air blankets, warmed infused fluids and protection of the head. (A litre of blood infused at 4°C can lower core temperature by 0.5° C.)

Direction the viva will take
You will be asked about mechanisms by which patients lose heat during anaesthesia.

Mechanisms of heat loss
- **Radiation:** this is the most important mechanism and may account for 50% or more of heat loss. The body is a highly efficient radiator, transferring heat from a

hot to cooler objects. The process is accelerated during anaesthesia if the patient is surrounded by cool objects and prevented from receiving radiant heat from the environment. Further heat loss will also occur if the body is forced to heat cold infused fluids up to 37°C.

- **Convection:** this accounts for up to 30% of heat loss. Air in the layer close to the body is warmed by conduction, rises as its temperature increases and is carried away by convection currents. The process is accelerated during anaesthesia if a large surface area is exposed to convection currents (particularly in laminar flow theatres).
- **Evaporation:** this accounts for some 20–25% of heat loss. As moisture on the body's surface evaporates, it loses latent heat of vaporization and the body cools. This is a highly developed mechanism for heat loss in health, but undesirable during surgery. It is accelerated during anaesthesia if there is a large moist surface area open to atmosphere (especially in major intra-abdominal surgery, intrathoracic surgery, reconstructive plastic surgery and major orthopaedic surgery).
- **Conduction:** this is not a significant cause of heat loss during normal circumstances, accounting for only 3–5% of the total. Heat loss by this mechanism increases during anaesthesia only if the patient is lying unprotected on an efficient heat conductor such as metal table.
- **Respiration:** heat loss occurs due to evaporation and the heating of inspired air. This amounts to around 10% of the total but it can be minimized during anaesthesia by the use of heat and moisture exchangers.

Further direction the viva may take

You may be asked about the management of severe hypothermia.

- The examiner is much less interested in the generic approach (investigation of any underlying cause after attention to Airway, Breathing and Circulation) than in specific details of rewarming.
- Passive warming is effective only when the patient's heat-generating mechanisms are intact. Moderate and severe hypothermia requires active warming. Techniques include the use of external heat sources (forced warm air blankets, radiant heaters) and internal warming. This can be via the use of warm intravenous, intragastric and intraperitoneal fluids, as well as by bladder irrigation via a urinary catheter. The most efficient, but most invasive method, of rewarming is cardiopulmonary bypass. This can raise the core temperature by around 1°C every 5 minutes. Although other extracorporeal systems such as haemofiltration units lack rapid flow rates, veno–venous systems using counter-current blood warmers can raise core temperatures by 2°C an hour. The rate of rewarming is important. While some believe that fast rewarming is preferable following rapid onset hypothermia (such as sudden immersion), it is more usual to raise the core temperature gradually, by 1–2°C an hour. Even slow rewarming is associated with significant problems, including persistent temperature variation between organs, reperfusion injury, and 'rewarming shock' as the patient vasodilates too rapidly for the rate of fluid replacement.

Humidification (of inspired gases)

Commentary

This is a standard subject. Artificial humidification of dry inspired gases is important in the context both of anaesthesia and intensive care, and so you will be expected to know about the different methods that are commonly used. Although the methods of measurement are of limited clinical relevance, they may still be introduced as a means of bulking out what is not a very complex topic.

The viva

You will be asked about the clinical importance of humidification, and the patients for whom it is particularly relevant.

- The consequences of failure to humidify gases include drying and keratinization of parts of the tracheobronchial tree, reduction of ciliary activity and impairment of the mucociliary escalator. In addition, there may be inflammatory change in the ciliated pulmonary epithelium, drying and crusting of secretions, mucus plugging, atelectasis, superimposed chest infection, and impaired gas exchange. Finally, heat loss may occur via latent heat of vaporization as dry anaesthetic gas is humidified in the respiratory tract.
- Particular patients at risk include those undergoing prolonged anaesthesia and those with pre-existing respiratory disease in whom the impairment of important pulmonary defence functions will be more significant. Those at the extremes of age are at risk (neonates, infants and the elderly), as are all intensive care patients.
- It is also of some importance to maintain the relative humidity of the operating theatre environment at an appropriate level. High humidity is uncomfortable, and low humidity increases the risk of static sparks.

You will then be asked about the physical principles and methods of humidification. Humidity is expressed in one of two ways.

- **Absolute humidity:** this is defined by the mass of water vapour that is present in a given volume of air. The SI unit is $g\,m^{-3}$. Absolute humidity is temperature-dependent: at 20°C it is 17 $g\,m^{-3}$, whereas at 37°C it is 44 $g\,m^{-3}$.
- **Relative humidity:** this is the ratio of the mass of water in a given volume of air to the mass of water in the same volume were it to be fully saturated. It is usually expressed as a percentage.

Methods of humidification

- **HME (heat and moisture exchange) filter:** This is a widely used method, which is passive, and which cannot therefore attain 100% efficiency, but which may reach 70%. The HME contains a hygroscopic material within a sealed unit. As the warm expired gas cools so the water vapour condenses on the element, which is warmed both by the specific heat of the exhaled gas and the latent heat of the water. Inhaled, dry and cool gas is thus warmed during inspiration, during which process the element cools down prior to the next exhalation. Problems include moderate inefficiency with prolonged use, increased dead space and infection risk.

- **Water bath (cold):** this system is passive, in that dry gases bubble through water at room temperature. It is inefficient (~30%) and becomes even more so as the loss of latent heat of vaporization cools the water further.
- **Water bath (warm):** this system is active, in that dry gases bubble through water which is heated, usually to 60°C (to inhibit microbial contamination). These can achieve efficiencies of greater than 90%. They are more complex and there is a risk of thermal injury to the patient (which is minimized by thermostats).
- **Cascade humidifier:** this is a variation on the warm water bath. Gas is allowed to bubble through a perforated plate; this process maximizes the surface area which is exposed to water.
- **Nebulizers:** these can also be used as active humidifiers. A high-pressure gas stream is directed on to an anvil and entrains water which then breaks into droplets. There are also ultrasonic devices in which water is nebulized by a plate that vibrates at ultrasonic frequencies. These are not in common use as humidifiers, because they can deliver gas with greater than 100% relative humidity and may therefore overload the pulmonary tree with fluid.
- **Droplet size:** droplets of 1 micron (μm) will be deposited in the alveoli. This is optimal. Smaller droplets may simply pass in and out with the respiratory cycle. Larger droplets (5 μm) risk being deposited in the trachea, which may help loosen secretions, but will not humidify the distal airways (nor deliver a drug dose effectively). Larger droplets still, of 20 μm and above, will not travel further than the upper airway and may condense out in the equipment tubing itself.

Direction the viva could take

You may finally be asked about methods of measuring humidity. In common with most other anaesthetists on the planet you will probably never have done this, and so you should not have to take this part of the subject very far.

- **Hair hygrometer:** the hair, which is linked to a spring and pointer, elongates as humidity increases. It is accurate between relative humidity measurements of about 30% and 90%.
- **Wet and dry bulb hygrometer:** this is a cumbersome technique. The temperature difference between two thermometers relates to evaporation of water round the wet bulb, which in turn relates to ambient humidity. The figure is calculated from tables.
- **Regnault's hygrometer:** this is a more accurate technique in which air is blown through ether within a silver tube. The temperature at which condensation appears on the outer surface is the dew point, the temperature at which ambient air is fully saturated. The ratio of the saturated vapour pressure (SVP) at the dew point to the SVP at ambient temperature gives the relative humidity. The result is determined from tables.
- **Transducers:** as a substance absorbs atmospheric water, there is a change either in capacitance or in electrical resistance.

- **Mass spectrometer:** this is very accurate and has a rapid (breath-by-breath) response time. The equipment is expensive.

Lasers

Commentary

The subject of lasers reappears in the exam mainly because of safety issues. In practice, and with one exception, these concerns are modest; clearly staff and patients must be protected from potential harm, but the actual precautions required to achieve that aim are not complex. The exception is in ENT surgery where there is risk of instant conflagration if a laser beam hits an unprotected endotracheal tube. This aspect of the subject will not, however, extend to 8 minutes of questioning, hence the need for you to familiarize yourself with aspects of the basic science.

The viva

You will be asked to define 'laser' and to describe how these instruments work.

- 'LASER' is an acronym: **L**ight **A**mplification by **S**timulated **E**mission of **R**adiation.
- A laser produces a non-divergent intense beam of light, which is of a single wavelength (is monochromatic).
- It is produced by directing an energy source such as an intense flash of light or a high-voltage discharge into a lasing medium. Atoms within the medium absorb the photons of absorbed energy, which drive their electrons to a higher energy level. As the excited atom falls back to its stable state, it emits a photon of energy. If this is reflected back to encounter another excited atom, then another photon will be emitted which is parallel to, and in phase with, the first. Multiple reflection by mirrors back into the lasing medium is used to generate a chain reaction which then produces an intense parallel beam of light.
- The wavelength of the light is dependent on the lasing medium that is used. The lasing medium may be a gas, such as carbon dioxide, argon or helium, a solid such as neodymium: yttrium-aluminium garnet (Nd:YAG) or a liquid. There are many varieties of laser; some relevant examples are outlined below.
  — *CO_2 lasers:* these produce infrared light (10 600 nm) whose energy is absorbed by water, which is vaporized. These lasers penetrate tissue no further than 200 μm and so are used for cutting superficial tissues. The beam simultaneously coagulates blood vessels.
  — *Argon:* blue–green argon laser light (480 nm) penetrates between 0.5 and 2 mm and is absorbed maximally by red tissues. It is used, for example, to treat diabetic retinopathy and skin lesions such as port wine birthmarks.
  — *Nd:YAG:* these lasers produce energy in the near infrared spectrum (1064 nm) and penetrate tissues deeply between 2 and 6 mm. The beam is invisible to the human eye and so is guided by a low-power laser light. At lower power it

denatures protein molecules; at higher power it vaporizes tissue and can be used for the surgical removal and debulking of large tumours.

— *Excimer lasers:* these are 'cold' ultraviolet lasers which do not heat tissues but which break chemical bonds. Their main use is in refractive corneal surgery.

Direction the viva may take

You will be asked about the practical safety implications for the use of lasers in theatre.

- The main danger is to the eyesight of theatre personnel. The non-divergent beam of laser light, even when reflected, may be focused on the fovea and cause irreversible blindness. Distance offers no protection. Other parts of the retina may also absorb the energy, as may the lens and the aqueous and vitreous humours. This does not apply to CO_2 lasers, which will not penetrate further than the cornea.
- Staff should be issued with goggles which protect specifically against the wavelength that is being generated, and, ideally, surgical instruments should have a matt finish to minimize the likelihood of reflection.
- There is a specific hazard associated with laser surgery to the upper airway. A normal PVC tracheal tube will ignite within a few seconds should it be exposed directly to a laser beam. Stainless steel foil has been used to protect tubes, but there are specially designed tracheal tubes available for use with laser surgery on the upper airway. Although these have flexible metal bodies (either stainless steel or aluminium), they still have cuffs and pilot balloons which should be filled with saline as a precaution. Surgical swabs or packs can also ignite, and so these must be kept moistened with saline.

Magnetic resonance imaging

Commentary

Magnetic resonance (MR) scanning has become the prime imaging technique for numerous soft tissue conditions, and for diseases which affect the CNS. But despite this status few anaesthetists have wide experience of anaesthetizing patients in this environment. The physics that underlies MR imaging (MRI) is also formidable. Why then does the topic continue to reappear in this part of the exam? It may be because the underlying science is elegant, and because the consequences of ignorance are potentially so disastrous.

The viva

You may be asked about the implications of delivering anaesthesia or sedation in an MR scanner.

- MRI requires the generation of very strong magnetic fields, typically up to 2.0 tesla. The devices use superconducting magnets which are cooled by immersion in liquid helium at a temperature of 4.2 Kelvin. It complements computerized tomography (CT) in providing high quality images of soft tissue.

- **Practical problems:** there are practical difficulties in relation to the physical environment. The patient is enclosed within a narrow tube to which access is limited. The scanner is noisy (>85 decibels) and some patients may be very claustrophobic. Scanning may be prolonged, with complex examinations lasting up to an hour.
- **Magnetic field:** at a magnetic field strength of approximately 50 gauss (indicated within the scanning room as a contour marked as the '50-gauss' line), all ferromagnetic items will be subject to movement and will also interfere with the generated image. Items typically affected include hypodermic needles, watches, pagers, stethoscopes, anaesthetic gas cylinders and ECG electrodes. If these items are close to the field they will become projectile objects.
- **Anaesthesia delivery:** anaesthetic machines which contain ferrous metals (there are non-magnetic machines and cylinders available) must remain outside the 50-gauss line. The machine requires very long anaesthetic tubing and long leads.
- **Anaesthetic monitoring:** the field may induce current within electric cabling. The consequent heating may lead to thermal injury. Long sampling leads for gas analysis extends delay. Standard ECG electrodes cannot be used. An oesophageal stethoscope may be useful. Pulse oximetry probes are non-ferrous, but a distal site should be used and cable should be insulated. Non-invasive blood pressure cuffs must have plastic connections as well as long leads to the machines, which must be outside the 50-gauss line. Gas analysis, airways pressure and respiratory indices are usually displayed at the anaesthetic machine and so again the main problem is delayed sampling time (up to 20 s) owing to long tubing.
- **Pacemakers:** cardiac pacemakers and implantable defibrillators require special consideration, as they will malfunction in fields over 5 gauss.
- **Infusion pumps:** these may fail if the field strength exceeds 30 gauss.
- **Implants and foreign bodies:** most patient implants (such as orthopaedic prostheses) are non-ferrous. Surgical clips and wires may be magnetic, but their presence does not usually contraindicate MR scanning as they become embedded in fixed fibrous tissue. Exceptions are intracranial vascular clips. Metal foreign bodies are likely to be ferrous. Non-ferrous items may heat.
- **Generic problems:** there are the generic problems of anaesthetizing patients in remote, unfamiliar and isolated areas. Patients are commonly children.

Direction the viva may take
You will then be asked details of the imaging technique itself.

- MRI is based on the principle that, when a cell nucleus with an unpaired proton is exposed to an electromagnetic field, it becomes aligned along the axis of that field. A charged and spinning nucleus generates a magnetic field and acts itself like a small magnet. The aligned nuclei can then be displaced by brief exposure to another magnetic field, generated at right angles to the first. This provokes the phenomenon of nuclear precession, in which the nuclei rotate around an axis different from that around which they are spinning. When the electromagnetic field is removed, the nucleus resumes its original position, and as it relaxes to this position it emits low radiofrequency (RF) radiation. This signal, which is very small, is converted by sophisticated computer technology into an image. The rate at which the nucleus relaxes to its original position varies with the nature of the tissue. (This explanation is simplistic, but this is the FRCA, not the FRCR, and it would be hard to explain why any more detailed exposition is necessary for the practice of anaesthesia.)

- MR reports usually refer to T_1 and T_2 views. 'T' is a relaxation time constant, T_1 being the image generated a few milliseconds after the electromagnetic field is removed, while T_2 is an image generated slightly later. Nuclei in hydrogen take longer to decay to their original position. In practice, this means, for example, that in a T_1 view, fluid will be dark (as minimal signal is generated), whereas in the T_2 view, fluid will be white.
- MRI requires the generation of very strong magnetic fields, typically up to 2.0 tesla. The tesla is the unit of magnetic flux density. Should you be asked; 1 tesla (T) is equal to 1 weber m^{-2}, a weber being the SI unit of magnetic flux. It is equal to the magnetic flux that in linking a circuit of one turn produces in it an electromotive force of 1 V as it is uniformly reduced to zero within 1 second. The Earth's magnetic field is approximately 1 gauss. 10 000 gauss equal 1 tesla. It will be a very odd examiner who really wants to know the answer to these questions, but you may as well be prepared.

Further direction the viva could take

- Should you have either exhausted the information above or struggled to provide the information, then you may be asked how you might set up an anaesthetic service for MR scanning. You may not have much time on this and so a few generic platitudes about the undesirability of a remote location, of the need for training, the use of protocols, and the importance of safety issues, should be enough to see you through.

Ultrasound

Commentary

The uses of ultrasound are widening for anaesthetists. Some intensivists are now performing their own ultrasound scans of the thorax and abdomen, while anaesthetists are using ultrasound not only to guide central venous cannulation and peripheral nerve blockade but also to derive perioperative information about cardiac function. As there are so many important clinical applications you will not become involved in mathematical discussions about the Doppler equation, but, as with all these physics-based questions, you will have to demonstrate that you know enough about the basic principles of ultrasound to inform your use of the devices.

The viva

You are likely to be asked about the clinical uses of ultrasound in intensive care and anaesthesia.

- **Critical care:** ultrasound scans of the abdomen and thorax can identify fluid collections, which can then be drained under ultrasound guidance. Cranial scanning is routinely used in neonatal intensive care to detect intraventricular haemorrhage and midline shift.
- **Central venous cannulation:** ultrasonic-guided cannulation is now routine, particularly for the internal jugular route.
- **Regional anaesthesia:** it allows more accurate placement of needles for local anaesthetic nerve blocks.
- **Air embolism:** the interface between air and blood generates a strong reflected signal, and a Doppler probe over the praecordium is sensitive enough to produce ultrasound images from bubbles as small as 2 μm in diameter.
- **Cardiac function:** echocardiography, either transthoracic or transoesophageal (TOE), can provide useful information about ventricular and valvular function.
- **Ultrasonic devices:** the principles of ultrasound can be used in gas flowmeters, in cleaning devices and in humidifiers.

Direction the viva may take

You will then be asked to describe the basic principles of ultrasound.

- **Principles of ultrasound:** sound waves which exceed the threshold of human hearing (around 20 000 Hz) are described as ultrasonic. Medical ultrasound uses frequencies of 2–15 MHz. These waves are generated by applying a high frequency alternating voltage to the two sides of a piezo-electric crystal transducer (which deforms when a voltage is applied to it). This changes the thickness of the crystal, which then emits ultrasonic radiation of the same frequency as the applied potential difference. The crystal also transduces the reflected waves back into an electrical signal from which a computer-generated cross-sectional image can be displayed. The signals are unable to penetrate bone or gas-filled structures, including the lung, and so ultrasound studies of these structures are not possible. Reflected signals are strongest from the interface between tissues of different density, such as air and blood, and when the structure being examined is perpendicular to the angle of the beam.
- **Images of tissues:** tissue that is highly reflective (hyperechoic) appears white. (Examples include bone and fascial planes.) Weakly reflected waves (hypoechoic) are darker. (Examples include muscle and fat.) Nerves can be either hyperechoic or hypoechoic. Blood does not reflect (anechoic) and so blood vessels appear black.
- **Frequency effects:** the higher the frequency the better the resolution of the image, but this is at the expense of tissue penetration. Lower frequencies will produce images from deeper structures but their definition is less good.
- **Attenuation of ultrasound:** this can be expressed as the 'half-power distance', which is the depth at which the sound is halved. This depth is 3800 mm for water

and less than 1 mm for air and lung. Sound is attenuated by bone (2–7 mm) and also by muscle (6–10 mm).

- **Velocity:** ultrasound moves through tissue at 1540 m s^{-1}. This rapid transmission and reception of pulses of sound allows the generation of dynamic images.
- **2-D images:** these are generated by probes which comprise an array of parallel piezo-electric elements that are activated in sequence, rather than simultaneously. This wavefront can, in practice, scan a 90° sector of tissue, with the reflected echoes processed into a two-dimensional picture.
- **Doppler effect and colour Doppler:** the Doppler effect (page 322) describes the change in the frequency of sound and ultrasound if either the emitter or the receiver is moving. Colour flow Doppler is able to display blood flow in real time, using three basic colours. Blood flow towards the transducer is red, while that away from the transducer is blue. It is obviously important not to assume that these colours indicate arterial and venous blood. The colour green can be added when blood flow velocity exceeds a preset limit. In areas of turbulent flow, such as may occur across a diseased cardiac valve, all three colours may be displayed.

Direction the viva may take

At some stage you will be given the opportunity to discuss TOE, oesophageal Doppler monitoring and/or regional nerve blockade in more detail.

- **TOE:** modern TOE probes allow 180° views of the heart, and the absence of large tissue masses between the probe and the myocardium allows for well-defined ultrasound images. It has specialist cardiac uses such as the assessment of valvular heart disease, the diagnosis of bacterial endocarditis, the identification of atrial thrombus and the investigation of congenital heart disease. It can identify aortic atherosclerosis, aortic dissection and disease, and can assess paracardiac masses. For the general anaesthetist and intensivist, its main value lies in the determination of left ventricular preload and function (both perioperatively and in intensive care), the diagnosis of acute left ventricular dysfunction and myocardial ischaemia, and the detection of air embolism. (Complications are mainly mechanical, and relate to the passage and presence of a firm probe within the thin-walled oesophagus with the consequent risk of perforation. The reported complication rate is very low; in one (early) series of 10 419 awake patients there were only two cases of bleeding.)
- **Oesophageal Doppler monitoring (ODM):** see page 324.
- **Regional nerve blockade:** it is likely that ultrasound-guided regional anaesthesia (UGRA) will be seen in due course as a technique that is faster, safer and more efficacious than those currently in use. The controlled trials to support this view may be a long time coming. As the complication rate of nerve blocks is already low, the numbers of patients required to demonstrate a difference are impractically large. Few would argue, however, with the intuitive proposition that if the needle tip is visible and if the local anaesthetic is seen spreading circumferentially around the nerve, then more successful and safer blocks seem likely. Nerve fascicles themselves are dark whereas supporting connective tissue tends to be brighter and more hyperechoic. This is a generalization because the varying structure of the fascia which invests a particular

nerve means that the same nerve may have a different ultrasound appearance along its course. Superficial nerves and plexuses are more suitable for UGRA than those sited more deeply. The sciatic nerve in the buttock, for example, is a large structure that is nonetheless difficult to identify because of attenuation of the beam by surrounding gluteal muscles. The advancing needles are best displayed if they are parallel to the probe face; at angles greater than 45° they become difficult to see. In central neuraxial techniques, UGRA is mainly useful for confirming the spinal level rather than as a practical aid to the performance of epidural or subarachnoid blocks.

Peripheral nerve location using a stimulator

Commentary

Most anaesthetists use peripheral nerve stimulators for regional nerve blocks. Ultrasound-guided nerve block is now part of mainstream practice, but for the time being at least, often in conjunction with a stimulator. Success in their use does to some extent depend on an understanding of how they function, but they are not especially complex devices and the viva may focus equally on clinical and practical aspects of their use.

The viva

You may be asked first about methods of identifying peripheral nerves as part of a local anaesthetic technique. Ultrasound may be your first choice (page 337), but you will be led rapidly to the complementary value of stimulators. If your familiarity with these devices is limited, then do not pretend otherwise; it is usually obvious to examiners when candidates lay claim to practical experience that they do not have.

- Nerve stimulators complement, but do not obviate, the need for accurate anatomical knowledge. The rationale for their use is twofold.
  - *Efficacy:* their use has been reported to double the success rate of some blocks (pre-ultrasound). Their value may in due course be reduced to that of providing confirmation that an ultrasound-guided needle is correctly placed.
  - *Safety:* their use removes the need to elicit paraesthesia. Paraesthesia occurs only when the advancing needle touches a nerve, and some chronic pain specialists believe that paraesthesia is associated almost invariably with later dysaesthesia.

Direction the viva may take

The questioning may then proceed to a discussion of the characteristics that are necessary for a nerve stimulator to be effective and safe.

- It should maintain a constant current despite the changes in resistance that the needle will encounter as it penetrates tissues of different densities. This is perhaps the most important characteristic. These resistances in the external circuit can vary from around 1 to 20 kΩ (kOhm), so were the device to deliver a constant voltage the current could vary 20-fold.

- It should have a linear output which can easily be varied.
- It should have a clear digital display across the current range from 0.1 to 5.0 mA.
- It should have a short pulse width of 50–100 s, which provides better discrimination of the distance between the needle and the nerve. The shorter the pulse width the greater the change in stimulation strength as the needle advances.
- It should incorporate an indicator that shows the integrity of the electrical circuit.
- It should be battery-operated (for patient safety), have a battery level indicator, low resistance clips and be robust.

Further direction the viva could take

You may then be asked about the practical considerations of using a stimulator.

- **Electrodes:** the negative electrode should be attached to the stimulator needle rather than the positive. In this situation, the current flow towards the needle produces an area of depolarization which readily triggers an action potential. This requires only 25% of the current that is needed if the polarity is reversed. If the anode is used, the current produces a zone of hyperpolarization immediately around the needle tip, with an area of depolarization encircling it.
- **Pulse duration – rheobase and chronaxy:** the rheobase is the minimum current required to stimulate a nerve, while the chronaxy is the duration of current stimulus required to stimulate that nerve at twice the rheobase. This has some clinical relevance because different nerves have different chronaxy. A motor fibres have shorter chronaxy (0.05–0.1 ms) than the fibres subserving touch and pain (A and C fibres with chronaxy of 0.15 and 0.4 ms, respectively). This means that, in an awake patient, it is possible to use a short pulse duration to stimulate motor fibres without eliciting pain.
- **Thresholds:** techniques vary; some anaesthetists start with a relatively high current of up to 2.0 mA, while others stay below 1.0 mA. As the needle approaches the likely site of injection, the current should be reduced to about 0.5 mA: at this stimulus the needle tip will be 1–2 mm from the nerve. If you are eliciting a vigorous twitch at much less than that current, at around 0.2 mA, then you will be very close to, or even in, the nerve.
- **Injection:** a small amount of local anaesthetic will abolish the twitch by physical displacement. This has been demonstrated experimentally using saline and air. If the twitch does not disappear on injection, it suggests that the needle may be intraneural and so should be withdrawn slightly.

You may also be asked about the characteristics of stimulator needles.

- **Insulated or non-insulated:** most needles are insulated (with Teflon coating) apart from the uncovered tip through which the current passes. You should be aware that non-insulated needles can also be used effectively because the current density remains greater at the tip of the needle than down the shaft. False positives are more common, however, because there can be some nerve stimulation at the level of the shaft.

- **Long bevel, short bevel or side-ported:** the choice of needle is contentious. A long-bevelled needle is sharp, penetrates tissues readily and so reduces the appreciation of fascial planes. Should it penetrate a nerve, however, the clean cut may actually cause less damage either than a short-bevelled (30°) or pencil-point needle with a proximal side hole. Increasing experience with ultrasound is showing that even when an effective twitch has been elicited these 'atraumatic' needles may deliver the local anaesthetic too far from the nerve. They may also produce a less clear ultrasound image.
- **Sizes:** there are numerous sizes, depending on the manufacturer, but common lengths include 30, 50, 90, 100 and 150 mm. Most are 22G.

Electrical safety

Commentary

In general, patients are well protected from electrical danger, and for most anaesthetists this topic will remain only theoretical. Electricity does appear as a subject but its main application, apart from biological potentials, relates to safety. The viva may start with the effects of electricity on the human body and then move on to the means whereby these risks to the patient can be minimized.

The viva

You will be asked about the effects of electric current in the body.

- **Effects of electricity:** at 1 mA a subject will feel tingling and at 5 mA definite pain. At 15 mA there is tonic contraction of muscles, which at 50 mA involves all the muscles of respiration. At 100 mA ventricular fibrillation supervenes.
- **Electrocution:** this can happen should a patient become part of an electrical circuit. The main problem is the fibrillatory potential of the current, which, if applied externally, need reach only 50–100 mA. Such current disrupts the normal function of cells, causing muscle contraction, respiratory paralysis and ventricular fibrillation. The current frequency is also important, with 50 Hz (the frequency of alternating current (AC) in the UK) being optimally lethal. AC at 50 Hz can generate high voltages economically and can readily be transformed, but it will interfere with ion flux across all cell membranes and force ions in both directions. (The ion pump can cope better with direct current (DC) voltages.) Higher frequencies are much less dangerous and above 100 Hz have no fibrillatory potential. In electrocution there is additional thermal injury, caused as the electrical energy dissipates through tissues. The severity of the electrical burn is directly proportional to the current density and its duration of application.

You will be asked about the electrical risks to patients and how they are minimized, but it may helpful to familiarize yourself with some basic electrical terms.

- **Electricity:** this is the flow of electrons, which is driven by potential difference (the voltage) through a conductor past a given point per unit time. This current is measured in amperes.
- **Resistance:** this is the resistance along a conductor to the flow of current. It is not frequency-dependent. Resistance is measured in ohms.
- **Ohm's law:** this states that the electrical potential $(V) =$ current $(I) \times$ resistance (R).
- **Impedance:** the impedance is the sum of all the forces impeding electron flow in an AC circuit. Unlike resistance, it is dependent upon frequency and includes resistors, capacitors and inductors. (Insulators are high-impedance devices; conductors are low-impedance devices.) Impedance through capacitors and inductors is related to the frequency at which AC reverses direction. Impedance is also measured in ohms (volt/ampere).
- **Lethal current:** the relationships described above explain how dangerous currents can be generated. Ohm's law determines the magnitude of the current that flows, $I = V/R$. An individual standing on an antistatic floor may have an impedance of $20 \text{ k}\Omega$ or more and so, should he touch a live enclosure, the current flow will be $240/20\,000$ or 12 mA. Wet hands or fluid on the floor may reduce the impedance to $2 \text{ k}\Omega$, and so the current, $240/2000$, becomes potentially lethal at 120 mA. This is not enough to blow the fuse and the circuit remains live.

Direction the viva will take

You will be asked about the risks to patients within the operating theatre and how they can be minimized.

A patient can become part of an electrical circuit in two ways.

- **Direct connection (resistive coupling):** if any part of the body is directly in contact with an electricity source or with an earthed object, then current may pass through the patient to earth. This can be caused either by faulty equipment or by leakage currents. As all electrical equipment is at a higher potential than earth, current seeks to flow to earth through a circuit of which a patient may form part. Medical equipment is well insulated and these leakage currents are usually small, but they do still carry the risk of microshock (see below).
- **Indirect connection (capacitive coupling):** in some circumstances, the body can act as one plate of a capacitor. If DC is applied to a capacitor such as a defibrillator, current continues to flow only until the positive plate reaches the same potential as the electrical source. If, however, AC is applied then the plates alternate polarity at the same frequency as the current. The repetitive pattern of charge and discharge sets up a current flow across the gap with the effective completion of the circuit. A patient on an operating table can therefore act as one plate of a capacitor while the theatre light with its 50 Hz AC supply forms the other.

Risks can be minimized by using appropriate (and well-maintained) equipment.

- **Identification:** equipment designed for medical use is generally of high specification with an identifier to show the grade of protection that it offers.

— *Class I:* it offers basic protection only. Any conducting part that is accessible to the user, such as the casing, must be connected to earth, and must be insulated from the main supply. (Such equipment has fuses on the live and neutral supply in the equipment, as well as on the live wire in the mains plug.)

— *Class II:* this equipment has reinforced, or double, insulation that protects all the parts that are accessible. It does not require an earth.

— *Class III:* this equipment uses safety extra low voltage (SELV) which does not exceed 24 V AC. There is no risk of gross electrocution, but microshock is still possible.

— *Type B:* such equipment has low leakage currents; 0.5 mA for class 1B, and 0.1 mA for class IIB.

— *Type BF:* type BF is the same as type B, except that the piece of equipment that is applied to the patient is isolated from all its other parts.

— *Type CF:* this is class I or II equipment which is considered safe for direct connection to the heart. Leakage currents are extremely low, being 0.05 mA per electrode for class ICF equipment and 0.01 mA per electrode for class IICF.

Other precautions

- **Common earth:** voltage differences between multiple pieces of medical equipment increase the risk of leakage currents which may flow from the higher to the lower potential via the patient. This risk is minimized if the equipment is connected to a common equipotential earth point via a single cable.

- **Isolated (floating) circuits:** in these circuits the equipment that is mains-powered is separated from the patient circuit by an isolating transformer (comprising primary and secondary coils that are insulated from each other). AC from the primary (earthed) mains supply induces current in the secondary coil which means that although the patient circuit is live, it remains earth-free.

- **Earth leakage circuit breakers (ELCB):** these devices do not protect against short circuits or overloading (appropriate fuses are still required) but they do cut off the electrical supply to faulty equipment in the presence of current leakage. There are different types, but in simplistic terms each consists of a tripping coil which, when activated by excessive current, trips a relay which interrupts the supply.

Further direction the viva could take

You may be asked about microshock.

- **Microshock:** gross electrocution by externally applied energy requires currents of around 100 mA, but very much lower currents in the region of 50–100 μA can induce ventricular fibrillation if they are applied directly to the ventricle. This rare phenomenon is known as microshock. It can occur only with a combination of factors that arise in specialized situations in which the patient accidentally becomes part of an electrical circuit. Microshock requires an electrical contact applied directly over a small area of the myocardium and which can be earthed through the patient. Faulty equipment, even with very low leakage currents, but which is connected to intracardiac devices such as pacing wires or catheters, is capable of delivering this microcurrent directly to the ventricle and inducing fibrillation. Someone holding a pacing wire in one hand while touching the leakage source with the other may inadvertently complete the circuit and electrocute the patient. The risk is lessened in this instance by wearing gloves, and in general by the use of earth-free mains supply.

Defibrillation

Commentary

This is primarily a question about the physics of electrical defibrillation. There has been recent interest in different waveforms, and this may extend the science questioning, but not so far that you will not be asked about the clinical implications. Resuscitation is a core anaesthetic skill and so you must ensure that your knowledge of the treatment algorithms is sound. Otherwise, what may seem like a throwaway query about the management of cardiac arrest could fail you, no matter how authoritatively you may have dealt with capacitance.

The viva

The examiner may introduce the subject by asking you to describe what happens when a heart is fibrillating.

- **Atrial and ventricular fibrillation:** in health the sinus impulse is conducted evenly and concentrically to all parts of the atria and thence to the ventricles. When atrial fibrillation (AF) supervenes, the excitation and recovery of different parts of the atria becomes uncoordinated, with various areas at different stages of excitation and recovery. It is similar with ventricular fibrillation (VF). The changing amplitude of the ECG reflects electrical activity, but depolarization is chaotic and unable therefore to generate any cardiac output.
- **Effects:** in AF there is loss of the atrial contribution to ventricular filling, which is usually around 20%. In addition, the risk of thrombus formation is substantially increased. A fibrillating ventricle produces no cardiac output.
- **Causes:** these are numerous and the examiner will not want you to do more than suggest the most significant. Common causes of AF include ischaemic heart disease and acute critical illness, particularly sepsis. (Other cited causes such as mitral stenosis and thyrotoxicosis are very rare.) VF is caused by myocardial disease, both ischaemic and myopathic, by hypoxia, by profound hypothermia, by electrolyte imbalance, by some drugs and by electrocution.

Direction the viva may take

You may then be asked about the electrical (not the pharmacological) management of fibrillation.

- **AF:** refractory AF is treated by the application of a DC shock, which is synchronized to the peak deflection of the 'R' wave of ventricular depolarization on the ECG. The

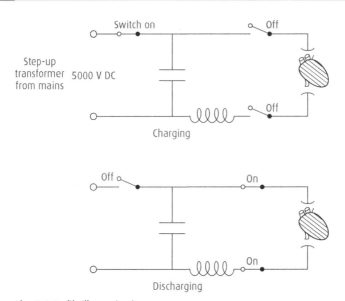

Fig. 5.8 Defibrillator circuit.

risk of inducing VF is very high during repolarization (as shown by the 'T' wave on the ECG). This is why the 'R-on-T' rhythm is particularly dangerous.

- **VF:** this can be treated either by mechanical defibrillation or electrical defibrillation. The application of mechanical energy in the form of a praecordial thump (sometimes known as 'thumpversion') may convert VF to a viable rhythm only if it is applied early. It normally achieves only around 5–10 joules of mechanical energy. In electrical defibrillation, a defibrillator delivers a charge across the chest which causes simultaneous depolarization of myocardial cells. If the procedure is successful, there is a short refractory period after which there is resumption of normal pacemaker activity with myocardial contraction and a stable rhythm.

The viva will then move on to the electrical principles underlying defibrillation and you may also be asked to draw and explain the basic circuit and its components (Figure 5.8).

- **Capacitance:** a capacitor consists of two plates that are separated by an insulator and which will store electrons after the application of a potential difference. Capacitance is the ability to hold electric charge. Its units are coulombs, C. One coulomb is the amount of electric charge which passes a point when a current of 1 A flows for 1 s.
- **Defibrillator circuit:** a potential of between 4000 and 6000 V is applied across the capacitor to produce a store of electrons. (The selected voltage is varied by means of a variable transformer.) When the defibrillator is activated this stored charge is released as a pulse of current across the patient's heart. This stored energy is by convention expressed in joules rather than volts. (One joule is the work required to move a charge of 1 C through a potential difference of 1 V ($J = V \times C$).) Not all of this energy

is delivered; the inductance coil (inductor) in the output circuit decelerates the rapid discharge of the capacitor to give a shock that is slowed to 4–10 ms. This duration gives the optimal chance of synchronous myocardial depolarization. (The displayed energy is that delivered, not that stored.)

- **Impedance:** the efficiency of the applied shock is greater if transthoracic impedance is minimized by the use of conductive gels, firm paddle pressure, and by defibrillation from front-to-back rather than from sternum to apex. (Impedance is the sum of all forces impeding electron flow in an AC circuit.)
- **Waveforms:** the current pulse described above is monophasic, travelling in the positive direction only. A monophasic pulse can have two waveforms (exponential current decay and a damped sine wave), which are of similar efficacy. In a defibrillator that uses a biphasic waveform, the current is reversed halfway through the discharge to move both in a positive and a negative direction. (There are also two biphasic waveforms: truncated exponential decay and rectilinear.) Biphasic shocks are not only more effective than monophasic, but they also cause less myocardial injury. Their use is now becoming widespread.

Surgical diathermy

Commentary
Diathermy is used widely and is in essence a surgical instrument. The anaesthetist, unfair though it seems, may in practice be blamed should a patient suffer a burn owing to malpositioning of the plate. Diathermy may also interfere with monitors and can disrupt pacemaker function, and so it is a topic on which some basic knowledge is expected.

The viva
You may be asked about the risks of diathermy.

- There is a risk of thermal injury at the site of the indifferent electrode (the diathermy plate) which must be in close and even contact with a large area of skin, ideally an area that is well perfused and so which will dissipate heat. Adhesive and conductive gels are useful. If the area of contact is small, the current density increases to the point at which a burn is probable.
- Thermal injury at a metal contact site may occur if the plate is detached or malpositioned. The diathermy current may flow to earth through any point at which the patient is touching metal (such as the operating table, lithotomy poles or ECG electrodes) and cause a burn.
- The plate should not be placed over an area where there is a metal prosthesis in place (usually the hip). Metal has a low resistance in comparison with tissue and so the current will flow preferentially through the prosthesis, generating a potentially dangerous current density.

- The instrument may be activated when it is not in contact with the tissue to be cut or coagulated.
- The circuit may be completed via a route that does not include the indifferent electrode; this may also result in a burn.
- Alcoholic skin preparation solutions have ignited after diathermy activation.
- Diathermy may interfere with cardiac pacemaker function. The indifferent electrode should be sited as far distant as possible from the pacemaker, and bipolar diathermy should be used wherever possible. If the use of unipolar diathermy is unavoidable, it should be deployed in short bursts. Cutting diathermy causes more of a problem than coagulation.
- Diathermy may interfere with monitoring devices. This problem can be minimized by the use of electrical filters.
- Diathermy may lead to ischaemia and infarction of structures supplied by fine end-arteries. Classic examples include the penis (hence unipolar diathermy must be avoided in circumcision) and the testis, which has a vulnerable vascular pedicle.

Direction the viva may take

You will then be asked about the physical principles.

- Diathermy is used widely in surgical practice, both for coagulation and for cutting, and relies on the heat generated as an electric current passes through a resistance that is concentrated in the probe itself.
- Heat generation is proportional to the power that is developed, typically 50–400 W. Heat is proportional to I^2 (current)/A (area).
- A high-frequency sine waveform is used for cutting, typically 0.5 MHz.
- A damped waveform is used for coagulation, typically 1.0–1.5 MHz.
- High frequency is necessary because muscle is very sensitive to DC and to AC at low frequencies. Mains frequency is low, at 50 Hz, which is a frequency that is particularly efficient at precipitating VF. Very high-frequency current has minimal tissue penetration and passes across the myocardium without ill effect.
- Burning and heating effects can occur at all frequencies.
- There are two types of diathermy:
  — *Unipolar:* there are two connections to the patient; the neutral (or indifferent) patient plate, and the active coagulation or cutting electrode. Current passes through both, but the current density at the active electrode is very high and generates high temperatures. At the patient plate, the current density is dispersed over a wide area and heating does not occur. The patient plate and hence the patient, is kept at earth potential, which reduces the risks of capacitor linkage (in which diathermy current may flow in the absence of direct contact). Modern diathermy machines incorporate isolating capacitors to minimize the problem. An alternative is to use an earth-free or floating circuit.
  — *Bipolar:* in this instance the current is localized to the instrument; it passes only from one blade of the forceps to the other. Bipolar diathermy uses low

power, and this limits its efficacy in the coagulation of all but small vessels. The circuit is not earthed.

Biological potentials

Commentary

It is difficult to make the topic of biological potentials overtly clinical and the questioning is likely to revert quite rapidly to the equipment that is necessary for their capture. It may seem as though the subject has no obvious narrative and the viva may feel unstructured. There should be sufficient information in the simplified details below to allow you to discuss it convincingly.

The viva

You will be asked how biological potentials are generated and to give some examples.

- There is a negative resting potential across the membrane of excitable cells of around 90 mV. When the interior depolarizes, an action potential is generated that leads to a wave of depolarization that spreads along a neuron or across a contracting muscle. These electric potentials are transmitted through overlying tissues and can be detected by electrodes on the skin.
- Biological potentials differ both in magnitude and in frequency. The signals are also greatly attenuated as they pass through tissue. The myocardium generates local potentials at the skin of only around 0.5–2.0 mV with a frequency range of 0.5–100 Hz. The brain produces much smaller potentials of some 50 μV with a more restricted frequency range of 1–60 Hz. Muscle potentials range from 100 μV up to 30 mV depending on the size of the motor unit and with a wide frequency range of between 1 and >1000 Hz. (These potentials are detected by the ECG, the EEG and the EMG, respectively.)

Direction the viva will take

You will then be asked how these signals can be captured, amplified and displayed.

- **Detection:** the small electrical potentials are detected by skin electrodes. These are not simply passive devices and their characteristics are important. When metal contacts an electrolyte solution, it forms an electrochemical half-cell which generates a potential. This potential may not only be detected by the amplifier but can also alter the characteristics of the electrode in a process known as polarization. This distorts any signal being captured. The problem is largely theoretical because modern electrodes whose surfaces use a metal which is in contact with one of its own salts (such as Ag: AgCl) do not cause polarization, and they produce a stable electrode potential that does not distort recordings.

- **Amplification:** these small potentials require amplifiers with a high degree of discrimination, which can minimize distortion by electrical noise emanating either from the patient or from the environment. It is easy to see how the potential differences produced by the heart beat could interfere with the much smaller differences produced by cerebral neuronal activity, and how both could be swamped by AC mains voltage at 50 Hz. Typically, biological amplifiers are differential; that is, they measure the difference in electrical potential between two sources. Any input that is common to both is eliminated, while the difference in input to both is amplified. This capacity of a differential amplifier to eliminate the signals that are common to both inputs is known as the common-mode rejection ratio (CMRR). (It is defined as the ratio of the magnitude of the differential gain to the magnitude of the common mode gain. For a biopotential amplifier, the CMRR should be at least 1000:1.) The design of amplifiers is such that they can exploit the dissimilarities between biological potentials. The ECG signal is many times larger than that of the EEG but it is in phase. Highly discriminating instruments are able to attenuate in-phase signals and amplify out-of-phase signals, thereby ensuring that the EEG can be recorded free from interference. Similarly, the generally much higher frequency of muscle potentials can also be eliminated. (Modern instruments offer multiple filters for signal processing.) In addition to a high CMRR, the amplifier should have a high input impedance (>5 ohms). In combination with good electrode contact and minimal attenuation of the input signal, this ensures both truer recording of the potential and protection of the patient from electrocution. (In modern equipment both the CMRR and input impedance are much higher than the figures quoted.) Amplifiers must also have the appropriate bandwidth; that is, the ability to amplify the signal constantly across the range of frequencies that are involved. They also require adequate gain so that very small biological potentials can be captured. (Gain is the ratio of the voltage at the amplifier output to the voltage at the signal input.) Some instruments can demonstrate drift; this is a change in amplifier output even while the input potential remains constant. This is a function of the alteration in resistance of semiconductor materials in response to temperature changes. It is less problematic in amplifiers designed for AC potentials.
- **Recording and display:** there are a number of historical and rather cumbersome devices based on galvanometers which the viva should bypass. They are adequate for recording slow analogue signals but not for those of higher frequency. These signals are best displayed by a cathode ray tube (CRT). The cathode produces a stream of electrons which passes between two sets of charged plates before striking a phosphorescent screen. The charged electrons will be repelled from the negative plate and attracted to the positive with the degree of deflection being proportional to the charge. The x axis plates move the electron beam horizontally while the y axis plates move it vertically. As the beam reaches the right hand side of the screen, the charge reverses and restores it to the left. The beam has negligible inertia and thus the CRT has a very high frequency response suitable for the display of all biological potentials.

Osmosis

Commentary

This is a fairly circumscribed topic which fits readily into the time frame of this viva. Although its main interest lies in clinical disorders which disrupt plasma osmolality, you will probably spend more time on the basic definitions and concepts, none of which is that complicated.

The viva

You may be asked about conditions that result in derangements of osmolality.

- **Syndrome of inappropriate antidiuretic hormone (ADH) secretion (SIADH):** this is defined by the non-osmotic release of ADH with consequent water retention and hypotonicity. Its causes are numerous, but include intracranial tumours and pulmonary malignancy and infection. Treatment is via water restriction and, in chronic cases, with the use of demeclocycline (a tetracycline) which blocks ADH action in the kidney.

(You may at this stage be asked to outline the importance of ADH.)

- **ADH:** this increases conservation of water and sodium in the distal renal tubules via a mechanism mediated by cAMP. Osmoreceptors in the supraoptic nuclei of the hypothalamus have a mean threshold of 289 ± 2.3 mosmol kg^{-1}. Above this plasma level, ADH release is stimulated. (The kidneys should be able to produce a urine osmolality of at least 1000 mosmol kg^{-1}.)
- **Diabetes insipidus (DI):** this also has many causes and can be neurogenic (with deficiency of ADH synthesis or impaired release) or nephrogenic (with renal resistance to the action of ADH). It is characterized by massive diuresis and hypovolaemia. Neurogenic DI is treated with desmopressin (an ADH analogue) in a dose tailored to allow a mild diuresis to avoid the complication of water intoxication. Chlorpropamide potentiates the effects of endogenous ADH and also sensitizes distal tubules.
- **Glycine intoxication (TUR syndrome) with hyponatraemia:** this may follow excessive absorption of irrigating fluid during transurethral procedures (usually prostatectomy). Treatment is with administration of normal saline and judicious diuretic. Rapid restoration of normal sodium (for example, by the use of hypertonic saline) is associated with central pontine myelinosis.
- **Water intoxication:** this follows excessive intake of water, usually self-inflicted (29% of the finishers in one Hawaiian Ironman Triathlon were hyponatraemic), but is also associated with iatrogenic infusion of large volumes of glucose solution. The decrease in plasma osmolality inhibits ADH secretion, but it can still cause potentially fatal electrolyte disturbance.
- **Hyperosmolar states:** the commonest hyperosmolar state is that of hyperglycaemic non-ketotic hyperosmolar coma, secondary to type 2 diabetes and

precipitated by any dehydrating illness or reduction in insulin activity. (The serum osmolarity is typically >320 mosmol kg^{-1}.) Hyperosmolarity can also be iatrogenic following, for example, the administration of mannitol to neuro-surgical patients.

Direction the viva may take

You will be asked about the underlying scientific principles, starting with a definition of osmosis and osmotic pressure.

- **Definition:** osmosis describes the process of the net movement of water molecules due to diffusion between areas of different concentration.
- **Osmotic pressure:** an effective concentration gradient of water can be produced between two compartments separated by a semi-permeable membrane (permeable to water but not to solute). The movement of water into such a compartment will increase the pressure and/or volume of the compartment. This movement can be opposed by increasing the pressure in the compartment, and the pressure needed to prevent osmosis is defined as the osmotic pressure exerted by the solution. (If one compartment contains 22.4 litres and 1 mol of solute at 0°C it will exert an osmotic pressure of 1 atmosphere, or 101.325 kPa.)
- **Calculation of osmotic pressure:** the van't Hoff equation is based on the recognition that dilute solutions behave in a similar way to gases, hence: osmotic pressure $= n$ (number of particles) $\times$ (concentration/molecular weight) $\times$ R (universal gas constant) $\times$ T (absolute temperature).
- **Measurement of osmotic pressure:** this is measured by an osmometer, which utilizes one or more of the colligative properties of a solution. (These depend on the osmolarity and are depression of freezing point, elevation of boiling point, reduction in vapour pressure and exertion of osmotic pressure.) Osmometers utilize the fact either that 1 mol of a solute which is added to 1 kg of water will depress the freezing point by 1.86°C, or that the molar concentration of a solute causes a directly proportional reduction in the vapour pressure of the solvent (Raoult's Law). (Such devices have the advantage of requiring smaller samples than the freezing point osmometer.) The measurement of change of 1 mosmol requires apparatus capable of recording a temperature change of 0.002°C.
- **Osmolarity and osmolality:** osmolarity is the number of osmoles (or mosmoles) of solute per litre of solution, Osm l^{-1}, and is influenced by temperature. Osmolality is the number of osmoles per kilogram of solution, Osm kg^{-1}, and, because it is temperature-independent, removes a source of potential inaccuracy.
- **Estimation of osmolality:** the plasma osmolality can be estimated from a simple formula which sums the major solutes: $[2 \times Na^+] + [Glucose] + [Urea]$. The plasma osmolality is kept constant in health, at around 290 mosmol kg^{-1} H$_2$O. More than 99% of the osmolality of plasma is due to electrolytes, with the contribution of plasma proteins (the oncotic pressure) being less than 1%. (1 mosmol is equivalent to 17 mmHg or 2.26 kPa.)
- **Oncotic pressure:** the oncotic pressure is the contribution made to total osmolality by colloids (hence the alternative term 'colloid osmotic pressure', COP). The plasma oncotic pressure, at 25–28 mmHg, is only about 0.5% that of total plasma osmotic

pressure, but it is significant because it is the major factor in the retention of fluid within capillaries. Albumin is responsible for about 75% of the total COP.

- **Measurement of oncotic pressure:** the colloid osmotic pressure can be measured by an oncometer, which comprises a semi-permeable membrane which separates the plasma sample from a saline reference solution. The change to the oncotic pressure can readily be transduced and measured.
- **Tonicity:** in contrast to osmolality, which measures all the particles in a solution, tonicity refers only to those particles which exert an osmotic force. Urea and glucose are freely permeable and so are not included. (The exception is in diabetes mellitus when glucose does not pass into cells and so becomes osmotically active. Urea can exert a local osmotic effect because it does not cross the blood–brain barrier and so a high urea may cause intracranial dehydration and a reduction in ICP.)

Parametric and non-parametric data

Commentary
Statistics questions usually start quite simply and frequently end up simply, for the reasons outlined in the introduction. It may feel as though you are just being asked to give a series of definitions, but the examiners will be using your answers to discern whether or not you do understand the basic differences between types of data. You might at some stage be given a straightforward theoretical trial to discuss, but you will not be expected to perform any statistical calculations. The viva may divert to include meta-analysis or the design of clinical trials.

The viva
You will be asked to describe the difference between parametric and non-parametric data, and during the course of that description, to explain the terms that you are using.

- **Parametric data:** these are quantitative data that have a normal (Gaussian) distribution. In such a distribution the mean (average of all the results), the median (the value above and below which contains equal numbers of results) and the mode (the most frequently occurring value) are all the same. The variation around the mean is given by the variance, σ^2, the square root of which is the standard deviation (SD), σ.
- **Non-parametric data:** these do not have a normal distribution and the typical bell-shaped curve is replaced by one which may, for example, be skewed in either direction or may be bimodal (with two peaks). The data can sometimes be transformed mathematically so that they assume a normal distribution and can be analysed by parametric tests. This may be desirable because parametric statistical tests are more powerful than non-parametric.

- **SD:** this provides a convenient way of describing the spread around the mean, with 68% of a population falling within ±1 SD, 96% within ±2 SD, and 99% within ±3 SD of the mean. The information can be expressed the other way round, namely that 95% of the values will be included within 1.96 SDs of the mean.
- **Standard error of the mean (SEM):** this is used to determine whether the mean of the sample reflects the mean of the population. It is calculated by dividing the standard deviation by the square root of the degrees of freedom minus 1 ($SEM = SD/\sqrt{n-1}$). In effect, it is the SD of the mean, thus 68% of sample means lie within ±1 SE of the true population mean, 96% within ±2 SE, and 99.7% within ±3 SEs.
- **Confidence limits:** this concept is linked to the SEM. A sample mean will lie beyond 1.96 SEs only 5% of the time, and so we can be 95% confident that the sample mean does reflect the population mean. They have the advantage that they are expressed in the same units as the measurements, rather than as a probability value.
- **Parametric tests:** these include Student's t-test and analysis of variance (ANOVA). ANOVA and not the t-test should be used if there are more than two groups. The data are considered paired if they derive from the same patient. For example, blood pressure measurements before and after laryngoscopy would be analysed using a paired t-test. If different but very well matched patients are entered into separate limbs of a trial, then paired statistical tests may also be used.
- **Non-parametric tests:** these are applied to quantitative data which do not have a normal distribution. These include the Wilcoxon signed rank test for paired data and the Mann–Whitney U test for unpaired data. If there are more than two groups, then the corresponding tests are the Friedman (paired) and Kruskal–Wallis (unpaired).
- **Qualitative data:** these data (for example, ASA grades, pain scores, operation type) are usually analysed using the Chi-squared test.

Direction the viva may take

You may be asked what statistical tests you might use in a particular trial; for example, in a comparison of two anti-hypertensive agents.

- These are quantitative not qualitative data, and are likely to be normally distributed. (There are formal tests for normality, but if the mean and median are the same and the range of measurements spans around 5 SDs, then the data are probably parametric.)
- The data may be unpaired if two groups of patients are being studied, but will be paired if the anti-hypertensive drugs are being given sequentially to the same individuals.
- An appropriate test, therefore, would be Student's t-test (paired or unpaired as above), or ANOVA (also paired or unpaired).
- A P value of less than 0.05 may be the level at which the null hypothesis is disproved (i.e. confirming that there is a difference between the treatments), but

this means nevertheless that there is up to a 5% probability that this observed difference could have arisen entirely by chance. This is the type I or alpha error (false positive).

Further direction the viva could take
The discussion may widen to include the potential errors in data interpretation from clinical trials, meta-analysis and levels of evidence.

- **Trial data:** see page 356.
- **Meta-analysis:** this is a technique that aggregates the data from a number of individual randomized controlled clinical trials (RCTs) with the aim of confirming or refuting an effect that the smaller studies have been unable to do. It combines trials which individually may have been too small to demonstrate a significant difference.
    - *Advantages:* meta-analysis can produce a conclusion (synthesis) from a number of trials which may even have had contradictory findings. The power and significance of the overview can be increased by this synthesis of the individual results, and may allow a definite conclusion to be drawn even when individual studies do have contradictory findings. The technique requires inclusion of all relevant RCTs, which are scored according to their methodology.
    - *Problems:* meta-analyses are the tools of statisticians and epidemiologists and are not without drawbacks. They are subject to 'publication bias' since negative studies are much less likely to be published than positive ones. They may also be affected by double counting, which may occur when the same data are incorporated into more than one trial report. Their credibility is also tested severely if the populations in the RCTs are different. The Cochrane Injuries Group Albumin Reviewers concluded in 1998 that albumin increased mortality in critically ill patients. The patient populations were very disparate and even included neonates, and subsequent subgroup analysis suggested that in some of the groups albumin actually improved survival. Even if the populations are similar, the trial designs may be very different, with matched subgroups being too small to permit formal meta-analysis.
- **Levels of evidence:** these have been defined as follows.
    - *I:* evidence from at least one review of multiple RCTs.
    - *II:* evidence from at least one well designed RCT.
    - *III:* evidence from well designed trials without randomization or matched controls.
    - *IV:* evidence from well designed non-experimental studies from more than one group.
    - *V:* opinions based on clinical evidence, on descriptive studies, or on the reports of expert committees.
    - *Recommendations:* these are linked to levels of evidence: **A**, level I studies; **B**, level II or III studies, **C**, level IV studies; **D**, level V evidence or inconsistent or inconclusive studies of any level.

Clinical trials: errors in interpretation of data

Commentary

This is not a question about flaws in the design of clinical trials, but about potential problems with statistical analysis. Many of the terms and definitions are similar, and do need precise enunciation so as to avoid confusion of both candidate and examiner. This is one of the areas in which a slow careful delivery is interpreted as clarity of thought and so you may even find the viva drawing to a close before you know it.

The viva

You may be asked initially about the basic types of error. You could start by explaining the null hypothesis, because it is integral to a discussion of type I and II errors, and you will almost certainly be asked about it at some stage of the viva.

- **Null hypothesis:** this is the assumption made at the start of any investigation, that there is no difference between the populations, treatments and samples that are being compared. Tests of statistical significance aim to disprove the null hypothesis at a given level of probability. This is usually 0.05 (which means that there is a 5% likelihood of the difference occurring purely due to chance).
- **Types of error**
  - *Type I or α error:* in this case the null hypothesis is wrongly rejected, and a difference is found when there is none. This is a false positive. The likelihood of a type I error is reduced by requiring a higher probability value (making P smaller), by increasing the sample size, or both. By convention, a 5% probability of making a type I error is accepted, and the confidence level is given by $(1-\alpha)$.
  - *Type II or β error:* in this instance the null hypothesis is wrongly proved, and so no difference is found when one does in fact exist. This is a false negative. Type II errors are easier to avoid than type I, and their commonest cause is a sample size that is too small. They may also occur if there is a wide variation in the study population or if differences that may be clinically significant are quantitatively quite small. Type II errors are linked with the power of the study. More leniency is allowed in respect of type II errors, such that a 10% or 20% probability of an error is accepted. A study is adequately powered, therefore, if β is equal to or less than 0.2.
- **Power:** the 'power' of a study is the measure of its likelihood of detecting a difference between groups if a difference really does exist. It is also defined by $(1-\beta)$ where β is the probability of a type II error. The power of a trial is the probability of avoiding a type II error, and so it is clear that underpowered studies may reject treatments that in fact may be effective. The determination of the numbers needed is also a reflection of the minimal clinically important difference, which is set by the investigator. It is probably not important, for example, to detect a 5% reduction in systolic blood pressure, but it may be very important to

identify a 5% reduction in mortality. Were a study to miss such a fall in mortality then it might lead to the abandonment of a therapy that might save 50 lives for every 1000 patients treated.

Direction the viva may take

By way of an extension to the preceding discussion you may be asked about ways of quantifying the value of a clinical test.

- **Sensitivity:** this is a measure of how good is a clinical test at excluding false positives, and is defined by the proportion of positives that are correctly identified by the test. It is determined by the proportion of patients who test positive in relation to the numbers who actually are positive.
- **Positive predictive value:** this is an alternative means of determining whether an abnormal result predicts a genuine abnormality. It is defined by the numbers of patients who both test positive and who are genuinely positive as a proportion of the total of correct positive tests.
- **Specificity:** this is a measure of how good is a clinical test at excluding false negatives, and is defined by the proportion of negatives that are correctly identified by the test. It is determined by the proportion of patients who test negative in relation to the numbers who actually are negative.
- **Negative predictive value:** this is an alternative means of determining whether a normal result precludes a genuine abnormality. It is defined by the numbers of patients who both test negative and who are genuinely negative, as a proportion of the total of correct negative tests.
- **Statistical and clinical significance:** it is erroneous to equate statistical with clinical significance. Statistics are essentially measures of probability; clinical judgement must thereafter inform their use.

Miscellaneous science and medicine

Mechanisms of action of general anaesthetics

Commentary

This has been the focus of fundamental research which this viva will not have time to explore in depth. The subject matter is complex and although selective effects on CNS proteins appear to offer the most complete explanation, much remains unexplained. If you can give a reasonably plausible summary of the main points, then you should have done enough to pass.

The viva

You will be asked about the theories that have been advanced to explain the action of general anaesthetics.

- Compounds that cause reversible insensibility range from xenon, which is chemically unreactive and whose structure could not be simpler, to barbiturates and phenols, whose structures are both complex and dissimilar. This makes the search for a unifying theory of action with particular emphasis on a specific structure–activity relationship more difficult.
- **Meyer–Overton hypothesis:** Meyer and Overton (separately) were the first to relate the potency of anaesthetic agents to their lipid solubility. They argued further that the onset of narcosis was evident as soon as the particular substance had attained a certain molar concentration in the lipids of the cell, and that the lipid layers of the cell membrane represented the main site of action. Much early research was based on the hypothesis that disruption of the lipid bilayer affected the function of membrane proteins and mediated an interruption of neuronal traffic. As a unifying theory however, it was undermined by the observations that temperature rises

disrupt lipid membranes without inducing a state of general anaesthesia, and that there are many compounds with high lipid solubility which exert no anaesthetic effect. None the less, there remains a clear relationship between anaesthetic potency and lipid solubility which any theory of action must accommodate.

- **Clathrate theory:** it was proposed that anaesthetic agents form hydrates (clathrates) and from these microcrystals which aggregate in cell membranes to affect their function. At body temperature, however, very high pressure is needed for clathrate formation and this alone makes the hypothesis unsustainable.

- **Pressure reversal:** it was discovered that anaesthesia induced with halothane in tadpoles and in mice could be reversed by subjecting them to pressure, a process which was assumed to restore the normal configuration of the cell membrane. The pressures required to reanimate these creatures, however, were in excess of 50 atmospheres, and so the volume expansion theory is also untenable.

- **Voltage-gated ion channels:** general anaesthetic agents appear to exert minimal effect at voltage-gated ion channels.

- **Transmitter-gated ion channels (TGIC):** ligand-gated membrane ion channels have been the focus of most recent investigations. They include the γ-hydroxybutyrate (GABA$_A$) receptor, as well as 5-HT$_3$, acetylcholine, glutamate and glycine receptors. As membrane-bound proteins, these receptors contain integral anion-conducting channels, in which function is altered by the allosteric effects of a number of disparate compounds.

- **GABA$_A$:** GABA$_A$ is the major inhibitory neurotransmitter receptor system (accounting for around 30% of all inhibitory synapses), which makes it a prime candidate for a major site of action of general anaesthetics. Experimental work confirms that various compounds, including volatile and intravenous induction agents, enhance the ability of GABA to open the GABA$_A$ receptor ion channel. Almost all general anaesthetic agents, with the exceptions of xenon and ketamine, appear to influence the GABA$_A$ receptor at therapeutically relevant concentrations. The receptor consists of a pentameric arrangement of different subunits around the central ion channel pore. There are 18 subunits (α_{1-6}, β_{1-3}, γ_{1-3}, δ, ε, π, ρ_{1-3}) and a total of around 30 receptor isoforms. Complex research techniques have shown that single amino acid substitutions within the receptor subunit have a marked influence on anaesthetic effect, which confirms the highly specific interaction of drug and receptor. In respect of benzodiazepines, for example, it appears as though the α_1 subunit mediates sedation and amnesia, whereas the α_2 subunit is responsible for anxiolysis. (This is already more detail than you are likely to need.)

- **Glycine receptors:** the glycine receptor is the spinal cord and brain stem analogue of the GABA$_A$ receptor of the brain. This too contains an integral chloride channel and is affected by general anaesthetic agents.

- **5-HT$_3$ and neuronal nicotinic acetylcholine receptors:** general anaesthesia affects cationic currents through these receptors, but further than this the function of these central receptors is not fully understood.

- **Glutamate receptors:** these consist of the N-methyl-D-aspartate (NMDA) and non-NMDA receptor classes, which comprise the primary excitatory neurotransmitter system in the brain. Inhibition of their function is therefore consistent with a theory of general anaesthesia. Ketamine, xenon and nitrous oxide all inhibit the NMDA receptor. The non-NMDA glutamate receptors are divided into various subclasses (AMPA and kainate), which are both strongly affected by ethyl alcohol but not by volatile anaesthetics.

- **Conclusion:** those who searched originally for a unifying theory of general anaesthetic action could not have envisaged the research techniques that have begun to identify the highly complex structures of CNS receptors. Although many details remain to be elucidated, it now seems clear that the spectrum of altered physiological states which is characterized by anaesthesia is mediated by highly specific interactions of anaesthetic compounds with receptor proteins.

Direction the viva may take

Once you have explored some of the concepts outlined above there is nowhere much for the questioning to go, and so the viva may well move on. If you find yourself discussing individual anaesthetic agents then it is likely that either you, the examiner, or possibly both, have exhausted all mutual knowledge of the subject.

Jaundice

Commentary

In routine practice it is rare to encounter deeply jaundiced patients. The outline science of the topic will occupy part of the viva, and its relevance to clinical medicine is obvious. Hepatic disease is a large subject, but you will be expected to recall the important implications for anaesthesia, among which are the hepatorenal syndrome and coagulopathy.

The viva

You may be asked about the perioperative implications of jaundice.

- **Aetiology:** the cause is important because of accompanying morbidity; cirrhosis, for example, may be associated with alcoholic cardiomyopathy.
- **Coagulopathy:** the liver synthesizes many of the protein clotting factors, including prothrombin (factor II) and the other vitamin K-dependent factors (VII, IX and X). Jaundice may be associated with derangements of coagulation.
- **Myocardium:** bile salts can depress the myocardial conduction system and cause significant bradycardia.
- **Renal system:** anaesthesia in the presence of liver dysfunction can be followed by the hepatorenal syndrome, in which acute renal failure may supervene in the immediate postoperative period. The cause remains unknown, although it is presumed to be due to a hepatic endotoxin that the damaged liver can no longer contain. Management recommendations include the use of generous fluid therapy with the use of mannitol to enhance urine output. The risk is particularly great if bilirubin concentrations exceed 180 μmol l^{-1}.

- **Infective hepatitis:** anaesthesia in the acute phase is invariably deleterious to hepatic function. Theatre staff must also be protected against the risks of contamination.
- **Drug elimination:** the reserve even of the damaged liver is great, but anaesthetists should be aware that the normal mechanisms by which drugs are excreted may be impaired. Cytochrome P450 enzymes are converted to the inactive cytochrome P420. Hypoproteinaemia may increase the proportion of free active drug.
- **SpO$_2$ monitoring:** the absorption coefficient of bilirubin is similar to that of deoxygenated haemoglobin, and so SpO$_2$ will read artificially low.
- **Postoperative jaundice:** causes de novo include haemolysis following blood transfusion, and adverse drug reactions. All volatile anaesthetics are metabolized in the liver, and halothane hepatitis is a well recognized entity. The use of halothane is now negligible in the UK, but hepatitis of unknown aetiology has been reported rarely following the use of enflurane, isoflurane and sevoflurane.

Direction the viva may take

You will be asked to discuss the aetiology of jaundice.

- Jaundice (icterus) is the yellowing of skin, sclera and mucous membranes which occurs as a result of the accumulation of bilirubin (either free or conjugated) in the blood. The normal bilirubin concentration is less than 17 μmol l^{-1} and jaundice is not usually detectable clinically until it reaches around 35 μmol l^{-1}. (Some authorities say 50 μmol l^{-1}.)
- Bilirubin is formed from the breakdown of haemoglobin in the reticuloendothelial system. The polypeptides of the haemoglobin molecule (the 'globin') are separated from the haem moiety, which in turn is catabolized to biliverdin. Haem is an iron-containing porphyrin derivative. Biliverdin is converted to bilirubin prior to excretion in bile.
- Fat-soluble unconjugated bilirubin binds to albumin in the circulation and is transported to the liver, where it dissociates prior to conjugation with glucuronic acid. As the water-soluble bilirubin diglucuronide it is excreted via the bile canaliculi. A small amount gains access to the circulation to be excreted in urine.

Causes of jaundice

There are four potential causes of hyperbilirubinaemia. It may be caused by excess production, by defective uptake into hepatocytes, by deficient intracellular binding or conjugation, and by problems with secretion of bilirubin into the biliary system.

- **Increased bilirubin production:** the major cause is haemolytic anaemia. Free bilirubin concentrations rise, but rarely exceed 50 μmol l^{-1} because the liver has substantial reserve capacity to handle the excess.
- **Decreased hepatic bilirubin uptake:** diminished intake of bilirubin into hepatocytes occurs in Gilbert's disease, which causes unconjugated non-haemolytic hyperbilirubinaemia. It can also occur during the resolving phase of viral hepatitis. Free bilirubin concentration is rarely >50 μmol l^{-1}.
- **Defective bilirubin binding or conjugation:** this is characteristic particularly of premature neonates whose enzyme systems may be immature. It also occurs in rare

(and usually fatal) diseases such as Crigler–Najjar syndrome. Free bilirubin concentrations rise.

- **Diminished secretion into the biliary system:** there are both extrahepatic and intrahepatic causes of a rise in conjugated bilirubin concentrations. Biliary outflow may be obstructed by gallstones (common), and by biliary and pancreatic carcinoma (rare). Intrahepatic cholestasis is associated with numerous conditions. It occurs in infective and alcoholic hepatitis, in severe cirrhosis of the liver, and as a result of primary biliary cirrhosis and sclerosing cholangitis. Cholestasis can occur in pregnancy (it is usually mild and is of unknown cause) and can be drug-induced. Implicated agents include oral contraceptives, anabolic steroids, sulphonamides and some neuroleptic agents, including chlorpromazine and haloperidol.
- These causes may combine: hepatocellular damage for example, increases serum bilirubin by all four mechanisms.

Latex allergy

Commentary

Latex allergy was first recognized in the late 1970s, since which time the use of latex in the surgical environment has become ubiquitous. In the last decade it has been identified as a cause of anaphylaxis, and it has been suggested that, because of prolonged exposure to latex-containing products, as many as 10% of healthcare workers may be sensitive. It is an important cause of unexplained intraoperative collapse, and so you will be expected to have an understanding of the problem and its management.

The viva

You will be asked to describe latex allergy.

- Latex is natural rubber produced from the milky sap of the rubber plant (*Hevea brasiliensis*). It comprises not only proteins but also lipid and carbohydrate molecules. It is the soluble proteins that cause severe allergic responses.
- The reactions to latex products include simple irritant contact dermatitis, and allergic contact dermatitis, which is a type IV T cell-mediated hypersensitivity reaction to the chemicals used in manufacture. The potentially fatal response to latex exposure is a type I IgE-mediated hypersensitivity reaction. Sensitized individuals produce IgE antibodies to latex proteins which, on re-exposure, may lead to an anaphylactic reaction with massive histamine release from mast cells and basophils (page 397).

Direction the viva may take

You may be asked how you would identify patients at risk, and about their peri-operative management.

- **Identification:** type I hypersensitivity is best diagnosed by skin-prick testing. As long as the testing solutions contain a range of specific latex allergens, this has a sensitivity of 97% and specificity of 100%. Radioallergoabsorbent tests (RAST) may identify latex-specific IgE, but have a 25% rate of false positive and false negative results. In the absence of such evidence the diagnosis is clinical. There may be a history of sensitivity to rubber products; also at risk are individuals who have been exposed repeatedly to latex products. Healthcare workers, patients undergoing repeated urinary catheterization, and patients who have undergone multiple surgical operations are included in this group. The patient may have a history of atopy and multiple allergy. There is cross-reactivity with a number of foods, among them kiwi fruit, avocado, papaya and chestnuts. Patients may also describe allergy to poinsettia plants.

- **Perioperative management:** all latex-containing products must be identified and avoided. Latex is ubiquitous and is found in trolley mattresses, pillows, TED stockings (those for the lower leg are latex-free), surgical gloves, elastic bandages, urinary catheters and surgical drains. Anaesthetic equipment which may contain latex includes the rubber bungs in some drug vials, which should therefore be removed before they are made into solution, some giving sets, blood pressure cuffs, face masks, nasopharyngeal airways, breathing systems and electrode pads. Recognition of this problem, however, has meant that latex-free equipment is now so widely available that many hospitals no longer need a separate trolley or box containing specific items for the latex-allergic patient. Some units insist that such patients should be placed first on a list to minimize the risk of exposure to airborne latex particles released during previous surgical procedures.

Further direction the viva could take

You may be asked how you would recognize and treat an anaphylactic reaction. Your management of this emergency must be accurate and safe.

- **Diagnosis:** in an established anaphylactic reaction the patient will be hypotensive, with angio-oedema or an urticarial rash, and have severe bronchoconstriction. Hypotension is commoner as a main feature than bronchoconstriction, but the latter may be much more refractory to treatment. Only one system may be involved, and few patients will manifest the full range of clinical features. The onset of an anaphylactic reaction can sometimes be heralded by more subtle signs such as sneezing or coughing, and by the slower development of cutaneous signs. (Reactions to latex usually occur at least 30 minutes into surgery.)
- **Management:** after discontinuing contact with the trigger substance, management can follow the **A**irway, **B**reathing, **C**irculation algorithm. The patient should be given 100% oxygen and positioned supine with the legs and pelvis elevated to enhance venous return. The mainstay of treatment is adrenaline, which can be given initially in a dose of 0.5 mg (0.5 ml of 1:1000) by intramuscular injection into the lateral thigh. Anaesthetists are likely to prefer intravenous administration; typically 50–100 μg over a minute and repeated according to response. Severe cases may need adrenaline by infusion at a rate of 100 μg min^{-1}. Secondary treatment can include corticosteroids, antihistamines and bronchodilators, although these are much less important than adrenaline, which is potentially life-saving.

Brain stem death testing

Commentary

Testing for brain stem death is long established, but still excites debate. The residual controversy may greatly trouble the relatives of a patient who may be brain-dead, and so it is of crucial importance that you understand the neurological basis of the tests sufficiently well to be able to answer any question that they might wish to ask.

The viva

You will be asked to describe the criteria for brain stem death testing.

- **Definition:** brain death describes the situation in which a patient has undergone the irreversible loss of any capacity for consciousness, together with the irreversible loss of the ability to breathe.
- **Preconditions:** before testing can be considered, there are preconditions that must be satisfied, the most important of which is that there must be a definite diagnosis of the cause of the brain damage. The patient should also be in an apnoeic coma, with a Glasgow Coma Score of 3 (no eye opening, no verbal response and no localization of pain).
- **Children:** theoretically, the clinical criteria are the same in children, although there are enough concerns about their applicability to make this a very difficult area. In neonates, for example, CNS immaturity raises doubts about the validity of brain stem death tests, and there is much anecdotal evidence of children who have recovered substantial neurological function despite severe insult and prolonged coma.
- **Exclusions:** the patient's temperature must be at least 35°C. There should be no residual depressant drugs in the system, which in practice may mean substantial delay until clearance can be assured. Neuromuscular blockade should be excluded (where appropriate) by using a peripheral nerve stimulator. There must be no endocrine or metabolic disturbance that may contribute to continued coma, and there should be no possibility that impaired circulatory function is compromising cerebral perfusion. A high $PaCO_2$ can obtund cerebral function, and so must be kept normal (for that patient).
- **The tests:** these are carried out by two doctors, both of who have been registered for more than 5 years, and one of whom must be a consultant. Two sets of tests are performed, although there is no set interval between them. In practice, they are usually done a few hours apart. There has never been a reported case of a patient who initially satisfied the criteria for brain stem death and who subsequently failed to do so. The tests aim to confirm the absence of brain stem reflexes, and examine those cranial nerves which are amenable to testing.
- **The cranial nerve reflexes**
    - *I:* the first nerve (olfactory) cannot be tested.

— *II:* the second nerve (optic), together with the parasympathetic constrictor outflow, is tested by pupillary responses to light (direct and consensual). Pupillary size is not important.

— *III, IV, VI:* the third, fourth and sixth nerves (oculomotor, trochlear and abducens) are not tested.

— *V, VII:* the fifth (trigeminal) and seventh (facial) nerves are tested first by the corneal reflex, and then by the response to painful stimuli applied to the face (supraorbital or infraorbital pressure), to the limbs (nail bed pressure) and to the trunk (sternal stimulation). It is because of the possibility of tetraplegia that a stimulus should be applied above the neck.

— *VIII:* the eighth nerve (auditory/vestibular) is examined by caloric testing. It is important to establish that both drums are visible and intact, after which 30 ml of ice cold water is instilled via a syringe. Nystagmus is absent if the patient is brain-dead. The assessment of doll's eye movements, to test whether the eyes move with the head (which is abnormal) instead of maintaining central gaze, is not part of the brain stem death tests as performed in the UK.

— *IX, X:* the ninth (glossopharyngeal) and tenth (vagus) nerves are tested by stimulating the pharynx, larynx and trachea. The patient should neither gag nor cough.

— *XI, XII:* the eleventh (accessory) and twelfth (hypoglossal) nerves are not tested.

- **Apnoea testing:** after ventilation with 100% oxygen for 10 minutes, the patient is disconnected from the ventilator. Oxygen saturation is maintained thereafter by apnoeic oxygenation via a tracheal catheter. In the apnoeic patient, arterial CO_2 rises at a rate of about 0.40–0.80 kPa per minute depending on the metabolic rate, and so it may take some time to reach the arterial blood gas level of 6.6 kPa required by the testing criteria.

Direction the viva may take
You may be asked about potential pitfalls.

- With the preconditions satisfied and the tests performed with scrupulous care, there should be none. There are, however, some conditions of which those carrying out the tests should be aware.
- There are a number of lesions of the brain stem which may closely mimic irreversible brain death. These include severe Guillain–Barré and Miller–Fisher syndromes, Bickerstaff's brain stem encephalitis, and ventral pontine infarction associated with the locked-in syndrome. Brain stem encephalitis is characterized by acute progressive cranial nerve dysfunction associated with ataxia, coma and apnoea. There is no structural abnormality of the brain, but the picture is one of brain stem death. It is reversible. Bilateral ventral pontine lesions may involve both corticospinal and corticobulbar tracts, leading to tetraplegia and the 'locked-in' syndrome. Patients are unable to speak or produce facial movements. They can usually blink and move their eyes vertically, and because the tegmentum of the pons is spared they remain sensate, fully conscious and aware. It is the stuff of nightmares, and recovery from the locked-in syndrome is unknown.

Further direction the viva could take

You may be asked about any further confirmatory tests that can be undertaken.

- Auditory, visual and somatosensory evoked potentials can be used, as can the EEG and cerebral angiography. None of these is required in the UK.
- It is unlikely that you will be asked about management of the ASA 6 patient for organ retrieval. Clearly the potential donor organs must be oxygenated and well perfused, and this may require some haemodynamic manipulation. The problem arises with the question of 'anaesthesia'. The legal time of death occurs when brain stem death is confirmed, and so logically a dead patient cannot require anaesthesia (except perhaps for muscle relaxants to prevent spinal reflexes). However, there are those who believe brain stem death testing to be little more than a pragmatic way of providing donor organs for transplant, and some anaesthetists appear to share enough residual unease about the process to make them give a general anaesthetic. The philosophical questions that this raises are interesting and important, but the clinical science viva is probably not the best place to explore them.

You might also at some stage be asked about pupillary and eye signs (in general).

- **Pupillary signs:** lateral herniation of the tentorium as a result of increased ICP can compress the oculomotor (III) nerve with ipsilateral papillary dilatation. This may also be accompanied by ptosis and motor paralysis of the extraocular muscles (apart from the superior oblique and lateral rectus muscles which are supplied by cranial nerves IV and VI, respectively). Central tentorial herniation can cause miosis (due to diencephalic damage). If there is midbrain compression, the size of the pupils may remain in the mid-range, but they are unresponsive. Pinpoint and unreactive pupils may signify pontine haemorrhage.
- **Eye signs:** raised ICP obstructs CSF flow in the optic nerve sheath with the development of papilloedema. The lateral rectus is also affected because of the displacement of the sixth cranial nerve (abducens) during its long intracranial course. (As it leaves the posterior margin of the pons, it is crossed by the anterior inferior cerebellar artery. Cerebellar displacement may cause compression of the nerve, paresis and failure of lateral gaze.)

Haemofiltration

Commentary

Haemofiltration (HF) is a common intensive therapy intervention. Many patients require a period of renal support and you are expected to be familiar with its principles. Remember again that if your examiners do not work in intensive care units, then your experience and knowledge may be more recent than theirs.

The viva

You may be asked first about the indications for HF. The list is not long and so you will rapidly move on to the principles underlying the technique.

- **Indications:** these include acute renal failure (ARF) accompanied by a metabolic acidosis, hyperkalaemia or uraemia. Isolated uraemia is a problem usually only when the urea concentration is high enough to cause clinical symptoms such as vomiting, diarrhoea, pruritus or mental disturbance. HF is also used to manage volume overload and to clear some drugs and poisons from the circulation. HF can be used in the management of severe hypothermia; veno–venous systems using counter-current blood warmers can raise core temperatures by up to 2°C per hour.

Principles of haemofiltration

- The filters used in HF are sometimes referred to colloquially as 'kidneys', which reflects their role as literal renal substitutes.
- In the normal kidney the glomerulus filters water, ions, negatively charged particles of molecular weight of less than 15 000 and neutral substances of molecular weight up to about 40 000. Renal corpuscular channels have negatively charged pores, which oppose the passage of negatively charged plasma proteins such as albumin.
- Normal glomerular filtration rate (GFR) is $125 \, \text{ml} \, \text{min}^{-1}$ ($7.5 \, \text{l} \, \text{h}^{-1}$).
- Tubular reabsorption reduces the filtrate of $180 \, \text{l} \, \text{day}^{-1}$ to about $1 \, \text{l} \, \text{day}^{-1}$, and salvages many of the filtered ions and other particles (diffusion and mediated transport). Tubular secretion is the means whereby larger molecules and protein-bound substances (such as drugs and toxins) are eliminated.
- In the HF system, arterial pressure (which may be pump-assisted) delivers a flow of up to $100–200 \, \text{ml} \, \text{min}^{-1}$ to the semi-permeable membrane in the filter. Water and low molecular weight substances (up to 20 000) cross the membrane (which is acting as the 'glomerulus').
- Urea and creatinine will be removed, as will electrolytes and some drugs and toxins. Plasma proteins and all formed blood components remain within the circulation.
- Tubular reabsorption is mimicked by the direct infusion of balanced electrolyte solution, with concentrations adjusted as necessary. The volume infused will depend on the clinical situation. If the patient is not volume-overloaded, then infusion will be at the same rate as the filtration rate, plus a component for maintenance fluid. If fluid removal is indicated, then negative balance is easily achieved by decreasing the infusion rate.
- HF is an efficient means of treating fluid overload, but in comparison with the kidney is very inefficient at removing solute. Very high volumes of ultrafiltrate (upwards of $15 \, \text{l} \, \text{day}^{-1}$) are required to remove urea, creatinine and other products of metabolism.
- Haemodiafiltration is much more efficient at removing solute. A dialysis solution is passed across the filter in a counter-current fashion so that solute can be removed both by convection (as in HF alone) and by diffusion.

Direction the viva may take

You may be asked about potential complications of the therapy.

- **Fluid mismanagement:** very large volumes are both filtered and infused, and the potential scope for error is high.
- **Coagulation problems:** blood clots in extracorporeal circulations and produces diffuse thrombi on the artificial surfaces unless the system is anticoagulated, usually with heparins or prostacyclin. Inadequate coagulation leads to problems with the circuit (the 'kidney' fails), but not the patient. An iatrogenic coagulopathy, however, may be much more hazardous.
- **Other complications**
  — *Air embolus:* this is always a potential danger with the use of relatively complex extracorporeal circuits.
  — *Heat loss:* this is caused by the large fluid shifts.
  — *Disconnection:* HF requires wide-bore dedicated arterial and venous lines.
  — *Filter failure.*

Blood groups

Commentary

The subject of blood groups might appear on its own linked to a clinical question about acute haemolytic reactions; alternatively, it may arise as part of a general discussion of the complications of blood transfusion (pages 371–373). The importance of the topic is self-evident, and so examiners could well assume that your knowledge of the clinical aspects is secure. The viva may start with a discussion of transfusion reactions before continuing with the science of the ABO blood group typing system. After the relatively straightforward concepts of the major types, the subject becomes too complex to explore in a short viva, and the questioning is likely to revert to clinical aspects.

The viva

You may be asked first what would make you suspect that a patient was having an immediate transfusion reaction and how you would manage it.

- The acute antigen–antibody reaction can start after transfusion of only very small volumes of blood. The donor cells are destroyed by antibodies in the recipient plasma, with haemolysis; this leads in some cases to intravascular fibrin deposition, disseminated intravascular coagulation and renal failure. If the patient is conscious then the relatively non-specific symptoms include dyspnoea, loin and chest pain, headache, nausea and vomiting. The patient may become pyrexial, may have rigors, can develop an urticarial rash and usually becomes hypotensive. In the anaesthetized patient, most of these features are lost apart from the possible urticaria and hypotension. As the reaction continues the patient may develop haemoglobinuria and a coagulopathy.

- **Management:** after stopping the transfusion, management is directed mainly towards standard cardiorespiratory support with airway intervention, fluids and inotropes as indicated. It is important to maximize renal perfusion because the risk of ARF is high. Acute haemolytic reactions due to ABO or rhesus incompatibility are very rare (10 cases were reported to Serious Hazards of Transfusion (SHOT) in 2005) and occur usually as a result of human error.

Direction the viva will take

You will then be asked to describe the major blood groups.

- The red cell membrane contains various blood group antigens, or agglutinogens. These are complex oligosaccharides which vary in their terminal sugar molecule (*N*-acetylgalactosamine in group A, and galactose in group B).
- The most important of many variants are the A and the B antigens. These are inherited as Mendelian dominants which allows separation of individuals into one of four main types: group A, which have the A antigen; B, which have the B antigen; AB, which carry both antigens; and group O which carry neither. Red blood cells of all types also carry an H antigen which also differs in the terminal sugar residues.
- Antibodies against these red cell agglutinogens are known as red cell agglutinins, and these are formed early in life. Individuals do not necessarily require exposure to blood; antigens that are related to A and B are found in gut bacteria and even in some foods, and so neonates develop early antibody responses. Type A individuals develop anti-B antibodies; type B develop anti-A antibodies; type AB develop neither, while type O develop both. Type O blood will therefore agglutinate (clump) blood of all other types, while group AB will agglutinate none. Thus AB is the universal recipient and O the universal donor. Around 45% of individuals in the UK have the blood group O; 40% group A; 10% group B; and 5% group AB.
- **Other agglutinogens:** there are a large number of systems of which the rhesus is the most significant. (Others, amongst many, include the Lutheran, the Kidd and the Kell systems.) The rhesus factor comprises C, D and E antigens, of which D is the most important, being by far the most antigenic. Eighty-five per cent of the Caucasian population and 99% of the non-Caucasian population are D-rhesus-positive. In contrast to ABO antigens, individuals do require exposure to the D antigen in blood to develop antibodies, and this happens either by transfusion or by exposure of the maternal circulation to small amounts of fetal D-positive blood. This is significant for subsequent pregnancies should a mother be rhesus-negative but carrying a rhesus-positive fetus. Maternal antibodies will cross the placenta to cause haemolytic disease of the newborn. Hence the importance of administering rhesus immune globulin in the postpartum period to prevent the mother forming active antibodies.

Further direction the viva could take

You may be asked how you can reduce the requirement for banked (stored) blood. There are a number of techniques which can minimize exposure to allogenic blood with its attendant risks (adverse reactions, infection and immunomodulation).

- **Autologous donation:** patients donate 450 ml (1 unit) of blood up to twice a week, but more commonly weekly, up to 72 hours before surgery. Iron supplementation is routine. The production of endogenous erythropoietin is enhanced during twice-weekly donation, but is more modest if donation is less frequent. The procedure is useful for patients undergoing surgery with anticipated major blood loss. Units stored should be matched against likely usage, but wastage is high (around 50%).

- **Acute normovolaemic haemodilution:** whole blood is removed from the patient and replaced with crystalloid and/or colloid solutions prior to the anticipated blood loss. Blood is then reinfused as appropriate, but in the reverse order of collection, because the first unit collected has the highest haematocrit and the greatest concentrations of platelets and clotting factors. The technique is conceptually attractive, but mathematical modelling demonstrates that the actual volumes of saved blood are relatively small (amounting to the equivalent of 1 unit of packed cells). For example, it has been calculated that a patient from whom 3 units totalling 1350 ml are withdrawn prior to a blood loss of 2600 ml will require only about 215 ml less allogenic blood than otherwise would be the case.

- **Perioperative autologous blood recovery:** intraoperative cell-saver devices can be very efficient, saving the equivalent of up to 10 units hourly should massive transfusion be necessary. Its cost-effectiveness is disputed, and some prospective trials in major vascular patients have demonstrated that it does not reduce the requirement to give allogenic blood. It can, however, provide blood rapidly, which may be one of its major benefits. Postoperative reinfusion of blood collected from drains is used after orthopaedic surgery, but the blood so collected has a low haematocrit of around 0.20, is partly haemolysed and may be rich in cytokines. Its benefits are debated.

Complications of blood transfusion

Commentary

The most recent Serious Hazards of Transfusion (SHOT) Report identified 609 adverse events and five deaths out of a total of 3.1 million blood components that were issued by the BTS. At that time (2005) the reporting system was still voluntary and so this incidence of 0.02% is an underestimate. It is clear none the less that administration of blood and blood products is very safe. Their rarity notwithstanding, anaesthetists should be familiar with the complications of transfusion, and you should be able to give a reasonable overview of the main problems.

The viva

You will be asked about the complications associated with blood transfusion.

- **Transfusion-related acute lung injury (TRALI):** there were two deaths attributed to TRALI in the 2005 report, which makes it numerically the most significant complication. Of 23 suspected cases, 6 were described as 'probable', which confirms the diagnostic uncertainty of the condition. TRALI presents with an acute respiratory distress syndrome either immediately or within 6 hours of transfusion. The plasma of donor blood can contain leucocyte antibodies which target recipient neutrophils. Within the pulmonary microvasculature there is destruction of capillary endothelium by oxygen free radicals and proteolytic enzymes, with resultant exudation of fluid and proteinaceous material into the alveoli and the development of pulmonary oedema. The same phenomenon can occur in the absence of measurable leucocyte antibodies but in the presence of some other trigger in donor plasma. This is referred to as non-immune TRALI (mortality is lower). TRALI is more likely in response to blood products with a high plasma component such as fresh frozen plasma (FFP), platelets and cryoprecipitate, and especially if the donor is female. (Human leucocyte antigen antibodies are commoner in multiparous women.) The risk is reduced by leucocyte depletion and by the use of male donors.

- **Acute haemolytic reactions:** an acute antigen–antibody reaction is initiated by ABO or rhesus incompatibility (page 370). Donor cells are destroyed by antibodies in the recipient plasma, with the resultant haemolysis leading in some cases to intravascular fibrin deposition, disseminated intravascular coagulation and renal failure. Ten such reactions were reported in the last SHOT report, with one death.
- **Non-haemolytic (febrile) reactions:** these are common and are mediated by donor leucocyte antigens which react with recipient antibodies to form a complex that binds complement and releases pyrogenic inflammatory mediators such as IL-1 and IL-6 and TNFα. Cytokines can also be introduced directly into the circulation by contaminated residual leucocytes in platelet concentrates. Leucodepletion attenuates the risk.
- **Allergic and anaphylactic reactions:** allergic reactions to proteins in donor plasma are relatively common, are usually mild, and present with typical features of pruritus and urticaria. Anaphylactic reactions are rare, although one such fatal reaction to FFP was reported in the 2005 report.
- **Complications of massive transfusion:** the replacement of a patient's total blood volume within 24 hours (which is one simple definition of a massive transfusion) can affect their temperature, their biochemistry and their coagulation.
  - *Temperature:* blood infused directly from storage will be at around 4°C. One litre of unwarmed blood can lower core temperature by 0.5°C. The effects of perioperative hypothermia are well known and include reduced oxygen delivery (because of the leftward shift of the oxygen–haemoglobin dissociation curve), impaired wound healing, abnormalities of coagulation and increased infection rates. Hypothermia also slows enzymatic reactions so that metabolism of the citrate and lactate in stored blood is reduced.
  - *Biochemistry:* hyperkalaemia is rarely a problem because, although the potassium in stored blood can be many times higher than normal, once within the circulation intracellular re-uptake is rapid. However, if cold blood is infused quickly through a central venous cannula (in error) it will be cardioplegic. Stored blood contains citrate as an anticoagulant, which, when metabolized to bicarbonate in large amounts, can contribute to a metabolic alkalosis (which further impairs enzyme function).
  - *Coagulation:* plasma-reduced blood contains minimal coagulation factors which rapidly become depleted during massive transfusion. This dilutional coagulopathy

may be complicated by the onset of disseminated intravascular coagulation associated with persistent haemorrhage.

- **Immunomodulation:** the immunosuppressive effect of homologous blood was exploited deliberately in early renal transplantation to reduce rejection rates. It is now evident that transfusion suppresses IL-2 production, killer cell activity and macrophage function. It also lowers the CD4/CD8 cell count ratio (which is the ratio of T lymphocytes that express the C4 antigen to those that express the C8 antigen, and is an indicator of the overall level of immune suppression). This immunomodulation is associated with increased rates of metastasis and tumour recurrence following surgery for colonic and other cancers, with a heightened risk of postoperative infection, and with the activation of latent chronic viral infection (such as herpes simplex).

- **Transmission of infection:** bacterial contamination of blood and blood products is possible, and, because transfusion will ensure a large intravenous inoculum of pathogen, such contamination can result in fulminant septicaemia. (Gram-negative species thrive at the blood storage temperature of 4°C.) Viral contamination may be more insidious and there are many recipients who are now suffering the consequences of receiving blood that at the time was unknowingly contaminated with the hepatitis B and C viruses, and with HIV. Although blood is now screened for these viruses as well as T cell lymphotrophic virus, syphilis and cytomegalovirus, there remains a transmission window during which the donor may be infected but still seronegative. Prion diseases (such as variant Creutzfeld–Jacob disease) are more insidious still; the latent period may be very long and there are no diagnostic tests.

- **Graft-versus-host disease:** this is a very rare complication which can occur in recipients who are immunocompromised. Donor immune cells, particularly T lymphocytes, attack host tissue, which includes bone marrow stem cells. Ninety per cent of cases are fatal.

Cytochrome P450

Commentary

This is the kind of question that risks giving the College and its examinations a bad name. It is not as though cytochrome P450 is a single well defined entity; on the contrary, it comprises numerous key forms with yet further genetic variations. Nor is it a topic of searing anaesthetic relevance; certainly it is of academic interest, but ignorance of most of its functions is little impediment to the delivery of safe and sophisticated anaesthesia. However, as a subject that is perceived both as intellectual and topical it is no surprise to find it appearing in the Final FRCA. If the question is asked of you, just reproduce confidently some of what appears below (which itself is a substantial oversimplification of a complex and detailed topic), and you will almost certainly know more than your examiners. If, however, you should happen to be discussing this with an examiner whose special interest this happens to be, then do not worry. His or her specialist knowledge will inhibit their line of questioning because they will be conscious of their loss of objectivity regarding this particular subject.

The viva

There is no obvious starting point for this question because the science will need to precede the clinical aspects. You may just be asked what you can tell the examiner about cytochrome P450.

- **Description:** cytochrome or, more accurately, cytochromes P450 comprise a superfamily of enzymes which are concerned with the metabolism of a wide range both of endogenous and exogenous compounds. They contain a pigment (hence cyto*chrome*) and are characterized by maximal absorption in the presence of carbon monoxide, at 450 nm. This cytochrome–carbon monoxide compound is pink, which explains the 'P' in the nomenclature.
- **Biochemistry:** they are haem–thiolate proteins, and they act as mixed function mono-oxygenases, now known as 'Phase I enzymes' because they mediate the Phase I oxidative metabolism (mainly oxidation and hydroxylation) of numerous compounds.
- **Numbers:** in humans there are 18 families, 43 subfamilies and 57 enzymes, each encoded by a separate gene. This manifests as a wide variation in the susceptibility of different individuals to particular drugs and toxins. Despite these large numbers it is estimated that six main CYP enzymes are responsible for more than 90% of all drug oxidation.
- **Sites:** these ubiquitous microsomal enzymes are sited on the smooth endoplasmic reticulum of cells, but are found in highest concentrations in the liver and small bowel. Individual hepatocytes may contain several forms of the enzyme.
- **Nomenclature:** the enzymes are divided into main families according to similarities in their amino acid sequences (possessing 40% or more structural homology) and are named CYP1, CYP2 and so on. It is families CYP1, CYP2 and CYP3 which appear to be responsible for most drug biotransformation. These groups are then further classified into subfamilies (possessing 55% or more homology) which are described using capital letters following the family designation. Individual enzymes of the subgroup are designated using arabic numerals for example, CYP3A4: (CYP3 (family), A (subfamily), 4 (individual enzyme)).
- **Important subtypes:** the most abundant cytochrome enzymes are members of the CYP3A subfamily, which comprise 70% of the cytochrome enzymes in the gastrointestinal system, and 30% of those in the liver. The enzyme that metabolizes the greatest proportion of drugs in the liver is cytochrome CYP3A4. This enzyme and CYP3A3 are the major isoforms of the small gut, while the variant that is found in the stomach is CYP3A5. (This is absent in 70% of Caucasians but its functions are replicated in such cases by CYP3A4.)

Direction the viva may take

You may be asked about factors which influence the function of the cytochrome enzymes, particularly in respect of drug metabolism, because this is the area of potential relevance to anaesthetic practice.

- **Induction of enzymes:** as plasma concentrations of drugs increase, so enzyme synthesis may increase to match it, and numerous substances induce cytochrome P450. These include barbiturates, anticonvulsants, alcohol, glucocorticoids and some antibiotics. (This is a generalization because these agents induce different groups; alcohol, for example, induces CYP2E1. You will not be expected to recount this level of detail.) Tobacco, or at least its polycyclic aromatic hydrocarbons, is also a potent inducer of cytochrome P450 (CYP1A1 and CYP1A2), and this is of anaesthetic interest because smoking appears to confer a protective effect against postoperative nausea and vomiting (PONV). This may be because of the more rapid metabolism and elimination of volatile agents which are associated with PONV, although the hypothesis remains speculative. (Smokers also show less sensitivity both to the effects of aminosteroid neuromuscular blockers as well as to morphine, although probably not by mechanisms associated with cytochrome P450.)

- **Inhibition of enzyme action:** competitive inhibition occurs when two (or more) drugs are metabolized by the same enzyme. The process can be complex, with reversible and irreversible binding to the haem binding site, either by drugs or by their metabolites. Such interactions may have serious consequences. An example is the cardiac arrhythmias associated with the antihistamine terfenadine. The drug can lead to a prolonged Q–T interval with the development of torsade de pointes (a malignant form of ventricular tachycardia characterized by a changing QRS axis). Inhibition of CYP3A4 by substances as diverse as the antibiotic erythromycin or by the bioflavinoids in grapefruit juice may precipitate arrhythmias by inhibiting terfenadine metabolism. Terfenadine itself is a prodrug which is cardiotoxic, whereas its active metabolite is not. Drugs such as metronidazole and amiodarone inhibit CYP2C9, which is the enzyme involved in the metabolism of warfarin. Both can produce significant prolongations of prothrombin time. The analogous effects of cimetidine, which is a non-specific inhibitor of cytochrome P450, are relatively weak in comparison.

Mitral valve disease

Commentary

Valvular pathology is of clinical interest because of the risk that anaesthesia and surgery will cause perioperative decompensation. Mitral valve disease is a popular topic because it allows discussion of physiology and pharmacology applied to a fixed cardiac output state.

The viva

You will be asked about the clinical features and anaesthetic implications of mitral valve disease.

Mitral stenosis

- Mitral stenosis is almost always due to untreated rheumatic fever, usually following streptococcal infection. It is increasingly rare.
- **Pathophysiology:**
  — The pressure gradient across the narrowed valve is less reliable than estimations of valvular area, which is the key factor which determines flow. The cross-sectional area of a normal mitral valve area is 4–6 cm^2. Stenosis may be graded as mild (1.6–2.5 cm^2), moderate (1.1–1.5 cm^2) and severe (<1 cm^2). Between 2.5 and 4.0 cm^2 the narrowing is not clinically significant.
  — As the stenosis worsens, the left atrium dilates and hypertrophies and the contribution of atrial contraction to left ventricular filling becomes progressively more important, increasing from 15% up to 40%. Compensatory bradycardia allows sufficient time for diastolic flow across the stenosis. These factors explain why the onset of atrial fibrillation (AF) with the loss of this crucial contribution to left ventricular filling can be calamitous. In time, the increased left atrial pressure (LAP) is reflected in pulmonary hypertension and right ventricular overload.
  — As pulmonary venous pressure increases, symptoms will include dyspnoea on exertion, orthopnoea and paroxysmal nocturnal dyspnoea. Impaired exercise tolerance is a good guide to disease severity. Pulmonary sequelae of mitral stenosis may encompass reduced lung compliance and a rise in airway resistance, both of which increase the work of breathing. Gas exchange worsens with a widening of the alveolar–arterial oxygen difference (A–aDO$_2$).

Anaesthetic implications of mitral stenosis

- Mitral stenosis can lead to a fixed output state. Anaesthesia must minimize interference with compensatory mechanisms, because attempts to manipulate the cardiac output by the use of fluids or vasoactive drugs may prove fruitless.
- **Heart rate and rhythm:** bradycardia may allow increased stroke volume but at the expense of cardiac output; tachycardia will reduce stroke volume and also reduce cardiac output.
- **Maintenance of cardiac rhythm:** sudden onset of AF must be treated aggressively, with DC cardioversion if necessary, otherwise pulmonary oedema may develop. If AF is already present, the ventricular response rate must be controlled.
- **Circulating volume:** normovolaemia is important. If LAP drops because of reduced venous return then cardiac output will fall as flow across the stenotic valve decreases. Patients may also be very sensitive to increases in venous return: in severe stenosis cardiac output cannot change and pulmonary oedema may supervene.
- **Contractility:** effective myocardial contraction is important and depression must be minimized.
- **Systemic vascular resistance (SVR):** normal SVR ensures adequate coronary perfusion during diastole.
- **Pulmonary vascular resistance (PVR):** hypercapnia, hypoxia and acidosis will all increase PVR. Nitrous oxide further increases PVR in the presence of pre-existing pulmonary hypertension and so should be avoided.
- **Infective bacterial endocarditis:** see below.

- **Anticoagulation:** patients may be taking oral anticoagulants which may need to be changed to parenteral heparin during the perioperative period, depending on the surgery to be undertaken.

Mitral incompetence

- Mitral incompetence is commoner than stenosis. It is rheumatic in origin in around 50% of cases. Other causes include disruption of the chordae tendinae and papillary muscle supporting structures (this can follow myocardial infarction), and dilatation of the valve ring itself.
- **Pathophysiology**
  - During systolic left ventricular contraction there is regurgitant flow back into the left atrium in addition to forward flow through the aorta. This can be quantified by measuring the regurgitant fraction: up to 0.3 is classified as mild; a fraction of 0.6 or greater is severe.
  - This regurgitant flow leads to volume overload of left atrium and left ventricle. Although left ventricular end-diastolic volume (LVEDV) may increase fourfold, the function of the ventricle is usually well preserved because the larger volume of blood can be unloaded both through the aorta and the mitral valve, and so systolic ventricular wall tension is not high. In time, however, this process leads to an irreversible decline in contractile function.
  - The left atrium dilates, and AF may supervene, but this does not cause the critical decompensation in cardiac function that may be seen in mitral stenosis. Mitral incompetence does not in general impose large costs in terms of myocardial oxygen demand (owing to ventricular wall tension, contractility and heart rate). This allows some compensation by a relatively rapid heart rate, which reduces the time for further ventricular overload. The prolonged filling time associated with a bradycardia increases ventricular volume, may cause further functional dilatation of the annulus and with it a rise in the regurgitant fraction. The left ventricle also dilates, with an increase in LVEDV and pressure. Forward flow of blood into the systemic circulation depends on the relative impedances of the two parallel paths, and so is enhanced by low PVR.

Anaesthetic implications of mitral incompetence

- **Heart rate:** relative tachycardia is preferable to bradycardia because it reduces left ventricular overload. Bradycardia may increase ventricular filling and further dilate the valve ring.
- **Circulating volume:** patients may be sensitive to large rises in preload, because this will further distend the left atrium and predispose to pulmonary oedema.
- **Contractility:** myocardial depression should be avoided.
- **SVR:** the forward flow of blood is dependent upon low peripheral resistance. Vasoconstrictors should be used with caution.
- **Infective bacterial endocarditis:** mitral incompetence is more likely to be associated with infective bacterial endocarditis than any other of the valvular lesions, and antibiotic prophylaxis is recommended. Guidelines change and it is unlikely that you will be asked to discuss this in great detail, but you should have some idea of the current regimens. Typically, amoxicillin is given prior to surgery

(either 3 g orally 4 hours before, or 1 g iv at induction of anaesthesia), followed by intravenous or oral amoxicillin postoperatively. Patients who are allergic to penicillin can be given various drugs, including vancomycin, gentamicin and teicoplanin. The simplest regimen to remember is probably clindamycin, 300 mg by slow intravenous infusion at induction, followed by 150 mg iv or orally at 6 hours postoperatively. There is no evidence to support the routine use of antibiotic prophylaxis, and rumour has it that a working party due to report in 2008 may abandon the recommendation completely.

Aortic valve disease

Commentary
As with other cardiac valvular conditions, anaesthetic interest in aortic valve disease centres on the need to avoid perioperative decompensation. Like mitral pathology, it is a popular exam topic because it allows discussion of applied physiology and pharmacology.

The viva
You will be asked about the clinical features and anaesthetic implications of aortic valve disease.

Aortic stenosis
- Aortic stenosis may be caused by rheumatic heart disease, degeneration and calcification of the valve, either as a result of ageing, or in a congenitally abnormal (usually bicuspid) valve. The distinction between a 'stenotic' and a 'sclerotic' valve is artificial. Sclerosis does stenose the valve but rarely to a critical degree.
- **Pathophysiology**
  — Determination of the pressure gradient across the valve is less reliable than estimations of valvular area. The cross-sectional area of a normal aortic valve is 2.5–3.5 cm^2. An area < 1.0 cm^2 is an indication for immediate surgical valve replacement. At areas of < 0.7 cm^2, any demand for increased cardiac output, such as occurs during advancing pregnancy or during exercise, is likely to be associated with angina pectoris, syncope and sudden death. Clinical signs of the disease include narrowed pulse pressure (a value of < 30 mmHg suggests severe disease), and a coarse systolic murmur in the aortic area. Systolic blood pressure may be lower than expected because of the reduced cardiac output. The gradient may be misleadingly low in a patient whose failing left ventricle is unable to generate high systolic intraventricular pressures.
  — As narrowing progresses there is increased pressure loading on the left ventricle, which undergoes concentric hypertrophy. The hypertrophic left ventricle is less compliant, thus myocardial oxygen demand increases while supply falls. Systole through the stenosed valve is prolonged and so diastolic time during the cardiac cycle is proportionately reduced. The high intraventricular pressures almost

completely abolish systolic coronary flow. Diastolic subendocardial perfusion also decreases unless perfusion pressures remain high.

— The decrease in ventricular compliance and the loss of ventricular filling by passive elastic recoil means that the atrial contribution to filling becomes more important. It may in some cases be responsible for up to 50% of LVEDV. AF may lead to decompensation.

Anaesthetic implications of aortic stenosis

- Aortic stenosis leads to a fixed output state, which is maintained by compensatory mechanisms that may be disrupted by anaesthesia. Decompensated mitral stenosis manifests as heart failure; decompensated aortic stenosis may manifest as death. It is particularly important to maintain coronary perfusion during diastole.
- **Contractility:** effective contraction maintains cardiac output in aortic stenosis (as in all valvular lesions), and undue myocardial depression should be avoided. Increasing myocardial drive, however, does increase myocardial work and oxygen demand, and may precipitate subendocardial ischaemia.
- **Maintenance of SVR and diastolic blood pressure:** if SVR falls then coronary diastolic perfusion may fail, with disastrous consequences. Vasodilatation must be avoided and preload maintained to ensure flow across the stenotic valve. This has obvious implications for the use of the many anaesthetic agents which decrease SVR, including local anaesthetics used in neuraxial block. Cardiopulmonary resuscitation in the presence of aortic stenosis and left ventricular hypertrophy is rarely successful.
- **Heart rate and rhythm:** bradycardia will decrease cardiac output, but tachycardia is more detrimental because it limits the time for diastolic coronary perfusion. Arrhythmias, including AF, require urgent treatment, but myocardial depressants such as β-adrenoceptor blockers are better avoided.
- **Infective bacterial endocarditis:** prophylaxis is recommended (page 377).
- Patients with aortic stenosis can be difficult to manage. Severe cases presenting for non-emergency surgery should be referred to a specialist centre for consideration of aortic valve replacement. Otherwise, anaesthesia should include invasive monitoring of intra-arterial and central venous pressure, and it may be necessary to run a continuous infusion of vasopressor (such as noradrenaline) to ensure that SVR is maintained.

Aortic incompetence

- Aortic incompetence has numerous causes, most of them rare. There are infectious causes (bacterial endocarditis, syphilis, rheumatic fever), congenital abnormalities (bicuspid valve), degenerative and connective tissue disorders (Marfan's syndrome, Ehlers–Danlos), and inflammatory conditions (rheumatoid arthritis, systemic lupus erythematosus).
- **Pathophysiology**
  - The condition is usually chronic, although acute aortic regurgitation can occur with dissection or as the result of destruction of the valve by bacterial endocarditis.
  - The regurgitation during diastole of part of the left ventricular stroke volume decreases forward blood flow through the aorta. This results in continuous

volume overload of the left ventricle, which initially dilates to accommodate this extra volume. On the ascending part of the Frank–Starling pressure–volume curve, the increase in myofibril length improves the efficiency of contraction. With increasing dilatation the heart moves on to the descending part of the curve, at which point acute cardiac failure may supervene.

— Compensatory mechanisms act to reduce the volume of regurgitant blood. As with mitral incompetence, a regurgitant fraction of 0.6 or greater denotes severe disease. There is an increase in left ventricular size with eccentric hypertrophy. There is also an increase in ventricular compliance, which allows an increase in volume at the same pressure. This means that end-diastolic pressure is reduced, and with it ventricular wall tension which is an important determinant of myocardial oxygen demand. The left ventricular ejection fraction is maintained, since the stroke volume and LVEDV increase together.

— A rapid heart rate is advantageous, because it reduces the time for diastolic filling. LVEDV is decreased and so there is less ventricular overdistension.

— Lower SVR offloads the myocardium and ensures forward flow.

Anaesthetic implications of aortic incompetence

- **Preload:** normovolaemia should be maintained to ensure that the dilated ventricle remains well filled.
- **SVR:** this should be kept low so as not to increase the impedance to outflow with an increase in the regurgitant fraction.
- **Heart rate:** bradycardia increases the time for ventricular overdistension. A relative tachycardia will reduce the regurgitant fraction.
- **Contractility:** undue myocardial depression should be avoided.
- **Infective bacterial endocarditis:** prophylaxis is recommended as above.

Electroconvulsive therapy

Commentary

There are few shorter anaesthetics than those given for electroconvulsive therapy (ECT). This benefit is usually offset by the fact that the procedure is often undertaken in isolated sites with patients who may have relevant co-morbidity. The physiological effects may be transient but they can be extreme, and are effects of which you should be aware. (The ECT list may be one of those to which your rota organizer will gratefully allocate you as soon as you obtain the FRCA. You will feel happier if you do know something about it.)

The viva

After an introductory question about the nature of ECT and its indications (which are restricted), you may be asked briefly to describe the characteristics of the stimulation that is used.

- ECT, in which an electric shock is used to induce a grand mal convulsion, is an empirical and somewhat controversial treatment. Its use is now confined mainly to patients with refractory psychiatric disorders, particularly psychotic depression but also catatonia, mania and schizophrenia.
- A shock of about 850 mA is delivered across the cerebral hemispheres by a stimulator that delivers a pulsatile square wave discharge. Pulses of 1.25 ms at 26 Hz are delivered for up to 5 seconds.

Direction the viva may take

The more relevant and interesting aspects for anaesthetists are the physiological changes that accompany ECT, and the viva is more likely to concentrate on these. If you are struggling to retrieve this information, then just try to remember instead the effects of a grand mal fit.

- **Grand mal convulsion:** a short latent phase is followed by a tonic phase of general contracture of skeletal muscle which lasts around 15 seconds. This is succeeded by a clonic phase which lasts 30–60 seconds. The central electrical seizure (as demonstrated by EEG) outlasts the peripheral myoclonus.
- **Autonomic effects – parasympathetic:** the discharge is short-lived, but is associated with typical parasympathetic effects. Their most extreme manifestations include bradycardia and vagal inhibition, leading to asystole.
- **Autonomic effects – sympathetic:** as the clonic phase of the seizure begins there is a mass sympathetic response which peaks at around 2 minutes. Plasma adrenaline and noradrenaline levels at 1 minute exceed baseline by 15 and 3 times, respectively. Predictable effects include tachyarrhythmias and hypertension, with increased myocardial and cerebral oxygen consumption.
- **Cerebral effects:** the cortical discharge is accompanied by a large increase in cerebral blood flow, which may increase over fivefold, and cerebral oxygen consumption ($CMRO_2$), which may increase by four times. Intracranial pressure rises accordingly.
- **Musculoskeletal effects:** the grand mal convulsion is accompanied by violent contractions of all skeletal muscles, and has been associated with vertebral fractures and other skeletal damage. The Bolam principle, which has underpinned the law relating to medical negligence since 1957, followed from a case in which a patient suffered a dislocated hip during an unmodified convulsion associated with ECT.

Further direction the viva could take

You may be asked about complications of the procedure and finally about the anaesthetic implications.

- There are predictable complications associated with the convulsion, which include cardiac arrhythmias and hypertension. The risk of skeletal and tissue damage, for example to the tongue, is minimized by 'modifying' the convulsion with a small dose of suxamethonium. This attenuates the force of the muscle contraction on the skeletal system.

- ECT should not be used in patients who have suffered a recent cerebrovascular or myocardial event (within 3 months), who have a CNS mass lesion or have raised intracranial pressure. It should probably be avoided in patients with osteoporotic bone disease because of the risk of fractures, and should be used with caution in patients with glaucoma and severe ischemic heart disease. A symptomatic hiatus hernia does not contraindicate ECT but does mandate intubation following a rapid sequence induction.
- Anaesthetic implications relate to the physiological effects outlined above, together with the problems of anaesthetizing often elderly patients in remote locations.

Postpartum haemorrhage

Commentary

Deaths due to obstetric haemorrhage continue to feature in successive reports of the triennial Confidential Enquiry into Maternal Deaths in the UK. The absolute numbers are small, yet the preventable death of any young mother has an importance that is belied by the simple epidemiological statistics. This is a more clinically orientated question than many that appear in the clinical science viva, but it does aim to test that your knowledge of factors that predispose to postpartum haemorrhage (PPH) will allow you to manage it aggressively when it occurs.

The viva

You will be asked about the causes of PPH and its predisposing factors.

- **Incidence:** this depends on the definition of PPH. By convention PPH is defined as a blood loss of 500 ml within 24 hours of birth, but as 20% of women will lose that much this exaggerates the number who are at risk of significant haemodynamic disturbance. In the UK, this has been estimated at around 1400 cases a year.
- **Uterine causes:** the most important immediate cause is uterine atony. The placenta receives almost 20% of the cardiac output at term (600–700 ml min^{-1}), which explains why haemorrhage may be catastrophic. In the UK, uterine atony accounts for around one-third of all deaths associated with maternal haemorrhage. Other causes include uterine disruption or inversion, complications of operative or instrumental delivery, and retained products of conception. Retained placenta itself, although not invariably associated with bleeding, complicates some 2% of all deliveries. Abnormal placentation (placenta accreta, increta and percreta) occurs in 1 in 3000 deliveries.
- **Non-uterine causes:** the main causes are genital tract trauma and disorders of coagulation.
- **Risk factors**
  - *Uterine atony:* there is a strong association with augmentation of labour. It may also follow uterine overdistension by multiple births, by polyhydramnios and by

delivery of babies weighing greater than 4 kg. It is associated with protracted labour, with the use of tocolytic drugs and also with maternal hypotension. The relative ischaemia that may accompany uterine hypoperfusion or hypoxia will impair the ability of the uterus to contract effectively. There appears to be no link to multiparity.

— *Abnormal placentation:* a mother with an anterior placenta praevia overlying a previous Caesarean section scar has at least a one in four chance of placenta accreta.

— *Genital tract trauma:* this very vascular area may be damaged during delivery of a large baby, during delivery complicated by shoulder dystocia, or during a forceps delivery or vacuum extraction. Bleeding from the genital tract may be masked by normal post-delivery vaginal loss.

— *Coagulopathy:* this may be associated with abruption of the placenta (in 10% of cases), amniotic fluid embolism (up to 90% of cases), intrauterine death, pregnancy-induced hypertension (particularly HELLP syndrome) and Gram-negative septicaemia.

Direction the viva may take

The viva is likely to concentrate on the drugs that are used to treat uterine atony, as this is the most common cause (page 269).

Pre-eclampsia

Commentary

Pre-eclampsia complicates about 7% of all pregnancies in the UK, and is part of a spectrum of disease which includes HELLP syndrome, peripartum cardiomyopathy and possibly acute fatty liver of pregnancy. It is the second commonest cause of maternal death after thromboembolic disease. Patients with pre-eclampsia are more likely to require anaesthetic expertise than mothers with uncomplicated pregnancies, and so you need to be aware of its potential problems. If you have worked on a labour ward then you will have seen this condition, and your experience is likely to be more recent than many of the examiners, only a proportion of whom are obstetric anaesthetists. The viva will concentrate as much on the basic science as on the practicalities of managing these sick mothers.

The viva

You will be asked about the condition and its aetiology.

• The cause of pre-eclampsia remains unknown, but a simplification of the pathophysiology is summarized below. It is an ischaemic condition that can affect every organ system.

- The normal vasodilatation of vessels in the placental bed which normally occurs after the first trimester does not take place; the vessels instead become constricted and may develop atherosclerosis. Simultaneously, there may be evidence of endothelial abnormality and increased vascular reactivity.
- This primary endothelial damage leads to increased production of the vasoconstrictor thromboxane A_2 and decreased production of vasodilatory prostacyclin, which manifests as an increase in systemic vascular resistance. There may also be an increase in platelet turnover, together with abnormal cytokine release that can precipitate intravascular coagulation.
- This process can result in multi-organ failure, with fibrinoid ischaemic necrosis not only in the placenta but also in cerebral, renal and hepatic vessels. Microvascular thrombin is deposited throughout all vascular beds. This in turn can initiate primary disseminated intravascular coagulation.
- HELLP syndrome (described in 1982) is a variant of the parent disorder, which is characterized by **H**aemolysis, **E**levated **L**iver enzymes and **L**ow **P**latelets. There is hepatic ischaemia with periportal haemorrhage, which can proceed to frank necrosis. Microangiopathic haemolytic anaemia is accompanied by thrombocytopenia. Other parts of the coagulation process may be unaffected. Liver dysfunction is characterized by elevated transaminases (AST, ALT, and γ-GT), and renal impairment is manifest by elevated urea and creatinine, and, in severe cases, haemoglobinuria secondary to haemolysis. These complications may require critical care; although delivery initiates reversal of the disease, platelets may continue to fall for up to 72 hours.
- The aetiology of pre-eclampsia remains elusive. Uteroplacental inadequacy is one factor. This stimulates production of endogenous vasoconstrictors as a means of ensuring uteroplacental perfusion. The resulting hypertension is caused by circulating vasoactive humoral compounds that have been identified in blood, placenta and amniotic fluid. The vascular damage may be mediated via circulating immune complexes. The fetus is antigenic and it is believed that these immune complexes are the result of an inadequate maternal antibody response to what in effect is a foreign allograft.

Direction the viva may take

You may be asked about the clinical aspects of the condition.

- **Clinical features:** severe pre-eclampsia is characterized by hypertension (systolic blood pressure >160 mmHg, diastolic DBP >110 mmHg, and mean arterial pressure >125 mmHg), with proteinuria of >5 g in 24 hours. Patients may show renal impairment with oliguria (defined as output <500 ml in 24 hours), and they may complain of headache and visual disturbances. Distension of the liver capsule may cause epigastric and hypochondrial pain. Pulmonary oedema will impair gas exchange, and clotting may be deranged, particularly by thrombocytopenia. Hyperreflexia and clonus may presage the grand mal convulsions associated with eclampsia. Intrauterine growth retardation of the fetus is common.

Further direction the viva could take

You may be asked to discuss anaesthetic techniques for caesarean section, particularly regional versus general anaesthesia.

- The choice of anaesthetic technique for caesarean section in mothers with pre-eclampsia has been controversial. The potential airway and haemodynamic problems associated with general anaesthesia are well recognized, but the choice between spinal and epidural anaesthesia is contentious. Traditional teaching has it that well-controlled incremental epidural anaesthesia should be used to avoid the precipitous falls in blood pressure which, it is claimed, will accompany spinal anaesthesia. There is no evidence to support this; indeed, there are at least four recent studies which dispute the presumption that severe hypotension accompanies spinal anaesthesia in mothers with pre-eclampsia. There is even a well designed study now over 50 years old and unethical by current standards, which examined the effect of high spinal block on pregnant, pregnant hypertensive, and non-pregnant controls. Profound hypotension affected only those mothers without hypertension. This is not surprising given that humoral rather than neurogenic factors mediate hypertension in pre-eclampsia.
- **Fluids and vasopressors:** these patients have the typical intravascular depletion of a vasoconstricted hypertensive circulation. An infusion of up to $10 \, \text{ml kg}^{-1}$ is accepted practice. Hypertensive mothers are said to be much more sensitive to the effects of catecholamines and so, although there are little data, it is prudent to 'decrease the dose' of prophylactic vasopressors (although no one ever tells you by how much).
- **Other anaesthetic implications:** coagulopathy (which only complicates very severe cases) precludes neuraxial blockade. Treatment may include anti-hypertensive agents (such as labetalol) which can influence the response to epidural and subarachnoid block. Treatment may also include $MgSO_4$, which can potentiate neuromuscular blocking drugs. There may be renal dysfunction and these mothers can easily be fluid-overloaded to the point at which they develop pulmonary oedema secondary to leaky pulmonary capillaries. Laryngoscopy, tracheal intubation and extubation can provoke an extreme pressor response, with surges in systolic blood pressure which may exceed 250 mmHg. Pre-eclampsia is associated with laryngeal and upper airway oedema.

The complex regional pain syndrome

Commentary

Complex regional pain syndrome (CRPS) types I and II are important examples of neuropathic pain. The condition is seen almost exclusively in chronic pain management clinics and you may well have little direct experience of its main features and management. However, neuropathic pain complicates many disease states, is severe and difficult to treat, and remains incompletely understood. For this reason it continues to appear as a popular examination topic.

The viva

You will be asked to define the condition.

- **CRPS types I and II** are the names given to what were formerly known, respectively, as reflex sympathetic dystrophy and causalgia. In some, but not all cases, sympathetically maintained pain may be a prominent feature.
- **CRPS type I** (formerly known as reflex sympathetic dystrophy or Sudek's atrophy) is associated with injury to tissue – bones, joints and connective tissue, but not necessarily to nerves. The trauma may be relatively trivial, and is most commonly precipitated by an orthopaedic injury to a distal extremity such as the lower leg or wrist.
- **CRPS type II** (formerly known as causalgia), by contrast, is characterized by significant nerve injury without transection. It is more commonly associated with proximal nerves in the upper leg and upper limb. Most frequently affected are the sciatic, tibial, median and ulnar nerves.
- **Sympathetic mediation:** the subdivision into sympathetically maintained pain (SMP) or sympathetically independent pain (SIP) applies to both types.
- The pathophysiology of the disorders remains unclear, but it has both peripheral and central components. A chronic peripheral inflammatory process accompanies alterations of central afferent processing, such as 'wind-up', but the pain may also be maintained by efferent noradrenergic sympathetic activity as well as by circulating catecholamines. The upregulation of α_2-adrenoceptors in local axons makes them hypersensitive to both. There is usually no communication between sympathetic efferent and afferent fibres, but following injury it is apparent that modulation of nociceptive impulses can occur not only at the site of injury, but also in distal undamaged fibres and the ipsilateral dorsal root ganglion itself around which sympathetic axons may proliferate.
- Both CRPS I and II are examples of neuropathic pain, which are distinguished only by the nature of the injury and the fact that in type I there is more diffuse pain whereas in type II there may be more discrete localization to the distribution of a single nerve.

Direction the viva may take

You may be asked to describe the typical clinical features.

- Symptoms include burning and constant pain, allodynia (which is pain provoked by an innocuous stimulus and which occurs in about one-third of cases), hyperpathia (which is an abnormally intense painful response to repetitive stimuli) and hyperalgesia (which is an exaggerated pain response to a noxious stimulus).
- The pain is accompanied by signs of failure of autonomic regulation in the region affected. These include swelling and local oedema, temperature changes due to vasomotor instability, associated skin colour changes and abnormal sudomotor activity.

- There may be associated weakness and trophic changes, with loss of the normal healthy appearance of skin, which thins and becomes translucent; of hair and of nails. There is also focal atrophy of underlying tissue, including muscle, and this in turn may precipitate focal osteoporosis.

Further direction the viva could take
You are likely to be asked about treatments.

- **Early treatment and prevention:** there is some evidence from controlled trials that early stellate ganglion block following upper limb trauma prevents onset in some patients, as does treatment with ascorbic acid (vitamin C) which antagonizes oxygen free radicals.
- **Sympathetic block (diagnostic):** if this is effective it will both diagnose the presence of sympathetically maintained pain and initiate its treatment, although the evidence for benefit is disputed. Procedures include stellate ganglion block as above, lumbar sympathectomy and plexus blocks.
- **Sympathetic block (therapeutic):** a series of blocks may confer benefit which increases in duration after each one, or which may confer only temporary relief which finally disappears. Several agents have been used in intravenous regional anaesthesia (IVRA). These include guanethidine, clonidine and bretylium. Randomized controlled trials (RCTs) have demonstrated IVRA to be no better than placebo. Some patients may be considered for a permanent neurolytic procedure (best if performed within 12 months of injury), but symptoms can recur as early as 6 months.
- It has been recommended that all treatment be directed towards functional restoration, so any window during which analgesia is satisfactory should be used for rehabilitation and sensory desensitization. Physiotherapy is important to minimize functional disability.
- **Dorsal column stimulation:** spinal cord stimulation has been used both in CRPS types I and II. Low-frequency pulsed stimulation appears to be a successful method of attenuating the pain associated with CRPS type II. Results otherwise have been equivocal, partly because the frequency and duration of stimuli have varied significantly between studies.
- **Transcutaneous electrical nerve stimulation (TENS):** this may benefit some patients (unlike acupuncture, for which there is little evidence of efficacy).

If a patient shows little or no response to sympathetic blockade there are various treatments that can be tried, few of which have been the subject of controlled trials. Their diversity suggests that none is universally successful.

- **Free radical scavengers:** some evidence from RCTs does support the use of the oxygen free radical scavengers dimethyl-sulphoxide and N-acetylcysteine.
- **Membrane stabilizers:** trials have shown gabapentin to be useful. Evidence for the benefit of tricyclic antidepressants such as amitryptiline or membrane stabilizers such as phenytoin remains anecdotal but is based on a substantial body of clinical experience.

- **Calcium modulating drugs:** calcitonin and biphosphonates (both of which inhibit bone resorption) ameliorate symptoms in early CRPS. The mechanism is unclear as osteoporotic changes usually occur late.
- **Simple analgesics:** codeine, co-drugs and non-steroidal anti-inflammatory drugs may give some patients relief. There are no robust data to support their prescription.
- **Opiates:** these are said to be effective in the early stages of the condition.
- **Glucocorticoids:** these may help the acute inflammatory stages of the disease process.
- **NMDA antagonists:** there are reports that ketamine given by low-dose subcutaneous injection or infusion can be beneficial. Side effects associated with racemic ketamine have limited its use, but development of the S enantiomer may allow it to be evaluated more widely.
- **Capsaicin:** topical capsaicin depletes peptide neurotransmitters from primary afferents and may help some patients.
- **Psychotherapy:** as with most chronic pain states, this is a very important part of the multidisciplinary approach. (If you mention it too early, however, you do run the risk of appearing to give a generic and thereby less convincing answer.)

Diabetic ketoacidosis

Commentary

This will be as much a question about the pathophysiology of this medical emergency as its management. To discuss the formation of ketones you need to know some of the pathways of intermediary metabolism. Make sure at least that you can explain the final steps which lead to the characteristic metabolic acidosis. In practice, anaesthetists become involved only infrequently with cases of diabetic ketoacidosis (DKA) because although they require intensive management they rarely require intensive care. Examiners, however, will tend to assume almost unconsciously that because diabetes is so common you will therefore be familiar with all its uncommon complications.

The viva

You may be asked first to define DKA, to describe its clinical features and to outline your management.

- **Definition:** DKA is a serious complication of diabetes mellitus. It can occur both in type 1 insulin-dependent, and type 2 non-insulin-dependent disease, although it is more common in the former. It is characterized by the biochemical triad of hyperglycaemia, metabolic acidosis and ketonaemia, and is a manifestation of an extreme disorder of carbohydrate metabolism.
- **Presentation:** a typical patient will present with the symptoms and signs of diabetes mellitus, namely polyuria, polydipsia, pronounced dehydration and weight loss.

In addition, their mental state may be obtunded, and they may hyperventilate owing to the metabolic acidosis (Kussmaul breathing). Their breath is characteristically ketotic, owing to the exhalation of volatile acetone. Abdominal pain, diarrhoea, and nausea and vomiting may also be evident, most commonly in children. Dehydration of muscle, gastric stasis and paralytic ileus have all been advanced as possible causes for this, although the case is unconvincing.

Management

- **Precipitants:** there is always a precipitating cause of DKA. Disparate factors can be involved, some of which are amenable to treatment. Its onset can be provoked by infection, by inadequate insulin treatment, by alcohol abuse, trauma, myocardial infarction and by the use of certain drugs, amongst them β-adrenoceptor blockers, corticosteroids and thiazide diuretics.
- **Assessment:** initial assessment can broadly follow the Airway, Breathing, Circulation algorithm, with particular emphasis on the patient's mental state and their volaemic status. Dehydration is usually severe. There are various methods of determining the fluid deficit. An orthostatic rise in heart rate without a change in blood pressure indicates an approximate 10% decrease in extracellular volume or a deficit of about 2 litres. An orthostatic fall in mean blood pressure of 10–12 mmHg indicates a 15–20% deficit (3–4 litres), while supine hypotension suggests dehydration greater than 20% (4 litres or more). Known acute weight loss is a more accurate guide.
- **Investigations:** those specific to DKA should encompass arterial blood gases, plasma glucose, electrolytes, ketones and serum osmolality. Other investigations may include urinalysis, a full blood count and differential, blood and urine cultures, chest X-ray and ECG. The blood lactate is usually normal.
- **Treatment aims:** the goals are to restore normovolaemia and adequate tissue perfusion, to reduce plasma glucose and osmolality towards normal, to clear ketones at a steady rate, and to correct the deranged acid–base and electrolyte status.
- **Management – fluids and insulin:** management of DKA need not be complex and it need not be hurried; it may take 12–16 hours to get the condition well under control, and the metabolic acidosis may persist for some days. Initial resuscitation should be with NaCl 0.9% (unless the corrected Na^+ is greater than $150\,mmol\,l^{-1}$), given at a rate of 1.0–1.5 litres in the first hour. This can be reduced to $300–500\,ml\,h^{-1}$ thereafter, titrated against response. Some authorities advocate giving bolus intravenous insulin ($0.15\,units\,kg^{-1}$) followed by an infusion at a rate of $0.1\,units\,kg^{-1}\,h^{-1}$, while others recommend omitting the bolus dose. A rate of $0.1\,units\,kg^{-1}\,h^{-1}$ is adequate to obtain high physiological levels of insulin, and there is no evidence that an initial bolus dose has any influence on outcome.
- **Phosphate:** phosphate, like potassium, shifts from the intracellular to the extracellular compartment, while the osmotic diuresis contributes to urinary losses. During treatment of DKA the phosphate re-enters cells to unmask the total body depletion. There are theoretical problems associated with hypophosphataemia which include muscle weakness, haemolytic anaemia, cardiac depression and depleted 2,3-DPG, but there is no evidence that supplemental phosphate improves outcome in these cases. The mean phosphate deficit is around $1\,mmol\,kg^{-1}$.

- **Bicarbonate:** the administration of HCO_3^- remains contentious. Bicarbonate does not cross the blood–brain barrier and so, if given, it will worsen intracellular cerebral acidosis. It can also reduce extracellular potassium and may provoke cardiac arrhythmias. If the patient's pH is >6.8 there is no evidence of any outcome benefit.
- **Complications:** cerebral oedema can supervene if glucose concentration drops too fast. It may also follow excessive fluid therapy as well as the administration of bicarbonate.

Direction the viva may take

You may then be asked to explain its pathogenesis.

- DKA follows a decrease in the effective levels of circulating insulin, which is accompanied by an increase in the plasma concentrations of counter-regulatory stress hormones, including glucagon, catecholamines, cortisol and growth hormone.
- **Gluconeogenesis:** in the presence of insulinopaenia, hyperglycaemia occurs as a result of gluconeogenesis, accelerated glycogenolysis and impaired glucose utilization by peripheral tissues. Gluconeogenesis is enhanced by a large number of gluconeogenetic precursors, which include amino acids from proteolysis. Increased glycogenolysis in muscle also produces lactate (CH_3–CHOH–COOH), which is converted in the presence of lactate dehydrogenase to pyruvate (CH_3–C=O–COOH), whose concentration rises as a consequence of all these effects. Glycerol from increased lipolysis, mainly in adipose tissue, makes a small contribution, but there is otherwise no pathway of conversion of lipid to glucose. There is also an increase in the activity of a range of gluconeogenetic enzymes. (These are numerous, but as an example, catecholamines increase the activity of glycogen phosphorylase.) Of these various mechanisms which lead to hyperglycaemia, it is hepatic and renal gluconeogenesis which quantitatively are the most important.
- **Lipid and ketone metabolism:** pyruvate is at the gateway of the citric acid cycle (Krebs cycle, tricarboxylic acid cycle) of aerobic metabolism. Two molecules of pyruvate become incorporated into each molecule of acetyl-coenzyme A (acetyl-CoA), and so the concentration of acetyl-CoA increases. At the same time, insulin inhibits hormone-sensitive lipase, while counter-regulatory hormones, particularly adrenaline, activate it. There follows at least a doubling of the plasma concentrations of free fatty acids (FFAs), whose metabolic utilization also takes place via acetyl-CoA. When the pathways are saturated, excess acetyl-CoA condenses to form acetoacetyl-CoA. This is then converted in the liver (via a deacylase) to free acetoacetate, which in turn is a precursor of β-hydroxybutyrate, acetoacetate and acetone. These three compounds are known as ketone bodies. β-hydroxybutyrate and acetoacetate are the anions of the strong acids acetoacetic acid and β-hydroxybutyric acid. (β-hydroxybutyrate is the more important of the two, being three times as abundant.) The acids fully dissociate at body pH and are buffered. When the buffering capacity is exceeded, metabolic acidosis supervenes. (In health, ketones are a useful energy substrate, being utilized by brain, heart and muscle.)

Further direction the viva could take

You may be asked as a final point (and this will probably be an indication that you have answered the question well), whether DKA can develop in the presence of normal blood glucose concentrations.

- There is an entity described as 'euglycaemic ketoacidosis'. By 'euglycaemic', however, is meant a blood glucose of less than $16.7 \, \text{mmol} \, l^{-1}$, and so in some patients the sugar will still be relatively high. The key factor in its pathogenesis appears to be the patient's recent oral intake. If the patient is well fed, then liver glycogen stores are high and ketogenesis is suppressed. If the patient has been unable to eat, for example because of intractable vomiting, then glycogen stores are depleted and the liver is primed for ketogenesis.

Pain pathways

Commentary

The neuraxial processing of nociceptive afferent input is formidably complex, and many details both of anatomical pathways and of neurotransmitter systems have yet to be elucidated. You will not be able to take complete refuge behind that complexity, because it is obvious that pain management is a central part of anaesthetic practice. You will be expected to provide at least a simplified account of how a pain stimulus travels from the periphery to the centre, and how it may be modulated within the CNS. However, because the information does remain incomplete you may be able to satisfy the examiners with a relatively limited account. You would be able to suggest, for example, that a drug might exert its effects by activating descending inhibitory nor-adrenergic pathways. There is little danger of your being asked to develop this much further, because you might find yourself otherwise discussing some of the 20 or more neurotransmitters that are believed to act at the dorsal horn. Examiners will have neither the time, nor perhaps the inclination, to do so.

The viva

You will be asked to describe the route from painful stimulus to conscious perception.

- The primary afferent nociceptors comprise free, unmyelinated nerve endings that are responsive to mechanical, thermal and chemical stimuli. These are relatively, but not completely, specific. Mechanoreceptors and temperature receptors, for example, are nociceptors only above a certain threshold. Following tissue trauma, the release of chemical mediators initiates nociception while activating an inflammatory response.
- Stimulation of these nociceptive afferents leads to propagation of impulses along the peripheral nerve fibres to the spinal cord by two parallel pathways. The first is via myelinated A-δ fibres, of diameter 2–5 μm, and rapidly conducting at between 12 and 30 m s^{-1}. This type of pain is fast, localized and sharp, and provokes reflex withdrawal

responses. The second route to the spinal cord is via non-myelinated C fibres, of smaller diameter (0.4–1.2 μm) and which conduct impulses more slowly at between 0.5 and 2.0 m s^{-1}. C fibres mediate pain sensations that are diffuse and dull.

- The primary afferents terminate in the dorsal horn of the spinal cord. The cell bodies lie in the dorsal root ganglia. A-δ fibres synapse in the laminae of Rexed I and V, while the C fibres synapse in the substantia gelatinosa. (This comprises lamina II and a part of lamina III.) They relay with various classes of second-order neurons in the cord, some of which are 'nociceptive-specific', which respond selectively to noxious stimuli and are located in the superficial laminae, and others of which are 'wide dynamic range', are non-specific and are located in the deeper laminae.

- Most of the secondary afferents decussate to ascend in the lateral spinothalamic tract, although some pass up the posterolateral part of the cord. These fibres pass through the medulla, midbrain and pons, giving off projection neurons as they do so, before terminating in the ventral posterior and medial nuclei of the thalamus.

- From the thalamus there is a specific sensory relay to areas of the contralateral cortex: to somatic sensory area I (SSI) in the post-central gyrus, to somatic sensory area II (SSII) in the wall of the sylvian fissure separating the frontal from the temporal lobes, and to the cingulate gyrus, which is thought to mediate the affective component of pain. The separation between sensory–discriminative and affective areas of the cortex is likely to be an oversimplification.

- **Modulation:** one of the major complexities of pain pathways is the modulation of afferent impulses which occurs at numerous levels, including the dorsal horn where there is a complex interaction between afferent input fibres, local intrinsic spinal neurons, and descending central efferents. Afferent impulses arriving at the dorsal horn themselves initiate inhibitory mechanisms which limit the effect of subsequent impulses. As pain fibres travel rostrally, they also send collateral projections to the higher centres such as the periaqueductal grey (PAG) matter and the locus ceruleus of the midbrain. Descending fibres from the PAG project to the nucleus raphe magnus in the medulla, and to the reticular formation to activate descending inhibitory neurons. These travel in the dorsolateral funiculus to terminate on interneurons in the dorsal horn. These fibres from the PAG are thought to be the main source of inhibitory control. Descending inhibitory projection also derives from the locus ceruleus. The inhibitory activity mediated from the PAG is also stimulated by endorphins released from the pituitary and which act directly at that site.

- **'Gate' control:** this represents one aspect of modulation. Synaptic transmission between primary and secondary nociceptive afferents can be 'gated' by interneurons. These neurons in the substantia gelatinosa can exert pre-synaptic inhibition on primary afferents, and post-synaptic inhibition on secondary neurons, thereby decreasing the pain response to a nociceptive stimulus. The inhibitory internuncials can be activated by afferents which subserve different sensory modalities, such as pressure (A-β fibres). This phenomenon underlies the use of counter-irritation, dorsal column stimulation, TENS and mechanical stimulation ('rubbing it better'). Descending central efferents from the PAG and locus ceruleus can also activate these inhibitory interneurons.

- **Transmitters:** these are numerous. Excitatory amino acids such as glutamate and aspartate have a major role in nociceptive transmission at the dorsal horn, where there are NMDA, non-NMDA, kainite, glutamate, AMPA, neurokinin, adenosine, 5-HT, GABA, a-adrenergic receptors, and μ, κ and δ opioid receptors. The primary afferents release various peptides, among them substance P, neurokinin A and calcitonin gene-related peptide (CGRP). There are different neurotransmitters in the various descending inhibitory pathways, which include neuropeptides (enkephalins and endorphins) in the PAG, metenkephalin and 5-HT in the nucleus raphe magnus pathway and noradrenaline in the locus ceruleus descending pathway.

Direction the viva may take
In the light of the foregoing you may be asked to outline where in the neuraxis analgesic agents or techniques may work.

- The usual target for analgesics is via ligand–receptor blockade, and the large number of receptor types means that you will only be able to give one or two examples. Opioid receptors, for instance, are expressed in the cell body of the dorsal root ganglion and transported both centrally to the dorsal horn, and peripherally. There are also receptors at higher centres such as the PAG, and so opiates exert their actions at numerous sites in the CNS. Ketamine acts on the open calcium channel of the NMDA receptor, amitriptyline modifies descending noradrenergic pathways, clonidine acts at pre-synaptic and post-synaptic a_2-receptors, while NSAIDs predominantly have a peripheral action which attenuates the hyperalgesia associated with the inflammatory response. The future may lie in analgesics that will regulate gene expression and exert selective modification. (Leave this final flourish until the end otherwise your impressed and interested examiner might inconveniently ask for details.)

Spinal cord injury

Commentary
This question occurs more commonly in the exam than in most anaesthetists' clinical practice. Approximately two individuals are paralysed each day in the UK after traumatic spinal cord injuries. Anaesthetists may be involved in their immediate care, but the more difficult and, from the examiners' point of view, more interesting aspects of spinal cord injury, only occur once they have been transferred to specialist centres. Your own knowledge, as well perhaps as that of your examiner, is likely to be largely theoretical, and the emphasis of the viva will be on the applied anatomy and pathophysiology of the condition.

The viva
You will be asked about the immediate management of spinal cord injury.

- The clinical signs depend on the level of injury. Over 50% of spinal injuries occur in the cervical region because, in comparison with the thoracic and lumbar spines, it is mobile and unprotected. In adults, the fulcrum of the cervical spine is at $C_{5/6}$, which is the commonest site of cord damage. (In children the fulcrum is higher.) The remaining injuries are divided equally between the thoracic, thoracolumbar and lumbosacral regions. Injuries involving the cervical cord are associated with tetraplegia; those at T_1 and below result in paraplegia.

- High thoracic or cervical cord injury is associated with 'neurogenic shock' which denotes the hypotension and bradycardia consequent upon the loss of sympathetic efferent pathways. This haemodynamic instability can persist. A second phenomenon is that of 'spinal shock', which may last from 3 days to 6 weeks, during which all spinal cord reflexes are profoundly depressed or abolished.

- The early management of cord injury includes immobilization and a standard approach to airway, breathing and circulation. Tracheal intubation may be necessary if there is any suggestion of respiratory compromise, and patients with lesions at C_3,C_4 or C_5 are likely to have lost some or all diaphragmatic function. A lower cervical injury spares the diaphragm, but breathing is still affected. The expansion of the rib cage via the intercostals and accessory muscles of respiration is responsible for 60% of normal tidal volume. Lung capacities are reduced such that vital capacity is only 25% of normal. Ventilation may be impaired, leading to sputum retention and chest infection, which is the commonest cause of death in the first 3 months after injury. In the spontaneously breathing tetraplegic patient, it is the supine position that is associated with the greater diaphragmatic excursion. The circulation may not respond to fluid infusion, and both vasopressors and atropine may be necessary. Neurogenic pulmonary oedema occurs in more than 40% of cases (in some series), and overzealous fluid therapy will compound the problem.

- **Corticosteroids:** evidence from the North American Spinal Cord Injury study suggests that high-dose methylprednisolone $30\,mg\,kg^{-1}$ may be of early benefit if given soon after injury. Whether or not outcomes are improved remains disputed.

- **Suxamethonium:** within about 48–72 hours after the acute injury, there is proliferation of acetylcholine receptors in extrajunctional areas of the denervated muscle. Administration of suxamethonium results in a large efflux of potassium into the circulation. This dangerous hyperkalaemic response is proportional to the amount of muscle that is involved and may persist for as long as 9 months.

Direction the viva may take

You may be asked about the later problems that may occur after spinal injury, and in particular how they might complicate anaesthesia.

- When spinal reflexes start to return they are hyperreflexic. The normal supraspinal descending inhibition of the thoracolumbar autonomic outflow is lost and so there occurs a mass reflex sympathetic discharge in response to stimulation below the level of the spinal lesion. There are changes in denervated muscle as well as the development of collateral neurons in the various reflex pathways. With time, the threshold appears to drop, together with the spread of stimulation across reflex centres. This explains why the mass response may be provoked by relatively minor stimuli.

- Both cutaneous and visceral stimuli (particularly associated with bladder distension, other genitourinary stimulus, and bowel disturbance) can provoke this reflex response. It is confined to the area below the level of transection, where the autonomic nervous system is not subject to any inhibitory influences; proximally there is compensatory parasympathetic overactivity. It is rare in lesions below T_{10}.

- The clinical features of this response include muscle contraction and increased spasticity below the lesion. There may be vasoconstriction and severe hypertension that can be accompanied by tachycardia or compensatory bradycardia. Other cardiac arrhythmias may occur. Above the level of the lesion there may be diaphoresis and flushing. The more distant the dermatome that is stimulated from the lesion the more emphatic is the sympathetic response. Autonomic hyperreflexia is more pronounced the higher the lesion in the cord, and the more limited the capacity for parasympathetic compensation.

- Patients may require surgery following cord injury, and autonomic hyperreflexia will complicate anaesthetic management. Reflex discharges can be prevented reliably by neuraxial block, although if an epidural is used it is important to ensure that the sacral segments are anaesthetized. Dense subarachnoid anaesthesia will prevent hyperreflexia completely. Deep anaesthesia or the use of vasoactive drugs to treat developing hypertension are less successful.

Immunology (and drug reactions)

Commentary

This is potentially a huge topic but does include an aspect of particular interest to anaesthetists, namely severe adverse drug reactions. This is where the viva may well end up, but not before you have been asked to give an overview of the immune system. Detailed discussion of T lymphocyte function or of cytokines would itself consume the entire viva, and so questioning on these subjects will necessarily be superficial. The basic science emphasis, however, means that you must at least demonstrate familiarity with the major components of immunity.

The viva

You will be asked to describe the basic components of the immune system.

Innate or non-specific immunity

- The body has a number of non-specific defences against infection. These include the skin, the antimicrobial secretions of sweat, sebaceous and lacrimal glands, and the mucus of the gastrointestinal tract and the upper airway to which organisms may adhere. The acidic environment of the stomach is hostile, and the lower gut is populated with commensals which prevent the overgrowth of less benign species.

- Non-specific immune defences do not recognize the substance that is being attacked, and are activated immediately in response to potential threats, for example from infectious agents. These defences include the activation of the alternative complement pathway (see below), phagocytosis by neutrophils, macrophages and mast cells, and the inflammatory response itself.

- **Inflammatory response:** this allows cells and proteins to reach extravascular sites by increasing the blood supply by vasodilatation, by increasing vascular permeability, by encouraging the movement of various inflammatory cells to the site of injury, and by activating the immune system.
- **Leucocytes:** these comprise neutrophils (60–70% of the total), which are responsible for phagocytosis and inflammatory mediator release; basophils (1%), which are the circulatory equivalent of tissue mast cells; monocytes (2–6%), which function in the blood like macrophages; eosinophils (1–4%), which destroy helminths and other parasites, and which may mediate hypersensitivity reactions; and lymphocytes (20–30%). Most lymphocytes mediate specific immune defences, but NK (natural killer) lymphocytes bind non-specifically to tumour cells and to cells that are infected by virus.
- **Macrophages:** these are ubiquitous cells that are derived from monocytes. They destroy foreign particles by phagocytosis, mediate extracellular destruction via the secretion of toxic chemicals, and also secrete cytokines. These are a complex set of soluble protein messengers that regulate immune responses, and include the interleukins, tumour necrosis factor, colony-stimulating factors and interferons.

Acquired or specific immunity

- **Lymphocytes:** specific immunity involves recognition of cells or substances to be attacked, and lymphocytes are the mainstay of the specific immune system. B lymphocytes differentiate into plasma cells which synthesize and secrete antibody. T lymphocytes comprise helper cells (T-helper, *Th*) and killer cells (cytotoxic, *Tc*). NK cells are non-specific. *Th* cells produce a large number of cytokines in a process that links the innate and specific components of the immune system.
- **Antibodies:** these immunoglobulins are proteins which bind specifically with antigens, which contain two identical light and two identical heavy chains, and which are characterized as IgA, IgD, IgE, IgG and IgM. IgG is the most abundant, and is the only immunoglobulin which crosses the placenta.

Direction the viva may take

You may be asked about adverse reactions to drugs. Not all of the described hypersensitivity reactions are necessarily involved in drug reactions, but a summary is included for completeness. This is because whenever type I reactions are mentioned the examiners will want to see if you are familiar with the rest of the classification.

- **Hapten formation:** most drugs are of low molecular weight and are not inherently immunogenic; they can, however, act as haptens by interacting with proteins to form stable antigenic conjugates.
- **Hypersensitivity reactions:** these are abnormal reactions involving different immune mechanisms, often with the formation of antibodies. They occur on second or subsequent exposure to the antigen concerned. Four types have been described.

— *Type I (immediate):* this is the classic anaphylactic, immediate hypersensitivity reaction, which is mediated by IgE. IgE is synthesized by B cells on first exposure to the antigen and binds to mast cells. On repeated introduction, the antigenic drug–protein complex degranulates mast cells with the release of a number of preformed vasoactive substances. These include histamine, heparin, serotonin, leukotrienes and platelet-activating factor. (Mast cells are numerous in skin, the bronchial mucosa, in the gut and in capillaries.)

— *Type II (cytotoxic):* in this reaction, circulating IgE and IgM antibodies react in the presence of complement to mediate reactions which cause cell lysis. Such reactions can lead to haemolysis (caused, for example, by sulphonamides), thrombocytopenia (heparin, thiazide diuretics) and agranulocytosis (carbimazole, NSAIDs, chloramphenicol).

— *Type III (immune complex):* the reaction of antibody and antigen produces a circulating immune complex (precipitin), which deposits in small vessels, in the glomeruli and in the connective tissue of joints. These precipitins also activate complement via the classical pathway. Type III reactions underlie many autoimmune diseases, including rheumatoid arthritis and systemic lupus erythematosus (SLE).

— *Type IV (delayed):* this is the delayed hypersensitivity reaction, which is cell-mediated without complement activation and without the formation of antibodies. The reaction results from the combination of antigen with T (killer) lymphocytes and macrophages attacking the foreign material. This mechanism underlies the development of contact dermatitis. Granuloma formation in diseases such as tuberculosis and sarcoidosis is a result of a large antigen burden or the failure of macrophages to destroy the antigen. This 'granulomatous hypersensitivity' is also a type IV response.

- **Complement:** complement is an enzyme system consisting of 20 or more serum glycoproteins which, in combination with antibody, are activated in a cascade that results in cell body lysis. In summary, the complement system coats (opsonizes) bacteria and immune complexes, activates phagocytes and destroys target cells. The final pathway is the amalgamation of complement proteins C5–C9 into a complex that disrupts the phospholipids of cell membranes to allow osmotic cytolysis. The classical complement pathway is a specific immune response that is initiated by the reaction of antibody with complement protein C1 and its subcomponents. The alternative pathway is a non-specific response that can be activated in the absence of antibody, but in the presence, for example, of anaesthetic agents, drugs or bacterial toxins.

- **Anaphylactoid reactions:** clinically, these may resemble anaphylactic reactions, but they involve the direct release of vasoactive substances (histamine, serotonin) from mast cells or from circulating basophils, rather than release mediated via an antigen–antibody response.

Further direction the viva could take

You may be asked how you would investigate a suspected drug reaction. If you (or the examiner) have run out of things to say about immunity, then you may be asked to describe your management of a severe reaction.

- **Investigation of a reaction:** non-specific markers include urinary methyl histamine, which increases in the first 2–3 hours following a reaction, and mast cell tryptase. This enzyme is responsible for activating part of the complement cascade (it cleaves C3 to form C3a and C3b), and serum concentrations are elevated for about 3 hours after a reaction. A clotted blood sample should therefore be taken as soon as possible after emergency resuscitation and another 1 hour later. Patients can further be investigated by skin testing (at 6 weeks or longer after the event) and by assays of drug-specific antibodies using radioallergoabsorbent (RAST) tests.
- **Management of an anaphylactic or anaphylactoid reaction:** see page 364.

Sepsis

Commentary

The terminology of sepsis is confusing. Research papers which deal with the subject include as keywords 'sepsis', 'septic shock', 'sepsis syndrome' and 'systemic inflammatory response syndrome'. The examiner who is not an intensivist may share some of that confusion which the summary account below should allow you to dispel. The topic is very detailed and so a relatively superficial overview of some of the important mediators should be adequate. The clinical aspects are likely to concentrate on critical care management, and you should be familiar with its broad principles.

The viva

You may be asked what you understand by the term 'sepsis'.

- **Definitions:** *sepsis* is defined as infection (suspected or proven) together with a systemic inflammatory response syndrome (SIRS). Sepsis plus organ dysfunction is described as *severe sepsis*, and, if this is accompanied by hypotension unrelieved by fluid resuscitation, it is known as *septic shock*. (This nomenclature has mainly been useful in designing RCTs. In the viva it will be fine to discuss 'sepsis' as a single entity. Both you and the examiner will find it much easier.)
- **SIRS:** this comprises features of the inflammatory response in the absence of an identifiable pathogen, end-organ damage or the need for circulatory support. It is therefore distinct from sepsis and its variants. Once a pathogen has been isolated, then the working diagnosis in a patient shifts from SIRS to sepsis, severe sepsis or septic shock. Once end-organ damage supervenes the diagnosis becomes that of early multiple organ dysfunction syndrome (MODS). SIRS is defined by the presence of two or more of the following: temperature $>38°C$ or $<36°C$; tachycardia >90 beats min^{-1}; tachypnoea >20 breaths min^{-1} (or $PaCO_2$ $<4.3\,kPa$); white cell count $>12 \times 10^3\,mm^{-3}$ or $<4 \times 10^3\,mm^{-3}$.
- **The inflammatory response:** this is systemic rather than localized and is part of an exaggerated or uncontrolled host response to a pathological insult. It is highly

complex, comprising a sequence of reactions which involves not only the secretion of key signalling molecules such as the cytokines (protein immunoregulators that include interleukins IL-1, 5, 6, 8, 11 and 15, tumour necrosis factor, colony-stimulating factors, interferons and platelet-activating factor), but also the activation of complement. Other inflammatory mediators such as kinins and histamine lead to vasodilatation and increased capillary permeability, while leukotrienes stimulate inward granulocyte migration. In addition, there is an increase in acute phase proteins such as haptoglobin, fibrinogen and C-reactive protein (CRP). CRP activates monocytes, increases cytokine production and can activate the complement cascade. Other aspects of immune function, such as cell-mediated and humoral immunity, may also be mobilized.

- **Procoagulant–anticoagulant balance:** sepsis alters this balance in favour of procoagulant factors. Endothelial cells appear to upregulate tissue factor and thereby activate coagulation and the formation of microvascular thrombus. The anticoagulant factors suppress coagulation and enhance fibrinolysis. They include protein C, its co-factor protein S, antithrombin III and tissue factor-pathway inhibitor. All are decreased by sepsis.

- **Causes and clinical features:** the final common pathway to the inflammatory response can be triggered by numerous insults such as trauma, major surgery, and challenges to the immune system by various antigens, including infective agents and the transfusion of blood and blood products. Consistent with the diagnostic criteria above, patients typically exhibit a tachycardia, disturbed temperature regulation, tachypnoea, a narrowed pulse pressure secondary to the reduced effective circulating volume, and oliguria. The hypoperfusion is responsible for the lactic acidosis that is a typical feature of the condition. These clinical signs are relatively non-specific.

Direction the viva may take

You may be asked about the principles of management. Start with 'A, B, C' if you wish, but be aware that a generic account is unlikely to prove sufficient.

- **Early goal-directed therapy (EGDT):** see page 128. GDT may reverse tissue hypoxia and decrease the inflammatory and procoagulant response, and, if initiated early (within 6 hours), has been shown to improve survival.

- **Ventilation:** acute lung injury with capillary leak frequently complicates sepsis. Lung-protective ventilation reduces mortality (page 121).

- **Antibiotics:** empirical broad-spectrum antibiotics are usually necessary until a pathogen has been identified. Expert microbiological advice is helpful, particularly in respect of factors such as local patterns of antibiotic usage and bacterial susceptibility.

- **Activated protein C:** in septic patients with high APACHE scores (>25) and an increased risk of death, recombinant activated protein C decreases mortality rates. The same benefit is not apparent in less critically ill subjects at lower risk of death. Activated protein C has a spectrum of actions which include the proteolytic inactivation of clotting factors Va and VIIIa, and enhanced fibrinolysis via the inhibition of plasminogen-activator inhibitor synthesis. It also decreases cytokine production, leucocyte activation and apoptosis (programmed cell death) affecting lymphocytes and endothelial cells.

- **Glycaemic control:** sepsis is associated with insulin resistance and hyperglycaemia, whose adverse effects in critical illness are well established. It is procoagulant, induces apoptosis, impairs neutrophil function and delays wound healing. Insulin counteracts all these effects. Tight glycaemic control which maintains blood glucose levels at between 4.4 and 6.1 mmol l^{-1} reduces mortality rates in critically ill surgical patients. The same benefit has not been demonstrated in critically ill medical patients.

- **Vasopressin:** vasopressin deficiency and receptor downregulation occur commonly in sepsis, and vasopressin infusion improves haemodynamic indices and reduces concomitant inotrope requirements. This is at the expense in some patients of decreased cardiac output and gastrointestinal ischaemia. Hazards increase at infusion rates greater than 0.04 units min^{-1}.

- **Transfusion:** data are equivocal, but although severely anaemic patients should be transfused with red cells, the threshold appears to be low, with haemoglobin levels of between 7.0 and 9.0 g dl^{-1} being acceptable.

- **Renal replacement therapy (RRT):** there is little evidence that early RRT alters outcomes, but it clearly cannot be withheld from patients with acute renal dysfunction and deranged biochemistry.

- **Other drugs**
  - *Corticosteroids:* RCTs of high-dose early glucocorticoids have shown no improvement in survival.
  - *Nitric oxide synthetase inhibitors:* excess production of nitric oxide (NO) may be associated with the early vasodilatation and myocardial depression that is seen in septic shock, but NO synthetase inhibitors such as arginine derivatives increase mortality rates.
  - *Monoclonal antibodies:* there is no evidence of benefit from the use of monoclonal antibodies such as anti-TNF.
  - *Selenium:* there is some evidence that adjuvant treatment with high-dose selenium is associated with a reduction in 28-day mortality rates. Selenium is an important antioxidant whose levels fall in sepsis. It has a relatively narrow therapeutic index.

The arterial tourniquet

Commentary

The arterial tourniquet seems at first sight to be a mundane piece of equipment on which to be examined. Its use is so widespread that it is easy to become complacent. However, the tourniquet is associated with a range of potential complications, not all of which are immediately obvious and so you will need to show both that you are aware of these and that you are able to minimize the risks.

The viva

You may be asked first about the indications for, and contraindications to, the use of an arterial tourniquet.

- **Indications:** the arterial tourniquet is used primarily to produce a bloodless field for extremity surgery. It also allows intravenous regional anaesthesia (IVRA or Bier's block) and intravenous regional sympathectomy with drugs such as guanethidine. As part of the isolated forearm technique it has been used as a tool for researching anaesthetic awareness (page 286) and in specialist oncological centres for isolated limb perfusion with high dose chemotherapy for patients with localized soft tissue cancers.
- **Contraindications:** these are mainly relative. Tourniquets should be avoided in patients with major trauma to the operated limb, in patients with localized infection or tumour (both of which in theory can be disseminated), and in those with peripheral vascular disease (particularly affecting the leg). They should be used with caution in those with poor cardiac reserve or a fixed output state. Sickle cell disease has traditionally been viewed as an absolute contraindication, but a number of studies have reported uneventful use of tourniquets providing that the general principles of sickle cell management have been observed and the limb has been exsanguinated effectively. The ischaemic tissue nonetheless still provides the hypoxic, hypothermic and acidotic environment most likely to promote red cell sickling, and so the risk of using a tourniquet must be evaluated carefully. Pulmonary embolism may complicate their use in patients who are at high risk of venous thrombosis.

You will then be asked in more detail about the device itself and the physiological consequences and complications of its use.

- **Arterial tourniquet:** the system comprises a cuff, a gas source and a pressure gauge which keeps cuff pressure at a preset value. The limb can be exsanguinated using arterial pressure and elevation, a pneumatic air exsanguinator or an Esmarch bandage.
- **Mechanical pressure effects:** these affect skin, muscles, nerves and blood vessels. Skin is most likely to be damaged by the shearing stresses caused by a tightly wound Esmarch exsanguinator. These can generate pressures as high as 1000 mmHg and are more likely to cause nerve injury than pneumatic devices. The nerves under the cuff itself are also vulnerable; intraneural microvascular injury and oedema can lead to axonal degeneration. Injury is most likely at the edges of the cuff where shearing forces are highest. The radial is the nerve most at risk in the upper limb; the sciatic nerve in the lower. Muscles directly beneath the cuff are also subject both to pressure effects and to ischaemia. The spectrum of injury that has been reported includes persistent post-tourniquet weakness, swelling and discomfort (the 'tourniquet syndrome', which can last for some weeks), and compartment syndrome and rhabdomyolysis, both of which are very rare. Atheromatous vessels can be traumatized, particularly in the lower limb, and peripheral vascular disease increases the risk of thrombus formation.
- **Duration:** a safe limit has not been established, but a 2-hour tourniquet time is a commonly recommended maximum, both to limit direct pressure effects and the

potential damage to distal tissues owing to prolonged ATP depletion and progressive tissue acidosis. Risks are higher in the elderly, in those with peripheral vascular disease, and if the limb is injured. The cuff can be deflated periodically as long as a reperfusion time of at least 10 minutes is allowed. Pre-tourniquet cooling of the limb can double 'safe' tourniquet time, but in practice this is rarely done.

- **Systemic effects – inflation:** limb exsanguination is a form of rapid autotransfusion. A single thigh tourniquet, for example, may divert 400 ml of blood into the circulation. This sudden increase in blood volume is usually well tolerated, but it may threaten haemodynamic stability in patients with precarious cardiac function or a fixed output state such as mitral stenosis.
- **Systemic effects – deflation**
  - *Cardiovascular:* upon deflation of the cuff there is a fall in systemic vascular resistance, with decreases in arterial and central venous pressures as blood moves back into the now hyperaemic circulation of the reperfusing limb. This may last for 10–15 minutes.
  - *Respiratory:* as residual hypercarbic blood in the ischaemic limb rejoins the systemic circulation there is a brief increase in the expired CO_2 tension which peaks at around 1 minute. The $FeCO_2$ (fractional concentration of expired CO_2) can rise by as much as 2.5 kPa but falls to baseline levels within a few minutes.
  - *CNS:* this transient increase in $PaCO_2$ is associated with an increase in cerebral blood flow, blood volume and intracranial pressure. Although this is usually insignificant, it can be important in trauma patients with closed head injuries.
- **Metabolic changes:** accumulation of lactate and potassium proportional to the duration of ischaemia results in transient plasma rises during reperfusion and causes a mild metabolic acidosis that corrects within around 30 minutes. (The limb venous pH is typically 7.0 after 2 hours' inflation time.)
- **Coagulation:** increased platelet aggregation owing to tissue compression and catecholamine release is offset by enhanced systemic thrombolysis (caused by release of tissue plasminogen activator) after tourniquet deflation. Emboli formation during all lower limb surgery is common; however, there is a fivefold increase in the risk of large venous thrombosis in patients undergoing total knee replacement in whom a tourniquet is used.
- **Temperature changes:** heat transfer from the core to the exsanguinated area is negligible and so central temperature can rise. This process is reversed following cuff deflation. Redistributed blood loses heat to the cool limb, which quickly becomes hyperaemic. Transient temperature falls of up to 0.7°C have been reported.
- **Tourniquet pain:** in the awake patient this is a dull, poorly localized but intense discomfort that intensifies with time. In both awake and anaesthetized patients it is associated with hypertension and tachycardia. Pain may persist even in the presence of dense neuraxial or deep general anaesthesia. Its likely mechanism is complex. It will probably be enough for you to identify the fact that high pressure appears to prevent nerve conduction in fast A-δ pain fibres, while having less effect on the smaller non-myelinated slow conducting C fibres which continue to transmit cutaneous impulses.
- **Complications secondary to leakage:** faulty or incorrectly applied cuffs can allow unintended access of drugs to the systemic circulation during IVRA. This is

particularly dangerous with large volumes of local anaesthetic or with high-dose cytotoxic chemotherapeutic agents. Rapid injection through small syringes (which generate higher pressures than larger ones) may allow venous pressure to exceed cuff pressure.

Direction the viva will take

You will be asked finally how you can minimize the risks to the patient.

- **Safe practice:** much of this is common sense. Equipment must be well maintained. Occlusion pressures and tourniquet inflation time should be minimized. The gauge pressure can be misleading; what is important is the pressure per unit area. This will be higher in a narrow cuff, or in a large limb where the pressure will be greatest at its widest point. Ideally the cuff that is used should be conical, thus exerting pressure more evenly around the limb. At the least it must be the correct size. Inflation pressure need be little higher than that needed to occlude arterial flow. Some have recommended using Doppler probes to detect the loss of peripheral flow before inflation to 50 mmHg above that level. In routine practice the tourniquet is usually inflated to around 100–150 mmHg above the systolic pressure, with the higher pressures reserved for the lower limb. Finally, tourniquets must be protected from contamination.

Index

Index